FAO Food and Nutrition Series

HUMAN NUTRITION
IN THE
DEVELOPING
WORLD

by
Michael C. Latham
Professor of International Nutrition
Cornell University
Ithaca, New York, USA

FOOD AND AGRICULTURE ORGANIZATION OF THE UNITED NATIONS
Rome, 1997

David Lubin Memorial Library Cataloguing in Publication Data

Latham, M.C.
    Human nutrition in the developing world.
    (FAO Food and Nutrition Series No. 29)
    ISBN 92-5-103818-X
    ISSN 1014-3181

    1. Human nutrition
    I. Title   II. Series   III. FAO, Rome (Italy)

    FAO code: 80   AGRIS: S01

Contents

Foreword

Human nutrition in the developing world contributes to the continuing efforts of the Food and Agriculture Organization (FAO) to improve the nutritional status of all populations. It is produced to reinforce FAO's implementation of the recommendations of the International Conference on Nutrition (ICN), held in December 1992 in Rome. It provides detailed and amplified information on the major themes addressed during the ICN, in a simple and practical manner. The book draws from the earlier publication *Human nutrition in tropical Africa* (FAO, 1965; second edition 1979), presenting an expanded, up-to-date, global perspective.

FAO strongly emphasizes that food-based approaches are the only sustainable way to improve the nutritional status of all. In developing countries better development of agricultural resources can improve food supplies, employment and incomes and enable adequate diets. Even among low-income families, diets can be improved by properly combining foods that are commonly available. Every food can have an important function in the human diet.

This book provides sound science-based information on food, nutrients, the causes of malnutrition, nutritional disorders and their prevention. The information can be used by workers in the field and disseminated to assist the public in making informed food choices and appropriate decisions about diet. The publication will be especially useful for those working with rural populations.

While various aspects of human nutrition are covered in this text, special emphasis is given to applied and multidisciplinary approaches for the alleviation of malnutrition. These approaches should facilitate both intersectoral and multisectoral actions for promoting and protecting nutritional well-being among people in developing countries.

It is hoped that *Human nutrition in the developing world* will serve as a comprehensive introduction to nutritional problems in developing countries. The book is also designed as a useful reference for workers in agriculture, health, education and other fields who are seeking to promote simple, practical and affordable actions to solve nutritional problems in developing countries.

This book was made possible through Professor Michael Latham's prodigious work in preparing the basic text. We at FAO are extremely grateful to Professor Latham for sharing his vast knowledge of nutrition with all readers.

John R. Lupien
Director
FAO Food and Nutrition Division

Preface

This book is designed to cover the most important nutritional problems of developing countries and to suggest appropriate programmes and policies to address these. Good nutrition for all of humankind is a basic human right. This requires food security, good health and adequate care.

A bibliography is provided to bring some useful publications to the reader's attention; however, since this book is likely to be used by many persons who do not have easy access to good scientific, agricultural or medical libraries, the bibliography does not include journal articles, except for those that are cited in the text. For the same reason, the bibliography is not comprehensive; I can acknowledge in only a general way the many hundreds of books, journal articles, reports and pamphlets that I have consulted or those publications that have led to the total sum of knowledge that makes possible the preparation of a book such as this. Two books in the bibliography deserve special attention because they were most often consulted: Davidson and Passmore's *Human nutrition and dietetics*, a comprehensive textbook of nutrition; and King and Burgess' *Nutrition for developing countries*, a practical guide for nutrition workers dealing with problems in poor countries. Both are excellent publications.

I wish to acknowledge with gratitude some of the institutions that over many years have influenced my thinking on health, nutrition and development. These include Trinity College in Dublin, Ireland, where I studied medicine; the London School of Hygiene and Tropical Medicine, where I completed a degree in tropical public health; and Harvard University, where I attained a Master of Public Health degree and worked in the Department of Nutrition. However, it was more than nine years' experience working in the United Republic of Tanzania, both as a District Medical Officer and as Director of the Nutrition Unit in the Ministry of Health, that most enriched my knowledge of medicine, nutrition and life.

More than 25 years' service as Director and Professor of International Nutrition at Cornell University has provided me an unusual opportunity to work with a faculty with expertise in almost every aspect of nutrition, to learn from and to guide an extraordinary group of graduate students from all parts of the world and to be involved on the ground in a wide variety of nutrition activities in Africa, Asia and the Americas. These associations and experiences have been greatly rewarding to me and in different ways have influenced the content of this publication.

Acknowledgements

This book has benefited from the advice, support and assistance of many individuals, too many to acknowledge here. However, special mention is due to: Dr John R. Lupien, Director of the FAO Food and Nutrition Division, who encouraged me to write this book and who has been enormously supportive from start to finish, and whose staff has also provided invaluable advice; Dr M. Anwar Hussain of FAO, who spent long hours reviewing various drafts of the book and improving the text; Doreen Doty, who for some 20 years served as my Administrative Assistant, and who expertly did most of the word processing for the first and subsequent drafts of this publication; Rozanne Chorlton of Scotland, United Kingdom, who edited over half the chapters; Elisabeth Linusson, who assisted both with the selection of illustrations and with the bibliography; Valerie Stetson and other Cornell graduate students who assisted with the revision and rewriting of specific chapters; Viera Larsson, who provided drawings; Dr Carolyn Campbell, who gave final editing assistance; and Dr Lani Stephenson, who over many years has provided invaluable advice and support. The publication was edited in FAO by Andrea Perlis.

Part I
Causes of malnutrition

Chapter 1

International nutrition and world food problems in perspective

We, the Ministers and Plenipotentiaries representing 159 nations ... declare our determination to eliminate hunger and to reduce all forms of malnutrition. Hunger and malnutrition are unacceptable in a world that has both the knowledge and the resources to end this human catastrophe.

These are the opening sentences of the World Declaration on Nutrition produced by the FAO and World Health Organization (WHO) International Conference on Nutrition (ICN) held in Rome in December 1992. That important conference (Photo 1) reviewed the current nutrition situation in the world and set the stage for markedly reducing these unacceptable conditions of humankind. Reaching the ICN goal is possible. Most of the work will need to be done in the developing countries by their own people. However, cooperative work across nations and across disciplines is also essential.

This book is aimed to help move forward the noble objectives elaborated by the ICN. It is hoped that a comprehensive text that describes the nature of the problems, their causes and ways to deal with them can be helpful. A brief review highlighting international food and nutrition issues can help to bring the most important issues into perspective.

The ICN declaration goes on to state:
1. ... We recognize that globally there is enough food for all and that inequitable access is the main problem. Bearing in mind the right to an adequate standard of living, including food, contained in the Universal Declaration of Human Rights, we pledge to act in solidarity to ensure that freedom from hunger becomes a reality. We also declare our firm commitment to work together to ensure sustained nutritional well-being for all people in a peaceful, just and environmentally safe world.

2. Despite appreciable worldwide improvements in life expectancy, adult literacy and nutritional status, we all view with the deepest concern the unacceptable fact that about 780 million people in developing countries – 20 percent of their combined population – still do not have access to enough food to meet their basic daily needs for nutritional well-being.

3. We are especially distressed by the high prevalence and increasing numbers of malnourished children under five years of age in parts of Africa, Asia and Latin America and the Caribbean. Moreover, more than 2 000 million people, mostly women and children, are deficient in one or more micronutrients; babies continue to be born mentally retarded as a result of iodine deficiency; children go blind and die of vitamin A deficiency; and enormous numbers of women and children are adversely affected by iron deficiency. Hundreds of millions of people also suffer from communicable and non-communicable diseases caused by contaminated food and water. At the same time, chronic non-communicable diseases related to excessive or unbalanced dietary intakes often lead to premature deaths in both developed and developing countries.

THE SCALE OF THE PROBLEM

Protein-energy malnutrition (PEM), vitamin A deficiency, iodine deficiency disorders (IDD) and nutritional anaemias – mainly resulting from iron deficiency or iron losses – are the most common serious nutritional problems in almost all countries of Asia, Africa, Latin America and the Near East.

Nutrition and development: a global assessment, prepared by FAO and WHO for the ICN, reviewed all available current information on the prevalence of hunger and malnutrition and provided a global estimate for the various regions of the world. FAO updated the estimates of the chronically undernourished population of the world for the Sixth World Food Survey and in preparation for the World Food Summit (Table 1), and WHO updated the estimates for iodine, vitamin A and iron deficiencies in 1995 (Table 2). The figures suggest that one of every five persons in the developing world is chronically undernourished, 192 million children suffer from PEM and over 2 000 million experience micronutrient deficiencies. In addition, diet-related non-communicable diseases such as obesity, cardiovascular disease, stroke, diabetes and some forms of cancer exist or are emerging as public health problems in many developing countries.

While these numbers and trends are alarming, progress has been made in reducing the prevalence of nutritional problems, and many countries have been remarkably successful in addressing the issues of hunger and malnutrition. For the developing countries as a whole there has been a consistent decline since the early 1970s in the proportion and absolute number of chronically undernourished people. From 1969 to 1971 approximately 893 million people were chronically undernourished, compared with 809 million from 1990 to 1992; these figures represent a drop from 35 to 20 percent of the population of these countries. The current – and achievable – challenge is to build upon and accelerate the progress that has been made.

FAO and WHO data indicate improvements of the nutritional situation in Asia and Latin America from 1980 to 1990 but a deterioration in sub-Saharan Africa. Although the prevalence of underweight children remained virtually unchanged in sub-Saharan Africa during that decade (increasing from 29 to 30 percent), the prevalence rates are much better than in South Asia, where about 59 percent of children – almost twice the prevalence in Africa – were underweight in 1990 (Table 3). In the same year, in total numbers, five times as many children were underweight in South Asia (101 million) as in sub-Saharan Africa (19.9 million).

Many nutritional statistics show the numbers of persons who have overt evidence of a deficiency. However, "at risk" populations are not often identified. In nutrition, as in public health, people considered at risk of developing malnutrition should be among the primary concerns. Prevention becomes more feasible and cost effective if groups at risk are identified and the causes of malnutrition are clearly understood.

One of the most dramatic aspects of the global nutrition situation is the extent of famine, hunger and starvation. While good progress has been made in averting famine, especially in Asia, these horrifying conditions persist throughout the world. Their occurrence is commonly attributed to drought and other natural disasters, but war, civil unrest and political instability have far greater importance. In the mid-1990s, hunger and malnutrition resulting from civil strife are serious problems in many parts of the world including Europe (particularly former Yugoslavia), Asia (for example, Afghanistan), the Near East (Iraq)

TABLE 1
Prevalence of chronic undernutrition in developing regions

Region	Percentage of population			Number (*millions*)		
	1969-1971	1979-1981	1990-1992	1969-1971	1979-1981	1990-1992
Latin America and the Caribbean	18	13	14	51	46	61
Near East and North Africa	25	10	10	44	24	32
Sub-Saharan Africa	36	39	41	96	140	204
East and Southeast Asia	41	27	16	468	371	262
South Asia	33	33	22	233	297	250
Continental Africa	34	33	34	116	148	211
Developing regions	35	27	20	893	878	809

TABLE 2
Population at risk of and affected by micronutrient malnutrition (millions)

Region[1]	Iodine deficiency disorders		Vitamin A deficiency		Iron deficiency or anaemia
	At risk	Affected (goitre)	At risk[2]	Affected (xerophthalmia)	
Africa	181	86	31	1.0	206
Americas	168	63	14	0.1	94
Southeast Asia	486	176	123	1.7	616
Europe	141	97	–	–	27
Eastern Mediterranean	173	93	18	0.2	149
Western Pacific[3]	423	141	42	0.1	1 058
Total	**1 572**	**655**	**228**	**3.1**	**2 150**

[1] WHO regions.
[2] Preschool children only.
[3] Including China.

and most extensively Africa. Tragically, civil strife often affects not only the countries in turmoil but also those that provide hospitality to the refugees who flee their homes in terror. In mid-1994, the United Republic of Tanzania accepted about 500 000 refugees from Rwanda, most of them in less than one week. Their arrival more than doubled the population of the resource-poor region, which welcomed them as best it could. The influx placed overwhelming pressure on local resources and necessitated a major international effort to prevent an increase in nutrition and health problems among the

TABLE 3

Prevalence of underweight[1] children under five years of age, by region

Region	Percentage underweight			Number underweight *(millions)*		
	1980	1985	1990	1980	1985	1990
Sub-Saharan Africa	28.9	29.9	29.9	19.9	24.1	28.2
Near East/North Africa	17.2	15.1	13.4	5.0	5.0	4.8
South Asia	63.7	61.1	58.5	89.9	100.1	101.2
Southeast Asia	39.1	34.7	31.3	22.8	21.7	19.9
China	23.8	21.3	21.8	20.5	21.1	23.6
Central America/Caribbean	17.7	15.2	15.4	3.1	2.8	3.0
South America	9.3	8.2	7.7	3.1	2.9	2.8
Global (average percentage/ total number)	**37.8**	**36.1**	**34.3**	**164**	**178**	**184**

Source: UN ACC/SCN, 1992a.
[1] Underweight is defined as weight-for-age less than –2 standard deviations from the mean.

local people as well as to contain these problems among the refugees.

NUTRITION IMPROVEMENT: NATURE AND EVOLUTION

Data from around the world show that the causes underlying most nutrition problems have not changed véry much over the past 50 years. Poverty, ignorance and disease, coupled with inadequate food supplies, unhealthy environments, social stress and discrimination, still persist unchanged as a web of interacting factors which combine to create conditions in which malnutrition flourishes. However, what does change greatly is the approach to tackling malnutrition. Each decade or so witnesses a new dominant framework, paradigm, panacea or quick fix claímed to be capable of reducing the malnutrition problem greatly before ten years have passed.

During the 1950s and 1960s, kwashiorkor and protein deficiencies were seen as the major problems. Quick fixes such as

fish protein concentrate, single-cell protein or amino acid fortification and increased production of protein-rich foods of animal origin were the strategies proposed for the control of malnutrition in the tropics and subtropics.

During the late 1960s and 1970s, the term "protein-energy malnutrition" entered the literature. Increasing protein and energy intake by children was the solution, and nutrition rehabilitation centres and applied nutrition programmes (ANPs) were offered up as sure strategies.

The 1974 World Food Conference began a decade of macroanalysis which placed first nutrition planning and then nutritional surveillance among the dominant strategies for the countries most affected. Economists began to take over from nutritionists and paediatricians as the architects of new policies, with much talk about national food security and agencies such as the World Bank stressing income generation.

In 1985 the International Monetary Fund (IMF) began to push structural adjustment, and WHO and UNICEF reinvented ANPs, which they renamed Joint Nutrition Support Programmes (JNSPs). In the early 1990s the subject of micronutrients pushed PEM to the background, as nutritionists, international agencies and universities attempted quick fixes to control vitamin A deficiency, anaemia and IDD. The micronutrient wave has not yet crested, and very large sums of money are likely to be provided by the World Bank, the United States Agency for International Development (USAID) and others to address this "hidden hunger". This effort is, in part, a response to the goals set by the 1989 World Summit on Children and the 1992 International Conference on Nutrition, which include the virtual elimination of vitamin A deficiency and IDD before the turn of the century.

Increased funding is needed if improvements in nutrition are to be achieved. However, there is a danger that the limited resources available may be diverted towards the development of new quick-fix strategies for micronutrient deficiencies. Little, then, will remain for addressing the underlying and basic causes of malnutrition. The quick fix addresses only the immediate causes of a problem, scratching the surface and providing no sustainability.

It is well recognized that inappropriate development strategies also contribute to the underlying causes of hunger in many countries. Policy reform and the institution of appropriate development and macroeconomic policies are advocated by many economists to improve nutrition. The ICN also emphasized that developing countries must work to ensure that development policies and projects are designed to include nutrition improvement objectives. Furthermore, in the low-income food-deficit countries, where most of the world's malnourished people live, economic growth and poverty alleviation must be based on better development of agricultural resources and improvement of food supplies. This approach should promote sustainable development, expand employment opportunities and improve access to food by the poor. Free and fair trade is clearly important for stimulating economic growth, and the prices for primary and processed agricultural products must be adequate to ensure sustained development. The primary producers must receive fair prices for their products, labour and use of resources.

It has to be recognized that inappropriate application and transfer of technology and even aspects of certain development projects can have negative as well as positive consequences for health and nutrition in poor countries. It is important that such possible negative consequences be identified early and that measures be taken to offset and prevent them. It may be more important to enhance during project preparation those aspects that will have a positive impact for maximum nutritional benefits.

There is also a greater realization that the poor should be more involved in solving their own problems and that the causes of malnutrition and the different levels of society implicated vary from place to place. People should be able to ask appropriate questions relevant to their situation, at the national, local or even family level, and they should be aware of the multisectoral nature of the problem of malnutrition. They can then, together with persons from different disciplines, suggest actions that might be taken at different levels. During the past ten years a good deal has been written about local participation in development decisions and programmes. The innate wisdom of peasants, with regard to agriculture as well as other development-related matters such as health and nutritional status, has finally been widely acknowledged.

It has also been recognized that international and national policies and actions can influence nutritional status in the rural villages and city slums of developing countries. The State may determine taxes, control prices, run national institutions and oversee a legal system. Almost all of these factors influence, and some of them are influenced by, the formal and informal institutions in society. Clearly these institutions influence the causes of malnutrition. Thus the presence or absence, the relevance and the quality of formal local institutions such as agriculture advisory services, health centres, primary schools and community centres have a very important role in areas related to nutrition. But the more informal institutions can also have a role in influencing food, health and care. The most important of these is the family; others include groups of friends and religious, sporting or social groups.

The realization that malnutrition is not just a food problem has been appreciated for many years, but the concept of the importance of giving consideration to food, health, education and care is of more recent origin. It is vital that this thinking continue to develop and to move forward steadily, in the place of erratic leaps in pursuit of fashion or funding. For a healthy approach, in the next ten years, the achievements should be reassessed; old strategies that have sound logic and a successful record should be protected and supported, and new policies promoted only when needed. This approach is possible with both discipline and flexibility, and examples of its success are visible today.

A FRAMEWORK FOR CAUSES OF MALNUTRITION

Malnutrition or undesirable physical or disease conditions related to nutrition can be caused by eating too little, too much or an unbalanced diet that does not contain all nutrients necessary for good nutritional status. In this book the term malnutrition is restricted to undernutrition, or lack of adequate energy, protein and micronutrients to meet basic requirements for body maintenance, growth and development.

An essential prerequisite to the prevention of malnutrition in a community is the availability of enough food to provide for the nutrient needs of all people. For adequate food to be available, certainly there must be adequate food production or sufficient funds at the national, local or family level to purchase enough food. Availability of food, however, is just part of the picture. It is now recognized that malnutrition is only the overt sign, or symptoms, of much deeper problems in society.

Inadequate dietary intake and disease, particularly infections, are immediate causes of malnutrition. It is obvious that each person must eat an adequate amount of good-quality and safe food throughout the year to meet all nutritional needs for body maintenance, work and recreation, and for growth and development in children. Similarly, one must be able to digest, absorb and utilize the food and nutrients effectively. Poor diets and disease are often the result of insufficient household food security, inappropriate care and feeding practices and inadequate health care. It is now understood that good nutrition depends on adequate levels of all three of these factors.

Other factors can also contribute to unavailability or inadequacy of resources for afflicted families. Every rural community or society has certain natural or human resources as well as a certain potential for production. A host of factors influence what and how much food will be produced and how and by whom it will be consumed.

The proper use of resources may be

affected by economic, social, political, technical, ecological, cultural and other constraints. It may be affected by lack of tools or training to use them and by limited knowledge, skills and general ability to use the resources. The cultural context is of special importance for its influence, especially at the local level, on the use of resources and the establishment and maintenance of institutions.

Malnutrition may manifest itself as a health problem, and health professionals can provide some answers, but they alone cannot solve the problem of malnutrition. Agriculturists, and often agricultural professionals, are required to ensure that enough foods, and the right kinds of food, are produced. Educators, both formal and non-formal, are required to assist people, particularly women, in achieving and ensuring good nutrition. Tackling malnutrition often requires the contributions of professionals in economics, social development, politics, government, the labour movement and many other spheres.

PROMOTION AND PROTECTION OF NUTRITIONAL WELL-BEING: THE ICN APPROACH

The International Conference on Nutrition developed nine common areas for action to promote and protect the nutritional welfare of the population:
- improving household food security,
- protecting consumers through improved food quality and safety,
- preventing specific micronutrient deficiencies,
- promoting breastfeeding,
- promoting appropriate diet and healthy lifestyles,
- preventing and managing infectious diseases,
- caring for the economically deprived and nutritionally vulnerable,
- assessing, analysing and monitoring the nutrition situation,

- incorporating nutrition objectives into development policies and programmes.

Addressing issues under these themes facilitates the development of a common understanding of nutrition problems by various sectors and allows a more focused approach for working towards solutions. Taking this thematic approach to nutrition problems should ensure that each of the many facets of a problem are noted, which should allow each sector or agency to assess how it can best work for improvements. These issues are discussed in detail in Part V.

THE SIX Ps

By shedding the sectoral perspective and adopting a multisectoral, multidisciplinary one, it is possible to see the causes of malnutrition in a different guise and to focus the development of solutions less narrowly than in the past. Each case will be different, of course, and the extent to which one cause or one area of expertise predominates will vary with the circumstances. However, six determinants of malnutrition are especially important, although none is usually the only cause of malnutrition or the only discipline that needs to be involved in nutrition strategies.

These six determinants – the six Ps – are:
- *production*, mainly agricultural and food production;
- *preservation* of food from wastage and loss, which includes the addition of economic value to food through processing;
- *population*, which refers both to child spacing in a family and also to population density in a local area or a country;
- *poverty*, which suggests economic causes of malnutrition;
- *politics*, as political ideology, political choices and political actions influence nutrition;
- *pathology* which is the medical term

for disease, since disease, especially infection, adversely influences nutritional status.

Production

The production of food comes mainly from agriculture. Most countries have a ministry of agriculture and different kinds of agricultural staff whose contributions are very important to nutrition, but adequate national agricultural and food production does not guarantee good nutritional status for all people. As described in Chapter 2, there have been remarkable developments in agriculture in the past four decades. High-yielding varieties of the important cereals (rice, wheat and maize) have been successfully developed, and much progress has been made in increasing food yields per hectare of land. Some countries that are self-sufficient in their production of staple foods, however, still have the highest prevalence of malnutrition. Agriculturists and agriculture ministries have an absolutely vital role in improving nutritional status, but they cannot win the battle against malnutrition without action from other ministries and without other expertise. Other areas such as food safety, food losses and food storage influence the availability of food. Consideration has to be given to food demand as well as food production.

Preservation

Despite the remarkable progress made in increasing food production at the global level, approximately half of the people of developing countries do not have access to an adequate food supply. A substantial part of the food produced is lost, for various reasons, before it can be consumed. It has been estimated that about 25 percent of the grains produced are lost because of bad post-harvest handling, spoilage and pest infestation. Losses of easily perishable fruits, vegetables and roots have been

estimated to be about 50 percent of what is grown. After food reaches the home, about 10 percent is lost in the kitchen. Therefore, ensuring that appropriate measures are taken to prevent food losses during harvesting, transportation, storage, processing and preservation should be an integral component of any programme for the prevention of malnutrition and the improvement of the population's access to food in developing countries. Processing can also add nutritional and economic value to foods. Adequate measures for the provision of safe and quality food should also be taken.

Population

The population question and the relationship of fertility and the availability of family planning to nutrition are discussed in Chapter 5. The food available per person in a family, a district or a nation depends on the amount of food produced or purchased divided by the number of people who have access to that food. A family of eight that produces and purchases the same amount of food as a family of four has less food available per person. However, it also needs to be recognized that among producing families, larger family size can also lead to greater family productivity.

In some countries the population problem is considered to be of great importance, and overpopulation, family size and child spacing are considered important determinants of malnutrition. Demographers study population, and many countries have a government body, often in the ministry of health, responsible for family planning. Birth spacing may deserve a very high priority. However, as with production, it is naive to believe that in any country population control or successful family planning will by itself solve the problems of hunger and malnutrition.

Poverty

Poverty is often stated to be the very root cause of malnutrition. Certainly in most countries it is mainly, and sometimes only, the poor whose children suffer from severe or moderate PEM or show evidence of vitamin A deficiency. In contrast, nutritional anaemias and IDD may not be confined to the poor.

Economists are the professionals who study poverty and income and suggest economic solutions for problems of poverty which may be related to malnutrition. Most governments have a group of economists working in the ministry of finance and sometimes also in a ministry of economic planning.

The experience of many developing countries shows that a major reduction in poverty would have a significant impact on rates of PEM in most countries and communities. Efforts to reduce poverty, raise incomes, lower food prices and redistribute wealth, as well as a host of other economic policies, can have a major impact on nutrition. But just as agriculturists and demographers alone cannot solve the nutritional problems of a nation, so also economic actions alone do not usually rid a country or area of malnutrition. In some cases raised incomes have not resulted in major reductions in malnutrition and certainly have not led to its eradication.

Poverty takes many forms and is expressed in many ways. Inadequate household income is one manifestation, but poor communities and nations lack the wealth needed to build and support schools and training programmes, to improve water supplies and sanitation and to provide needed health and social services.

Politics

All countries have a mechanism to create and implement policies in spheres of development. The systems differ from one country to another, but agriculture, health, education, economic and other related policies strongly influence the well-being of the people, including their nutritional status. Some governments take their obligations seriously. If government leaders take the right to freedom from want seriously, then they also respect the right to freedom from hunger, freedom from lack of health services, freedom from poor housing and so on. These conditions, however, also depend on the resources of the country. The way in which political ideology can have a significant influence on malnutrition is probably through government acting to ensure some level of equity. Equity does not imply equality, it simply means a reasonable or relatively fair access of all people to the essential resources such as housing, education, food and health care. Policies directed towards improving access of women to resources for income generation, education and health care would particularly improve the nutritional welfare of the family and children.

Pathology

This sixth P connotes disease. Physiology refers to the normal functioning of the body and its organs and cells. Pathology refers to abnormal function and to disease. Much malnutrition in the world is caused or influenced not only by shortage of food, but by disease.

The relationship between malnutrition and infection has been extensively studied and documented. There is no doubt that common infections such as diarrhoea, respiratory disease, intestinal worms, measles and acquired immunodeficiency syndrome (AIDS) are important causes of malnutrition. These relationships are discussed in Chapter 3. In addition, certain non-infectious diseases may also be causes of malnutrition. Examples of these include a variety of malabsorption syndromes (conditions where the body does not absorb nutrients properly), many cancers and malignancies and some psychological illnesses.

Ministries of health and a variety of health personnel in the public and private sectors are responsible both for treatment of disease and for public health or preventive measures. In many countries the responsibility for government nutrition policies rests with the ministry of health, and often national institutes of nutrition fall under this ministry. Certainly health measures to prevent disease, especially infections, and also actions to provide medical care and appropriate treatment will help very much to reduce the extent of malnutrition in a country or a community. Health measures alone, however, have never been able to eliminate malnutrition totally.

A multidisciplinary perspective

This discussion of the six Ps, namely production, processing, population, poverty, politics and pathology, is designed to illustrate the complexity of both the underlying causes of malnutrition and the solutions. It illustrates that agriculturists, industrialists, demographers, economists, politicians and health personnel all have important roles in controlling malnutrition. It is also clear that no one ministry or single group of professionals is likely to eliminate hunger and malnutrition in society. Nutritionists, food scientists and others work across all these lines, and in a properly functioning national food and nutrition strategy they will collaborate with professionals in several of these disciplines as well as others. Achieving good nutrition may also require experts in anthropology, sociology and community development; it requires a good transport and marketing system; it benefits greatly from an education system that provides school for all, especially females, and

guarantees the highest levels of literacy; and it may involve many other actors. Nutrition strategies are truly multisectoral, which may sometimes present more difficulties at the national level than at the local or community level. Community participation, with the assistance of actors from different sectors including at least agriculture, health, community development and education, will often be needed to meet the challenge of good nutrition for all. The chapters in this book are designed to allow persons from different disciplines to understand the complexities of the nutrition problem but also to see that a variety of quite simple actions can contribute to improving nutrition.

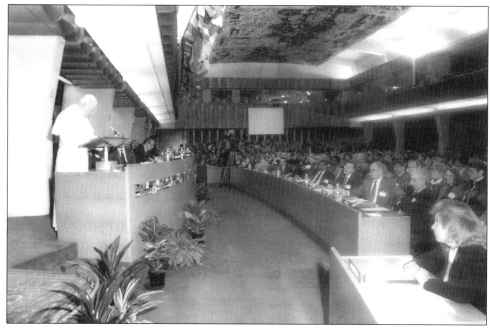

PHOTO 1
Pope John Paul II opens the International Conference on Nutrition

Chapter 2
Food production and food security

A national food policy should be a part of an overall nutrition strategy with household food security for all people as a central objective. Achieving food security includes ensuring:

- a nutritionally adequate and safe food supply at both the national and household levels;
- a reasonable degree of stability in the supply of food during the year and in all years;
- access by each household to sufficient food to meet the needs of all.

For all households to be food secure, each must have physical and economic access to adequate food. Each household must always have the ability, the knowledge and the resources to produce or procure the foods that it needs. Nutritionists stress also the need for the food to provide for all the nutritional requirements of the household members, which means a balanced diet providing all necessary energy, protein and micronutrients.

Beyond household food security is the need to encourage food distribution that ensures good nutritional status for all the members of the household. The right to an adequate standard of living, including food, is recognized in the Universal Declaration of Human Rights. National development policies should include food security as an objective, and achieving food security for all is an indication of success.

In nutrition there exists the paradox that while undernutrition leads to a serious set of health problems, overconsumption of food and of certain dietary components carries other risks to health. This book is particularly concerned with undernutri-tion. This chapter considers food security, at both the national and household levels, and food policy.

NATIONAL FOOD SECURITY

Food security is often defined as access by all people at all times to sufficient food required for a healthy and active life. It is now widely accepted that most of the undernutrition in developing countries is due to inadequate intake of both protein and energy and that it is often associated with infectious diseases.

In the past, protein deficiency was overemphasized as an important nutrition problem in the world. Commercial production of relatively expensive protein-rich foods, amino-acid fortification of cereal grains, production of single-cell protein and other ventures were offered as panaceas for the world's nutrition problems. These ventures only reduced the problem of protein-energy malnutrition (PEM) by a very small degree. Thus, in the context of combating malnutrition, attempts at making small changes in the amino-acid pattern of cereal grains by means of genetic manipulation are much less useful than increasing the yields per hectare of cereals and other food crops or enabling people to purchase the foods they need.

Satisfying the energy needs of a population, which should be the first goal of a food policy, has been a relatively neglected matter. In most populations where the staple food is a cereal such as rice, wheat, maize or millet, serious protein deficiencies seldom occur except where there is also an energy or overall food deficiency. The reason is that most cereals contain 8 to 12 percent protein and are often consumed with moderate quantities of legumes and vegetables. Protein deficiencies in people consuming these diets are mainly confined to very young children suffering increased nitrogen losses because of frequent infections. However, among populations whose staple food is plantain, cassava or some other food with a low protein content, protein intakes may be a problem for greater sections of the population.

A modest increase in cereal, legume, oil and vegetable consumption by children will greatly reduce the prevalence of PEM and growth deficits for children in developing countries, especially if combined with control of infectious diseases. Breast-feeding during the first few months of life can ensure an adequate diet, whereas bottle-feeding is a major cause of diarrhoea and nutritional marasmus (see Chapter 7).

Food availability (food supply)

To nourish a population adequately, there must be a sufficient quantity and variety of good-quality and safe food in the country. Therefore, in most low-income food-deficit countries a fundamental strategy of food policy is to improve and increase food production – a domain for agriculture experts. Clearly, decision-makers in the agriculture sector need to be aware of the nutritional needs of the population and to understand the nutritional implications of their actions.

Most food in the world comes from cereals. The second largest amount of food comes from root crops, followed by legumes or pulses. In round figures, the world produces about 2 000 million tonnes of cereals, 600 million tonnes of root crops and 60 million tonnes of pulses per year. In addition, about 85 million tonnes of fats and oils and 180 million tonnes of sugar are produced worldwide each year. Developing countries produce more of all

these items than do industrialized countries. In contrast, industrialized countries produce more foods of animal origin – meat, milk and eggs, for example – than do the developing countries.

In the last few decades, truly remarkable advances have influenced food production. Agricultural research has developed and made available new varieties of the main cereals: rice, maize and wheat. These new varieties produce much higher yields per hectare than the old varieties. Some have a shorter period between planting and harvesting, and some are relatively resistant to disease. However, most of these new varieties require increased fertilizer use. In addition, many of the improved rice varieties and some of the wheat and maize varieties require irrigation or more water. Both of these options may be economically unfeasible for most poor farmers. In general, cultivation of improved varieties is more suitable for large, economically comfortable farms with access to agricultural inputs. It should be a major agricultural policy objective to see that more resource-poor farmers have adequate access to such inputs.

The development of these new varieties – the green revolution – has allowed much higher yields of cereals for a given area of land. As population pressure increased on arable land, the green revolution offered an alternative to the old method of increasing production, namely expanding the area of land cultivated.

Average world food production has kept pace with or very slightly exceeded the increase in world population. In round figures, 2 700 kcal are available per person per day in the world. However, the figures vary among regions; the mean for industrialized countries is around 3 400 kcal, and that for developing countries is around 2 500 kcal. Of course, average availability figures for a country mask very large differences among groups of the population.

To improve nutrition, agricultural planners should aim to expand the production of currently grown staple cereals and legumes and should promote consumption of fruits, vegetables, oilseeds and livestock products or those of small animal husbandry. Where land pressures are a constraint, particular attention should be given to maintaining a proper balance between crops and livestock.

Some countries that were major food importers in the 1960s, such as India, are virtually self-sufficient in cereal production (mainly rice and wheat). Yet in India undernutrition and malnutrition remain highly prevalent. Other countries, such as Indonesia, have become self-sufficient in rice production and have significantly reduced the prevalence of malnutrition. Some countries are far from being self-sufficient in food production yet have far less malnutrition than countries like India. For example, many Caribbean countries have very low levels of PEM, and many have emphasized sugar production for export and chosen to pay to import much of their food. However, it should be pointed out that in environments with risky markets, joint promotion of both food and cash crops is required to achieve food security.

Developing countries should strive for integrated rural development combining sustainable agricultural development and the promotion of off-farm economic activities. Expanding agricultural efforts to increase and improve food production as well as to increase the income of rural families through greater production of cash crops is the job of most ministries of agriculture in developing countries.

Agricultural research in universities or in research stations is important to agricultural efforts. A good agricultural extension service can help farmers increase their productivity and make decisions about their farm practices. Agricultural research and extension, leading to higher levels of agricultural production, can have a major impact on nutrition, especially if improved production makes it easier for the poor to consume an adequate diet. Many textbooks examine how agriculture and food production are used to improve food intakes and nutritional status. They are essential reading for those who are interested in these aspects.

Local seasonal factors are very important influences on food supply. For example, rainfall patterns can give marked variations in food production within a year and between years. Food production can also be influenced by other factors such as pests, prices, availability of agricultural inputs and farmers' ability to procure them, political stability and peace. Climatic variations, especially rainfall (or its lack) and inclement weather, can lead to annual variations in food production. These variations may bring about complex food storage and management requirements (Photo 2). Seasonally high food prices may be tied to costs of storage and failure to manage public food stocks adequately.

Food storage limits and post-harvest losses due to insects, pests, moulds, bruising, high temperatures, etc. can seriously destabilize food supply. Yet even after production, harvest and storage are successfully accomplished, other factors can affect food supply. These include commercial food processing and industrialization; food marketing, including transport; policies related to importation and exportation of food, including food donated in multilateral or bilateral agreements; and external assistance and debt repayment.

Access to food (food demand)

Access to food, or food demand, is influenced by economic issues, physical infrastructure and consumer preferences.

Per caput incomes and food prices are important determinants of food demand.

Since the poor are the most vulnerable to food deficits and malnutrition, policies that increase their purchasing power will provide them with the potential to improve their nutrition. Therefore, increased employment and better wages become components of policies and programmes to improve nutrition. In many poor countries the minority of the working population are wage-earners and the majority are self-employed in agriculture. About 65 percent of the population in developing countries of Asia and Africa and about 35 percent in Latin America live in rural areas and rely on agriculture, fishing, animal production and forestry for food as well as for income to purchase food and other necessities. Assistance to help this group of poor farmers and rural workers increase their incomes and food productivity will have an effect similar to that of increasing the wages of the urban poor.

Food prices affect both supply and demand. Lower prices give farmers less revenue for their produce. If prices drop too low, farmers may not produce or sell at all. However, lower prices represent an increase in the purchasing power of the consumer. Lowering the price of a common staple food such as maize or rice is equivalent to raising the income of all those who purchase this food. Similarly, raising the price (a more common occurrence) is equivalent to lowering the income of those who purchase it.

Governments have various mechanisms at their disposal to help satisfy the needs of both producers and consumers. One of these is subsidizing food prices: the price paid to the farmer for a sack of maize or rice is raised while market prices for consumers are maintained, with the government paying for the difference between the two. Food price subsidies may be disastrous for the economy but politically expedient for the government. They

may help the poor to improve their nutrition.

Too often in the past, pricing policies and subsidies have been directed at foods consumed mainly by high-income groups and have thus had no beneficial effect on vulnerable groups. For example, price restrictions on meat, powdered milk or tinned baby foods or subsidies on beef or margarine would hardly benefit the poor at all, nor would they have important nutritional impact. Structural adjustment programmes put in place to mitigate severe economic crises often adversely affect the poor, particularly in the urban areas, through increased food prices. However, in many countries the majority of the rural poor are food producers, and structural adjustments may benefit them by raising their income from the sale of food produced and providing incentives to improve production efforts. By limiting inflation and reducing other macroeconomic distortions, structural adjustment programmes may benefit all population groups.

Food demand is also affected by consumer preferences, which can be shaped by cultural beliefs and practices or intra-household food allocation. An efficient infrastructure, including roads, railways, bridges and marketing facilities, is a determinant of the extent and success of food distribution to different segments of society. In the developing world and also in some industrialized countries, families living near food markets have a steady and easy access to cheaper foods and a more diversified diet, while people living far from markets usually have a rather narrow range of foods to choose from.

HOUSEHOLD FOOD SECURITY
Household food security is the ability of the household to secure enough food to provide for all the nutrient requirements of all members of the household. It is critical to link national food security and

household food security, because availability of food supplies in adequate quantity and variety is a necessary but insufficient condition for ensuring adequate access by all households in need. Furthermore, having adequate overall food supplies in households is a necessary but insufficient condition for ensuring nutritionally adequate consumption by all individuals within households. Clearly, the overall availability of food in a country, community or household is no guarantee of its equitable consumption.

Components of household food security
Household food security depends on a nutritionally adequate and safe food supply nationally, at the household level and for each individual; a fair degree of stability in the food availability to the household both during the year and from year to year; and access of each family member to sufficient food to meet nutritional requirements. (This last criterion includes not only physical access but also economic and social access to foods that are culturally acceptable.)

It is also important that the available food be both safe and of good quality. Attention to the food at every step of the food chain or food cycle is required to ensure its quality and safety. These steps include the cultivation of the food in the field (including protection against damage from pests or contamination with farm chemicals or pesticides); the harvesting, transport and storage of the food; processing and marketing; and finally the preparation and cooking of the food in the home and aspects of its consumption in the household. From the nutritionist's point of view, food losses and wastage along the chain are of great importance. However, important health concerns can also be raised if foods are not used correctly. An example is possible contamination, particularly from pesticides or other chemicals

used to enhance production or to control pests such as insects, fungi, bacteria and viruses, or from natural toxins.

Food quality and safety are also affected by food hygiene, food handlers, people involved in food processing, those retailing the food and finally practices in the home. Certain codes and government inspections may help ensure some degree of safety, and education and knowledge of food hygiene by all people will reduce the likelihood of contamination in the home. However, available facilities also influence food hygiene. Households that have poor facilities, no refrigeration, contaminated or inadequate water supplies or fuel shortages will find it more difficult to ensure food safety. See Chapter 33 for some ways to improve food safety and a discussion of food-borne diseases.

Another important aspect of food security is stability. The family or household must have the ability all year round to produce or procure the food its members require. The food must provide for all the family members' essential micronutrient and energy requirements, plus their wants, or desirable allowances, provided this does not lead to overconsumption. Of the greatest importance, especially when food or certain nutrients are available in marginal amounts, is proper distribution within the family to satisfy the special needs of children and females of child-bearing age.

Incomes received from cash crops or wage earnings and prices paid for purchased items influence a rural population's food security. Inadequate landholdings, landlessness, sharecropping and other causes of poverty are all potent causes of family food insecurity. For the one-third of the population of developing countries who live in urban areas, much of the food obtained is purchased. The household food security of the urban poor depends on incomes, prices and the need to spend earnings on other essentials such as housing and transport. Their food security can be threatened by increased prices, job loss, income reduction, rent increases, larger numbers of dependent persons (more children, or relatives moving into the household) and other factors.

In both urban and rural areas the food must satisfy not only the energy needs but also the micronutrient needs of each household member. Therefore, the food consumed by each person must be varied and its quantity must be sufficient. If this is not the case, micronutrient deficiencies may occur.

Household food insecurity

Malnutrition may result from inadequate food, inadequate health or inadequate care (see Chapter 1). Inadequate food, be it due to food shortages or to inappropriate consumer behaviour or intrahousehold distribution, is termed food insecurity.

Food insecurity at the household or individual level may be transitory, or short-term, because of a particular event of short duration. In these circumstances it results from a temporarily limited access to food. Chronic food insecurity is long-term, may have a more marked impact and may be more difficult to control. The intensity of either short-term or long-term food insecurity is also important. Food insecurity occurs in mild, moderate and severe forms, just as PEM does. The level of food insecurity may be related to the relative availability of food.

A "shock" often precipitates household food insecurity. The shock can aggravate poverty (suddenly making a poor family very poor) or adversely influence food production (suddenly threatening farm food availability). There are many different kinds of shock, for example, serious illness, which may result in loss of income in an urban family or reduced agricultural production in a farm family; loss of a rural

or urban job; farm production crises, such as failure of the rains; or a plague of locusts or some other agricultural catastrophe. Any crisis that has an adverse impact on the livelihood of the family may also result in household food insecurity.

Another important determinant of food insecurity is gender discrimination. Subordination of women in society, their overburdening and the greater difficulties faced by female-headed households contribute to food insecurity. Chapter 35 discusses ways to improve food security and reduce malnutrition in society.

FOOD POLICIES IN A DEVELOPMENT CONTEXT

Clearly, development strategies and interventions pursued by developed and developing nations have an impact on nutrition. For this impact to be positive, developed and developing countries must decide what "development" really means.

Too often in the past, development has been associated with industrialization and measured by the productive capacity and the material output of a country. Indicators of development were gross national product (GNP) or mean per caput incomes. Economists tended to view improved nutrition and health as welfare questions. However, it is now clear that economic development does not benefit everyone equally. The poor have often been bypassed, and improvements in the quality of life of most low-income families in many countries have not kept pace with the improvements in national economic figures. The purpose and the intended beneficiaries of economic development should be examined before the interventions begin. If development plans do not encompass improved health and better nutrition for people, then their worth must be seriously questioned.

Nutrition-positive development projects are those that will benefit a large segment of the population, help reduce inequalities in income distribution and be likely to improve the nutrition, health and quality of life of those currently deprived. Labour-intensive projects are often preferable to capital-intensive ones, and support for small farmers may be more useful in regard to nutrition than assistance for large estates. Small farmers and especially women farmers are the most disadvantaged and require the most help. They are also the ones who receive the least assistance, in terms of both extension services and access to credit. In many countries, too little of the national budget is devoted to support for agriculture, which is essential for social and economic development and for nutritional well-being.

Food policy should make marketing as logical, simple and well-organized as possible, with a minimum involvement of intermediaries, to help ensure that the producer gets a fair return for his or her produce and that the consumer pays the lowest reasonable price for his or her food. Cooperatives are one form of marketing that may benefit both producer and consumer.

Recently, both adequate food and good nutrition have been declared basic human rights. As discussed in Chapter 1, good nutrition goes beyond food rights, including also adequate care and adequate health. It has been suggested that household food security should be examined as part and parcel of a broader food and nutrition system. Food factors included in the system are food production and some of the influences on it; the transport system; the market and its relationship to exchange and storage; and finally household food availability and access. Most "food systems" do not give consideration to the health causes of malnutrition such as infections including diarrhoea and intestinal worms. They also do not include caring factors that may influence nutritional

status, such as breastfeeding, weaning and psycho-social stimulation. All of these factors are vital components of nutritional well-being. They are discussed in detail in other chapters of this book.

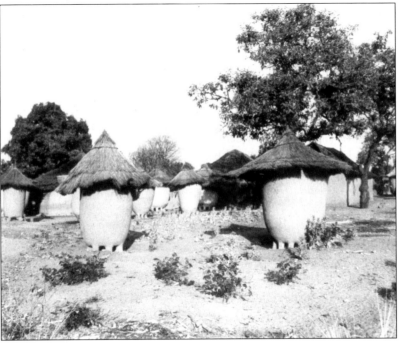

PHOTO 2
Village granaries in Côte d'Ivoire

Chapter 3
Nutrition and infection, health and disease

The interaction or synergism of malnutrition and infection is the leading cause of morbidity and mortality in children in most countries in Africa, Asia and Latin America. Viral, bacterial and parasitic infections tend to be prevalent, and all can have a negative impact on the nutritional status of children and adults. The situation was similar in North America and Europe from about 1900 to 1925; common infectious diseases had an impact on nutrition and produced high case fatality rates.

The synergistic relationship between malnutrition and infectious diseases is now well accepted and has been conclusively demonstrated in animal experiments. The simultaneous presence of both malnutrition and infection results in an interaction that has more serious consequences for the host than the additive effect would be if the two worked independently. Infections make malnutrition worse and poor nutrition increases the severity of infectious diseases.

EFFECTS OF MALNUTRITION ON INFECTION
The immune system
The human body has the ability to resist almost all types of organisms or toxins that tend to damage the tissues and organs. This capacity is called immunity. Much of the immunity is caused by a special immune system that forms antibodies and sensitized lymphocytes which attack and destroy the specific organisms or toxins. This type of immunity is called acquired immunity. An additional portion of the immunity results from the general processes of the body; this is called innate immunity.

Innate immunity is due to:
- resistance of the skin to invasion by organisms;
- phagocytosis of bacteria and other invaders by white blood cells and cells of the tissue macrophage system;
- destruction by the acid secretions of the stomach and by the digestive enzymes of organisms swallowed into the stomach;
- the presence in the blood of certain chemical compounds that attach to the foreign organisms or toxins and destroy them.

There are two basic but closely allied types of acquired immunity. In one of these the body develops circulating antibodies, which are globulin molecules that are capable of attacking the invading agents and destroying them. This type of immu-

---

Questions and answers

Why are the case fatality rates from measles often 200 times higher in poor, developing countries than in the industrialized countries? The main reason is that the malnourished child is often overwhelmed by the infection, whereas the well-nourished child can combat it and survive.

Why do so many cases of kwashiorkor develop following an infectious disease and so many cases of nutritional marasmus following gastro-enteritis? It is well established that infections result in increased nitrogen loss and that diarrhoea reduces the absorption of nutrients from the intestinal tract.

nity is called humoral immunity. Antibodies circulate in the blood and may remain there for a long time, so that a second infection with the same organism is immediately controlled. This is the basis for some forms of immunization, which are designed to stimulate antibody production.

The second type of acquired immunity is achieved through the formation of large numbers of highly specialized lymphocytes which are specifically sensitized against the invading foreign agents. These sensitized lymphocytes have the ability to attach to the foreign agents and to destroy them. This type of immunity is called cellular immunity. It is a highly complex system involving many different body organs (such as the spleen, thymus, lymph system and bone marrow) and also body fluids, particularly blood and its constituents and lymph.

The study of the complex system of immunity is termed immunology.

Effects of malnutrition on resistance to infection

A considerable amount of literature, documenting studies both in experimental animals and in people, demonstrates that dietary deficiency diseases may reduce the body's resistance to infections and adversely affect the immune system.

Some of the normal defence mechanisms of the body are impaired and do not function properly in the malnourished subject. For example, children with kwashiorkor were shown to be unable to form antibodies to either typhoid vaccine or diphtheria toxoid; their capacity to do so was restored after protein therapy. Similarly, children with protein malnutrition have an impaired antibody response to inoculation with yellow fever vaccine. An inhibition of the agglutinating response to cholera antigen has been reported in children with kwashiorkor and nutritional marasmus. These studies provide a fairly

clear indication that the malnourished body has a reduced ability to defend itself against infection.

Another defence mechanism that has been studied in relation to nutrition is that of leucocytosis (increased production of white blood cells) and phagocytic activity (destruction of bacteria by white corpuscles). Children with kwashiorkor show a lower than normal leucocyte response in the presence of an infection. Perhaps of greater importance is the reduced phagocytic efficiency in malnourished subjects of the polymorphonuclear leucocytes that are part of the fight against invading bacteria. When malnutrition is present, these cells appear to have a defect in their intracellular bactericidal (bacteria-destroying) capacity.

Although malnourished children frequently have increased immunoglobulin levels (presumably related to concurrent infections), they also may have depressed cell-mediated immunity. In a recent study, the extent of this depression was directly related to the severity of the protein-energy malnutrition (PEM). Serum transferrin levels are also low in those with severe PEM, and they often take considerable time to return to normal even after proper dietary treatment.

A quite different kind of interaction of nutrition and infection is seen in the effect of some deficiency diseases on the integrity of the tissues. Reduction in the integrity of certain epithelial surfaces, notably the skin and mucous membranes, decreases resistance to invasion and makes an easy avenue of entry for pathogenic organisms. Examples of this effect are cheilosis and angular stomatitis in riboflavin deficiency, bleeding gums and capillary fragility in vitamin C deficiency, flaky-paint dermatosis and atrophic intestinal changes in severe protein deficiency and serious eye lesions in vitamin A deficiency.

EFFECTS OF INFECTION ON NUTRITIONAL STATUS

Infection affects nutritional status in several ways. Perhaps the most important of these is that bacterial and some other infections lead to an increased loss of nitrogen from the body. This repercussion was first demonstrated in serious infections such as typhoid fever, but it has subsequently been shown in much milder infections such as otitis media, tonsillitis, chicken pox and abscesses.

Nitrogen is lost by several mechanisms. The principal one is probably increased breakdown of tissue protein and mobilization of amino acids, especially from the muscles. The nitrogen is excreted in the urine and is evidence of a depletion of body protein from muscles.

Full recovery is dependent upon the restoration of these amino acids to the tissues once the infection is overcome. This requires increased intake of protein, above maintenance levels, in the post-infection period. In children whose diet is marginal in protein content, or those who are already protein depleted, growth will be retarded during and after infections. In developing countries, children from poor families suffer from many infections in quick succession during the post-weaning period, and they often have multiple infections.

Anorexia or loss of appetite is another factor in the relationship between infection and nutrition. Infections, especially if accompanied by a fever, often lead to loss of appetite and therefore to reduced food intake. Some infectious diseases commonly cause vomiting, with the same result. In many societies mothers and often medical attendants as well consider it desirable to withhold food or to place the child with an infection on a liquid diet. Such a diet may consist of rice water, very dilute soups, water alone or some other fluid with a low calorie density and usually deficient in protein and other essential nutrients. The old adage of "starve a fever" is of doubtful validity, and this practice may have serious consequences for the child whose nutritional status is already precarious.

The traditional treatment of diarrhoea in some communities is to prescribe a purgative or enema. The gastro-enteritis may already have resulted in reduced absorption of nutrients from food, and the treatment may further aggravate this situation.

These are all examples of how illnesses such as measles, upper respiratory infections and gastro-intestinal infections may contribute to the development of malnutrition. The relationship of intestinal parasites, diarrhoea and measles to nutrition is discussed below.

Parasitic infections

Parasitic infections, particularly intestinal helminthic infections, are extremely prevalent and are increasingly being shown to have an adverse effect on nutritional status, especially in those heavily infected. Hookworms (*Ancylostoma duodenale* and *Necator americanus*) infect over 800 million people, mainly the poor in tropical and subtropical countries. They used to cause a prevalent debilitating disease in the southern United States. Hookworms cause intestinal blood loss, and although it appears that most of the protein in the lost blood is absorbed lower down in the intestinal tract, there is considerable loss of iron.

Hookworm disease is a major cause of iron deficiency anaemia in many countries. The extent of the loss of blood and iron in hookworm infections has been studied (Layrisse and Roche, 1966): daily faecal blood loss per hookworm (*N. americanus*) was reported to be 0.031 ± 0.015 ml. It was estimated that about 350 hookworms in the intestine cause a daily loss of 10 ml of blood, or 2 mg of iron. Infection densities much higher than this are not uncommon.

In Venezuela, where much of this work was done, iron losses greater than 3 mg per day often resulted in anaemia in adult males, and losses of half this amount frequently produced anaemia in women of child-bearing age and in young children.

Worldwide, roundworm (*Ascaris lumbricoides*) is among the most prevalent of intestinal parasites. It is estimated that 1 200 million people in the world (one-quarter of the world's population) harbour roundworms. The roundworm is large (15 to 30 cm long), so its own metabolic needs must be considerable. High parasite densities, particularly in children, are common in environments where sanitation is poor. Complications of ascariasis can develop, including intestinal obstruction or the presence of worms in aberrant sites such as the common bile duct. In some countries ascarids are a cause of surgical emergencies in children, and many with obstruction die. In the majority of children, however, when malnutrition is prevalent, deworming improves child growth.

Trichuris trichiura or whipworm inhabits the large intestine and infects about 600 million people worldwide. The worms are small and, in heavily infected children, may cause diarrhoea and abdominal pain.

Many children living in poor sanitary conditions are infected with several parasitic infections at the same time. In areas where infection with these three parasites is common and where malnutrition is prevalent, deworming of children leads to an improvement in growth, a reduction in the extent of malnutrition and an increase in appetite. It also positively influences physical fitness and perhaps psychological development.

Bilharzia or schistosomiasis infections are prevalent in some countries. They also contribute to poor nutrition, poor appetite and poor growth. The three organisms that cause schistosomiasis (*Schistosoma haematobium*, *Schistosoma mansoni* and *Schistosoma japonicum*) are flukes, rather than ordinary worms.

Somewhat less is known about the relationship between intestinal protozoal diseases and nutrition, but amoebas, causing serious dysentery and liver abscess, are highly pathogenic organisms, and infection with *Giardia lamblia* may cause malabsorption and abdominal pain.

The fish tapeworm (*Diphyllobothrium latum*) has an avidity for vitamin B_{12} and can deprive its host of this vitamin, with megaloblastic anaemia resulting. The fish tapeworm is common in people in only limited geographic areas, mainly in temperate areas and where undercooked fish is frequently consumed.

In many northern industrialized countries, farm animals and domestic pets such as dogs and cats are dewormed routinely. Much evidence suggests that pigs grow better when they regularly receive anthelmintics. Now that highly effective, relatively inexpensive and safe broad-spectrum anthelmintics such as albendazole and mebendazole are available, routine mass deworming should be introduced where parasitic infections are prevalent in humans and where PEM and anaemia are common. Similarly, routine efforts to treat children with schistosomiasis using metrifonate or praziquantel seem highly desirable both to rid children of potential serious pathology and to improve their nutritional status. More attention needs to be given to population-based chemotherapy for these infections along with intensification of public health and other measures to reduce their transmission, including improved sanitation and water supplies. Such efforts would improve the health and nutritional status of millions of the world's children.

Effects of diarrhoea

Many studies have indicated that gastrointestinal infections, and especially diarrhoea, are very important in precipitating serious PEM. Diarrhoea is common in, and often lethal to, the young child. In breast-fed infants there is often some protection during the first months of life, so diarrhoea is often a feature of the weaning process. Weanling diarrhoea is extraordinarily prevalent in poor communities throughout the world, both in tropical and temperate zones. The organism responsible varies and often cannot be identified. Diarrhoea was a major cause of mortality in children in industrialized countries up to the beginning of the twentieth century.

Several studies have shown that admissions of cases of malnutrition are greatly increased during the season when diarrhoea is most common. For example, in a report from the Islamic Republic of Iran, more than twice as many cases of PEM were admitted in the warm summer than in the cold winter. The incidence of diarrhoeal disease followed the same pattern.

Hospital and community studies indicate that cases of xerophthalmia and keratomalacia are frequently precipitated by gastro-enteritis, as well as by other infectious diseases such as measles and chicken pox. Xerophthalmia is the major cause of blindness in several Asian countries; it is also prevalent in certain parts of Africa, Latin America and the Near East.

Intestinal parasites may contribute to diarrhoea and to poor vitamin A status. The exact mechanism of this relationship has not been proved, but it is likely that many infections reduce vitamin A absorption and that some result in decreased consumption of foods containing vitamin A and carotene.

Diarrhoea can be fatal, usually because it can lead to severe dehydration (see Chapter 37). Diarrhoea, and the complication of dehydration, may be said to be a form of malnutrition. Dehydration is a "deficiency" in the body of water and mineral electrolytes, and providing adequate quantities of these cures the deficiency. The term "fluid electrolyte malnutrition" (FEM) has been coined for this condition. Provision of water and adequate minerals in home-prepared food, breast-feeding or administration of oral rehydration fluids is now the accepted treatment. Although these are forms of therapy or treatment, they are really refeeding and replenishment. However, prevention requires measures and interventions to reduce infections, poverty and malnutrition. These are essential if countries are to reduce the incidence of diarrhoea.

Fatality rates for measles and other infectious diseases

A dramatic illustration of the effect of malnutrition on infection is seen in the fatality rates for common childhood diseases such as measles. Measles is a severe disease with a case fatality rate of about 15 percent in many poor countries because the young children who develop it have poor nutritional status, lowered resistance and poor health. In Mexico the fatality rate for measles has been reported to be 180 times higher than that in the United States; in Guatemala, 268 times higher; and in Ecuador, 480 times higher. The decline in case fatality rates of measles in North America, Europe and other industrialized countries has been dramatic over the last century.

Differences in the clinical severity and the fatality rates of measles in developed and developing countries are due not to differences in virus virulence but to differences in the hosts' nutritional status. For example, during a measles epidemic in the United Republic of Tanzania that was causing considerable mortality among the children of poorer families, it was observed that fatalities from the disease were extremely uncommon in the children of families of moderate income, such as those of hospital employees. Measles is also related to vitamin A deficiency. It has been shown that providing vitamin A supplements to children with measles who have poor vitamin A status greatly reduces case fatality rates.

Immunization against measles is proving very effective, and in many countries measles incidence has been markedly reduced.

Other common infectious diseases such as whooping cough, diarrhoea and upper respiratory infections also have much more serious consequences in malnourished children than in those who are well nourished. Mortality statistics from most developing countries show that such communicable diseases are the major causes of death. It was observed in several African countries at the end of the Sahel famine that very few children were dying of starvation or malnutrition, but that deaths from measles, respiratory infections and other infectious diseases were still very much above pre-famine levels. It is clear that many, perhaps the majority, of these deaths were due to malnutrition. This may seem a moot point for a grieving parent, but for the policy planner and the public health official it is important to know to what extent morbidity and mortality rates are due to or related to undernutrition.

An inter-American investigation of mortality in childhood showed that of 35 000 deaths of children under five years of age in ten countries, in 57 percent of the cases malnutrition was either the underlying or an associated cause of death. Nutritional deficiency was the most serious health problem uncovered, and it was frequently associated with common infectious diseases.

HIV infection and AIDS

Perhaps no disease has a more dramatic and obvious effect on nutritional status than acquired immunodeficiency syn-drome (AIDS), the disease caused by the human immunodeficiency virus (HIV). In Uganda for many years the disease was called "slim disease" because extreme thinness was the main visible manifestation of the disease. Although the mechanisms by which AIDS leads to severe malnutrition have not been proven, there is no doubt that the disease and its associated opportunistic infections cause marked anorexia, diarrhoea and malabsorption as well as increased nitrogen losses. Some of the infections and conditions that are part of the AIDS complex of diseases were known to affect nutritional status long before the HIV virus was identified: tuberculosis has for many decades been associated with cachexia and weight loss, and malignancies such as sarcoma have long been known to result in wasting as they advance.

For a discussion of the relationship of AIDS to breastfeeding, see Chapter 7.

CHRONIC DISEASES AND OLD AGE

There is a relationship between certain chronic diseases and immune response. It has also been clearly shown that in old age immunologic response is reduced, and undernutrition worsens this decline. The association of diabetes with infections is well known, and it is clear that in diabetes there is often impaired cellular response. Other diseases, for example several cancers, may also be related to lowered immune response (see Chapter 23).

INTERVENTION STUDIES

There have been relatively few well-controlled intervention studies to demonstrate either the effects of improved diets on infection or the nutritional effects of control of infectious diseases. Research in the village of Candelaria in Colombia showed that diarrhoea declined sharply as a result of supplementary feeding of children. A similar study in a Guatemalan village illustrated a significant decline in morbidity and mortality from certain common illnesses following the introduction of a nutritious daily supplement for preschool children.

A classic study conducted in Narangwal in the Punjab region of India demonstrated the value of combining nutritional care and health care in one programme. Children were divided into four groups. One group was given dietary supplements, one group was given health care, one group received both the supplements and the health care, and the fourth group served as control. As far as nutritional status and certain other health parameters were concerned, the combined treatment gave the best results. Nutritional supplementation alone also had a major impact. In comparison with the control group, there was no improvement in the nutritional status of the group that received only medical care but no dietary supplements.

NUTRITION, INFECTION AND NATIONAL DEVELOPMENT

Clearly, the effects of nutritional status on infections and of infections on malnutrition signify a very important relationship. The majority of children in most developing countries suffer from malnutrition at some time in their first five years of life. The problems of infection and malnutrition are closely interrelated, yet programmes to control communicable diseases and to improve nutrition tend to be introduced quite independently. It would be much more efficient and effective if the twin problems were attacked together.

Success in improving the health and reducing the mortality of children is dependent both on control of infectious diseases and on improvements in the children's food intake and care. There is increasing evidence to suggest that parents are more willing to control their family size when the chances are good that most

children born will survive into adulthood. Consideration also needs to be given to providing a stimulating environment for the growing child.

The situation in the major industrial cities of Europe and North America a century ago was comparable to that in the poorest developing countries today. In New York City in the summer months of 1892, the infant mortality rate was 340 per 1 000, and diarrhoea accounted for half these deaths. Improvements in nutrition, through the use of milk stations, for example, and a reduction in infectious disease served to lower these mortality rates by half in a period of less than 25 years. In the United Kingdom at the beginning of the twentieth century, rickets, combined with infectious diseases, took a heavy toll in the insanitary, smoky slums of the industrial cities, and measles was very often fatal among children of poor families, presumably because of poor nutrition.

Malnutrition and infections combine to pose an enormous hazard to the health of the majority of the world's population who live in poverty. This ever-present hazard particularly threatens children under five years of age. Many of the children who suffer from both malnutrition and a series of infections succumb and die. They are continually replaced in answer to parents' strong desire and often real need to have surviving children. The children who live beyond five years of age are not mainly those who have escaped malnutrition or infectious diseases, but those who have survived. Seldom are they left without the permanent sequelae or scars of their early health experiences. They are often retarded in their physical, psychological or behavioural development, and they may have other abnormalities that contribute to a less than optimal ability to function as adults and possibly to a shortened life expectation. Other factors influencing the development of these children include a lack of environmental stimulation and a host of other deprivations related to poverty.

The challenge to health workers, development economists, governments and international agencies is how best to reduce the morbidity, mortality and permanent sequelae that result from the synergism of malnutrition and infection. The politicians must be persuaded that attention to these problems is not only highly desirable but politically advantageous.

The control of infectious diseases and projects aimed at providing more and better food for people are fully justified and important components of a development plan. By themselves they may contribute to increased productivity and better lives. An improved infant or toddler mortality rate, a lowered disease incidence and a better-nourished population are probably better indicators of development than national averages of telephones or automobiles per 1 000 families, or even than dollars or pesos per caput. Efforts for the control of infectious diseases and the improvement of nutrition both deserve a high priority in development plans and in international or bilateral assistance to low-income countries. They should be undertaken together because they will be mutually reinforcing and more economical if provided in a coordinated manner rather than separately. An allied issue is the need to provide a stimulating environment for the growing child.

Historical and epidemiological evidence suggests that reductions in infant and child mortality and improvements in health and nutritional status may be prerequisites to successful family planning efforts. Birth spacing deserves a high priority, especially where women are already overworked and undernurtured. Parents in all countries should receive assistance to help them achieve their desired family size.

Alarming as the situation of children's malnutrition and infection is, there is a general tendency to overlook the significance of these conditions in adults. Weakness, lethargy, absenteeism, poor productivity and stress can all have social and economic costs for individuals, families and communities.

There seems to be unassailable logic in recommending coordinated programmes that have three objectives: to control infectious disease, to improve nutrition and to make family planning services widely available. These three types of endeavour may themselves be synergistic.

Chapter 4
Social and cultural factors in nutrition

Social factors and cultural practices in most countries have a very great influence on what people eat, on how they prepare food, on their feeding practices and on the foods they prefer. Nonetheless, cultural food practices are very rarely the main, or even an important, cause of malnutrition. On the contrary, many practices are specifically designed to protect and promote health; providing women with rich, energy-dense foods during the first months following childbirth is an example. It is true, however, that some traditional food practices and taboos in some societies may contribute to nutritional deficiencies among particular groups of the population. Nutritionists need to have a knowledge of the food habits and practices of the communities in which they work so that they can help to reinforce the positive habits as well as strive to change any negative ones.

FOOD HABITS AND THEIR ORIGINS

All people have their likes and dislikes and their beliefs about food, and many people are conservative in their food habits. They tend to like what their mothers cooked for them when they were young, the foods that are served on festive occasions or those eaten with friends and family away from home during their childhood. The foods that adults ate without a second thought in childhood are seldom totally disagreeable to them in later life.

What one society regards as normal or even highly desirable, however, another society may consider revolting or totally inedible. Animal milk is commonly consumed and liked by many people in Asia, Africa, Europe and the Americas, but in China it is rarely taken. Lobsters, crabs and shrimps are considered delicacies and prized foods by many people in Europe and North America, but are revolting to many people in Africa and Asia, especially those who live far from the sea. The French eat horse meat; the English generally do not. Many people will delightedly consume the flesh of monkeys, snakes, dogs and rats or will eat certain insects, yet many others find these foods most unappealing. Religion may have an important role in forbidding the consumption of certain foods. For example, neither the Muslim nor the Jewish peoples consume pork, and Hindus do not eat beef and are frequently vegetarians.

Food habits differ most widely in regard to which foods of animal origin are liked, disliked, eaten or not eaten in a society. The foods in question comprise many of those that are rich in good-quality protein and that contain haem iron, both of which are important nutrients. People who do not consume these foods are deprived of the opportunity of obtaining these nutrients easily. On the other hand, those who overconsume animal flesh, some seafoods, eggs and other foods of animal origin will have undesirable amounts of saturated fat and cholesterol in the diet. Balanced consumption is the key.

Relatively few people or societies have strong negative feelings about consuming cereals, roots, legumes, vegetables or fruit. They may have strong preferences and likes, but most maize-eating people are also willing to eat rice, and most rice-eating people will eat wheat products.

It is often stated that food habits seldom or never change and are difficult to change. This is not true; in many countries the current staple foods are not the same as those eaten even a century ago. Food habits and customs do change, and they are influenced in many different ways. Maize and cassava are not indigenous to Africa, yet they are now major food staples in many African countries. Potatoes originated in the Americas and later became an important food in Ireland.

Food preferences are not made and abolished by whims and fancies, of course. More often the adjustments are generated by social and economic changes that take place throughout the community or society. The issue is often not what foods are eaten but rather how much of each food is eaten and how the consumption is distributed within the society or within the family.

The tendency of many wage-earners to spend almost all their wages within a few days of receiving them often results in a family diet of varying nutritive value. The family eats much better just after one payday than just before the next. Wages are often paid monthly, and there seems little doubt that a change to weekly payment of wages would improve the diet of wage-earners and their families.

The person who controls the family finances influences (intentionally or unintentionally) both the family diet and the food fed to children. In general, when mothers, rather than just fathers, have some control over finances, the family diet is likely to be better. When the mother has little control over family funds, dietary arrangements may become haphazard or even dangerous.

Nutrition education has been an important influence on food habits, and not always a positive one. Fortunately, the days are long gone when nutritionists promoted costly protein-rich foods to people who couldn't possibly afford them. Unfortunately, the tendency to single out foods or nutrients either to promote or to prohibit has not yet gone, nor has the tendency to try to teach by creating fear and taking the enjoyment out of eating. However, change always comes slowly and old habits die hard; people who were taught in these old ways are still responsible for feeding themselves and their families, and they may find it hard to change again.

NUTRITIONAL ADVANTAGES OF TRADITIONAL FOOD HABITS

The traditional diets of most societies in developing countries are good. Usually only minor changes are needed to enable them to satisfy the nutrient requirements of all members of the family. Although the quantity of food eaten is a more common problem than the quality, this chapter focuses on types of food and eating habits.

Eating certain protein-rich foods such as insects, snakes, baboons, mongooses, dogs, cats, unusual seafoods and snails is definitely beneficial. Another habit that is good nutritionally is the consumption of animal blood. Some African tribes puncture the vein of a cow, draw off a calabash of blood, arrest the bleeding and consume the blood, usually after mixing it with milk. Blood is a rich food, and mixed with milk it is highly nutritious.

A custom frequently found among pastoral and other peoples is the drinking of soured or curdled milk, rather than fresh. The souring of milk has little effect on its nutritive value but often substantially reduces the number of pathogenic organisms present. In communities where milking is not hygienically performed and where the containers into which the milk goes are likely to be contaminated, it is safer to drink sour rather than fresh milk. Boiled milk would be safer still.

Many societies, for example in Indonesia

and in parts of Africa, partly ferment foods before consumption. Fermentation may both improve the nutritional quality and reduce bacterial contamination of the food.

The traditional use of certain dark green leaves among rural peoples is another beneficial practice and should be encouraged. These leaves are rich sources of carotene, ascorbic acid, iron and calcium; they also contain useful quantities of protein. Non-cultivated or wild dark green leaves such as amaranth leaves as well as those from cultivated food crops such as pumpkin, sweet potato and cassava are much richer in vitamins than pale, leafy vegetables of European origin such as cabbage and lettuce. Well-meaning expatriate horticulturists in Africa have too often tried to get villagers to cultivate such European vegetables rather than their traditional vegetables.

Many wild fruits are rich in vitamin C; an example is the pulp within the pod of the frequently consumed baobab.

Traditional grain preparation methods produce a more nutritious product than does elaborate machine milling.

Some communities sprout legume seeds prior to cooking, which enhances their nutritive value, as does the soaking of whole-grain cereals before their processing into local beers and some non-alcoholic beverages. These seeds and grains usually have a high vitamin B content. Finally, it cannot be stressed too strongly that the traditional method of infant feeding – from the breast – is nutritionally far superior to bottle-feeding (see Chapter 7).

FOOD TABOOS

A number of food habits and practices are poor from a nutritional point of view. Some practices result from traditional views about food that are liable to change under the influence of neighbouring peoples, travel, education, etc. Other food practices are governed by definite taboos.

A taboo may be followed by a whole national group or tribe, by part of a tribe or by certain groups in the society. Within the society, different food customs may be practised only by women or children, or by pregnant women or female children. In certain cases traditional food customs are practised by a particular age group, and in other instances a taboo may be linked with an occupation such as hunting. At other times or in other individuals a taboo may be imposed because of some particular event such as an illness or an initiation ceremony.

Although these matters border on the realm of anthropology, it is important for a nutritionist to be familiar with the food customs of people in order to be able to improve their nutritional status through nutrition education or other means. Moreover, it is evident that anthropology and sociology are important to the nutrition worker who is either investigating or trying to improve the nutritional status of any community.

Some customs and taboos have known origins, and many are logical, although the original reasons may no longer be known. The custom may have become part of the religion of the people involved. For example, the Jewish taboo against pork was probably introduced to eliminate the prevalent pork tapeworm, which was thought to be sapping the strength of the Jewish people. Even though 2 000 years later it is now possible to eat pork safely, Jews still do not eat pork. Muslims share this view about pork. In neither case is this a nutritionally damaging taboo.

Many taboos concern the consumption of protein-rich animal foods, often by those groups of the community most in need of protein. A common taboo in Africa against the consumption of eggs is rapidly disappearing. This taboo usually applies to females, who are said to become sterile if they eat eggs. The psychological connection between human fertility and the egg is obvious. In other places the custom applies to children, perhaps to discourage them from stealing the eggs of setting hens, which would endanger the survival of poultry. Other customs, again often affecting women and children, concern fish. These customs may amount to a full taboo, although people not used to fish often dislike it merely because they find its smell distasteful or its appearance "snake-like". Many cultures have strong views about the consumption of milk or milk products.

The customs that prohibit consumption of certain nutritionally valuable foods may not have an important overall nutritional impact, particularly if only one or two food items are affected. Some societies, however, forbid such a wide range of foods to women during pregnancy that it is difficult for them to obtain a balanced diet.

Many of the nutritionally undesirable taboos that existed a quarter of a century ago have weakened or disappeared as a result of education, mixing of people from different societies and travel. Of those that remain, some food habits may seem illogical and their origins obscure, but it is not advisable for outsiders to try to alter ancient food habits without looking very closely into their origins. Moreover, it makes no sense to attempt to alter a habit that does not negatively affect nutritional status.

Nutritionally bad habits, like all other habits, are best changed by the people who have them. In this regard, influential local people, with the welfare of their fellows at heart, may join nutritionists and become part of an important alliance pledged to eradicating malnutrition. A speech by the president or a cabinet minister, the sight of a respected tribe leader eating some forbidden food and coming to no harm or the return to the village of educated and enlightened local people will prove much

more effective than the preaching or goading of an outsider.

CHANGING FOOD HABITS

In some parts of the world the staple foods are changing or have changed. Maize, cassava and potatoes, now grown in large amounts in Africa, originated outside the continent. Since none of these foods were eaten in Africa a few hundred years ago, it is clear that the food habits of millions of people have changed. Vast numbers of people in Africa have abandoned yams and millet for maize and cassava, just as many in Europe abandoned oats, barley and rye for wheat and potatoes. Food habits are still changing rapidly. The difficulty, of course, lies in trying to guide and foster desirable changes and to slow down undesirable ones.

It is often difficult to fathom what factors have been most important in stimulating or influencing changes in food habits. The rapid increase in bread consumption in many African, Latin American and Asian countries where wheat is not the staple food is understandable. It is at least in part a labour-saving phenomenon; bread is one of the first "convenience" foods to have become available. Before leaving home to go to work one can eat some slices of bread instead of the traditional breakfast of porridge, which requires preparation time and is unpleasant cold. Bread can be carried in the pocket and eaten during a break in the working day, or when travelling.

In most of the world the traditional main staple food has remained constant, irrespective of urbanization, modernization or even westernization. Thus in much of Asia rice remains the preferred staple food in rural and urban areas. Some people in Africa, such as the Buganda in Uganda and the Wachagga in the United Republic of Tanzania, continue to have a preference for plantains as their staple food. Maize-based products such as tortillas remain important in the diets of most Mexicans and many in Central America.

Changes in food habits are not just accidental, of course; they can be deliberately initiated. At community and family level, school-age children can be important agents for change. They are still forming their tastes and developing their preferences. If they are introduced to a new food they will often readily accept it and like it. School meals may usefully introduce new foods to children and thus influence food habits. This widening of food experience in childhood is extremely important. Children may influence the immediate family and later their own children to eat new, highly nutritious foods.

HARMFUL NEW HABITS

Not all change is desirable, of course, and not all new food habits are good. Chapter 7 describes in detail the harmful effects of the rapid spread of bottle-feeding using infant formula or animal milk in place of breastfeeding. This is an undesirable, relatively new food trend. Less attention has been given to the question of other baby foods that have been marketed and much promoted and advertised in developing countries. Locally available complementary or weaning foods, home-produced and traditionally fed, are often as or more nutritious than the manufactured baby foods, and they are always much cheaper. They are usually introduced gradually while breastfeeding continues well into the second year and beyond. Manufactured baby foods should only be promoted to those who are unable or unwilling to continue breastfeeding. They are safe and nutritionally adequate when prepared hygienically and in the right dilution. They are convenient for those who can afford to purchase them. However, such manufactured foods are expensive compared with local foods, and

for most families in developing countries, other than the very affluent, they may be a waste of money. For families who already have too little money to spend on food and other essentials, these foods are a very expensive way of buying the nutrients that they are advertised to contain.

Another particularly misleading type of advertising relates to the glucose products said to provide "instant energy". Energy is present in large amounts in nearly all the cheapest foods. Similarly, drinks advertised as "rich in vitamin C" are usually unnecessary, since few children suffer from vitamin C deficiency. Vitamin C can be obtained just as well from fruits such as guavas, mangoes and citrus, or from a range of vegetables.

The so-called protein-rich weaning foods are also much advertised. These are nutritionally good products, but they cost much more than protein-rich foods available in the market such as beans, groundnuts or dried fish, meat, eggs or milk. It usually costs much more to provide 100 g of protein from these commercially advertised products than, for example, from beans bought in the local market. The essential question is how a mother could best improve her child's diet if she had a little extra to spend. The answer would seldom be a manufactured baby food.

In some countries the staple food has remained unaltered, but the form in which it is preferred may have changed over the years. As described in Chapter 16, the rapid spread and popularity of highly milled rice in Asia had disastrous consequences and led to a high prevalence of beriberi, with much morbidity and many deaths. In many parts of the world highly milled cereals have replaced traditionally lightly milled and more nutritious wheat, rice and maize. In the United Kingdom and the Russian Federation, white bread has replaced brown or whole-grain breads, and in East Africa highly milled maize meal is often purchased and has replaced lightly milled maize flour. Urbanization, modernization and sophistication have often led to diets in which a greater percentage of energy intake comes from sugar and fats, and to increased consumption of salt. All of these are generally undesirable changes from a nutritional standpoint.

INFLUENCING CHANGE FOR THE BETTER

What can health workers or nutritionists in a community do about food habits, old and new? They can:

- protect, support and help preserve the many excellent existing food habits that are nutritionally valuable;
- respect the knowledge and customs of the people in the community in which they work;
- set good examples in their own households by adopting good food habits;
- influence respected local leaders to state publicly that they themselves have dropped undesirable food taboos, and arrange for them, when occasion arises, to eat "forbidden" foods in public;
- persuade people not to abandon good food habits under the influence of "sophisticates" back from the city who may try to discourage rural dwellers from eating nutritious traditional foods such as locusts or lake flies or to encourage the consumption and production of European-type vegetables in place of better traditional ones;
- explain the disadvantages of highly refined cereal flours if they have become popular in the area, and advocate the consumption of a range of cereals in the local diet;
- take the steps described in Chapter 7 to protect, support and promote breastfeeding and to eliminate all promotion of breastmilk substitutes;
- discourage poorer families from purchasing manufactured baby foods, and

encourage the use of locally available complementary foods;
- issue informational material to help stop the spread of bottle-feeding and the unnecessary purchase of expensive baby foods;
- strive, through civil service or local authority organizations, for the introduction of the payment of weekly wages instead of monthly wages to employees, and influence labour and trade union leaders to do the same;
- take steps to introduce good feeding practices in the local schools and other institutions.

Chapter 38 describes the use of social marketing and other well-tested nutrition education techniques that can help achieve some of these objectives.

Chapter 5
Population, food, nutrition and family planning

Many thinkers in the world and many who work in the development field believe that the world's population size and increase is its greatest problem and humanity's gravest threat. Clearly the ratio of the number of people to the amount of food available has an impact on nutrition, but how are the two caused to interact? Late in the eighteenth century the British political economist Thomas Malthus grimly speculated that population growth could soon outstrip food production and supply. Close to the end of the twentieth century this has not yet happened, but malnutrition is widespread.

Many books and journal articles address the enormously important questions of population, demography and family planning. These texts should be consulted by readers wishing to understand population issues in their entirety. This chapter briefly discusses some aspects of fertility and family planning as they relate to nutrition, and observes their importance for the world and particularly for the developing countries, where most population growth is taking place.

POPULATION GROWTH

World population is increasing at an alarming rate. Unless the rate of increase is slowed down in the next few decades, the world will face extremely serious problems. Figure 1 illustrates the rate of population increase over the last 2 000 years. The world population was around 250 million people 2 000 years ago. After taking 16 centuries to double to 500 million,

it then doubled in two and a half centuries to reach 1 000 million in 1850, and it doubled again in one century to reach 2 000 million people in 1950. Now the population of the world is doubling every 35 years; it reached 5 000 million before 1990.

Population pressure is most marked and is having a major impact in Asian countries

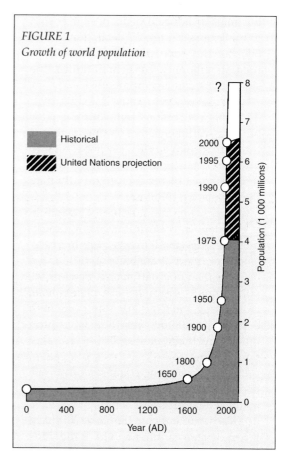

FIGURE 1
Growth of world population

such as Bangladesh, India and Pakistan. China has the largest population, but its government now manages to ensure that its people are reasonably fed. It has also recently managed to prevent any large increase in population.

Africa as a whole may not be overpopulated at present, but population density is putting pressure on land distribution in certain areas. In Kenya the population is increasing at about 3 percent per year. At this rate – among the highest in the world – the population will double in 25 years. The country may well have sufficient land, food-producing capacity and other resources to meet the demands of double or triple the present number of people. However, doubling food production is not enough. Kenya must also double the number of schools or school places, of hospitals or hospital beds, of houses and of all services in the 25 years that it will take for the population to double. Even then it will only have maintained the current level of development.

Each government must take its own decisions concerning population policy, but all governments must be aware that, if the nutritional status of people is to improve, the availability of food and services must increase more rapidly than the population (Photo 3).

Clearly when the number of people in a country, a community or a family increases, its food needs also increase. However, food availability is influenced by more than population size. Economics, politics and geography are factors, too. Hong Kong and the Netherlands are both densely populated, yet they have little hunger and their infant and child mortality rates are low.

In most developing countries – even the poorest – in Africa, Asia and Latin America, infant and young child mortality rates have declined markedly in the past 30 years. When women continued to have the same

number of babies and fewer died, family size increased.

In some countries, increased family size has also resulted from narrower spacing between pregnancies (partly because of a shorter duration of exclusive or nearly exclusive breastfeeding, as discussed in Chapter 7), younger age at first pregnancy and lack of knowledge about, or lack of availability of, family planning services. It is generally agreed that when the mother or the parents have confidence that most children born are likely to survive into adulthood, they are much more likely to consider and practise birth control.

Many of the more prosperous countries, particularly in Europe, have reached the stage of zero population growth, excluding growth from immigration. This means that the number of births per year nearly equals the number of deaths. In contrast, many developing countries have far more births than deaths and, consequently, rapidly increasing populations. However, several poor countries have reduced their rate of population increase, mainly through family planning methods.

URBANIZATION

Overall population growth is not the only demographic concern of many developing countries. The rapid increase in the percentage of people living in large cities is also a growing worry.

Population in urban areas has increased in part because of increased fertility rates, but migration from the rural areas to the cities is also a major cause. City dwellers in general are consumers, not producers, of food; as they become more numerous relative to the rural residents, the food production burden on the few becomes greater. In 1900 there were only four cities in the world with over 2 million residents; now there are over 100 such cities, as well as a number of megalopoli with over 10 million inhabitants.

The nutritional outcome of urbanization is on the whole positive. Urbanization, together with population growth and increasing incomes, contributes to tremendous increases in food demand and thus in the volume of food required, but also to varied and dynamic changes in dietary structure. The most significant dietary change caused by the urban migration has been the substitution of staple foods such as roots, tubers and coarse grains by other sources of energy such as highly milled cereals, sugar, soft drinks and other processed foods. In the urban environment, time constraints, availability of cheap, often subsidized processed foods and convenience of preparation are important considerations in influencing food consumption patterns.

The urban diet is generally more varied than the rural diet, mainly because of changes in non-staple foods. Fish, fresh vegetables, meat, poultry, milk and dairy products are consumed more often by urban people. Urban populations generally have lower energy intake than rural populations, but their physical activity may also be comparatively low. Consumption of animal protein, fat and vitamin A is higher in urban areas, and the iron consumed is better utilized. On the whole the diets of urban populations are more balanced than those of rural people.

A typical effect of urbanization is an increase in the amount of food eaten outside the home. Commercially prepared meals and other ready-to-eat foods are consumed from street vendors and food stalls. In many developing countries an informal sector for the sale of food has developed as a typically indigenous response to some of the food needs of the cities; this sector provides a cheap source of food and a significant source of income, particularly for women.

Urban nutrition is also affected by the fact that in most low-income urban households women work outside the home; as a consequence there has been an almost universal decline in breastfeeding in urban areas in all regions of the developing world, with a concomitant increase in the use of more costly breast-milk substitutes and commercial weaning foods (see Chapter 7).

On average, urban dwellers enjoy better nutritional status than their rural counterparts because of better health coverage and greater diversity in the diet. A more varied urban diet with minimal seasonal fluctuations confers important nutritional benefits. FAO data show that the incidence of child malnutrition, especially chronic malnutrition, is lower in urban areas. In Ghana, the weights of the adult urban population were found to be higher than those of the rural population. In general, urban areas also have lower morbidity and mortality rates, increased life expectancy, fewer children of low birth weight and fewer growth problems.

TECHNOLOGY

Despite rapid population growth, the world produced enough food in 1995 to feed adequately all the people on the globe – if the food were equitably distributed. Even if the population of the world doubles from the current 5 500 million to 11 000 million by the year 2030, the world's production will be capable of feeding all those people. Beyond that level, unless population growth stabilizes, serious shortages of food could result. Unlimited population increase on a planet of finite size is impossible; before too long the world would have standing room only, and each inhabitant one square metre of space.

It is a credit to agricultural advances and the skills of farmers that food supplies have increased to meet population needs. Many countries have achieved increased production levels not by expanding the land under cultivation, but by increasing the yields of cereals and other important crops per hectare farmed. This trend will have to continue. In addition, processing and marketing of foods must be improved.

REPRODUCTION AND NUTRITIONAL STATUS

In most developing countries the mean age of first menstruation is 12 to 24 months later than in industrialized countries. Menarche usually occurs about 12 months after the year with the greatest growth spurt (also known as peak height velocity). The onset of menses signals the beginning of a female's ability to become pregnant. It is almost certain that undernutrition delays the onset of menses. In this way poor nutrition influences human fertility.

Starvation and severe undernourishment, as in food shortages or famines resulting from drought, war or other factors, will usually result in cessation of menstruation in women of child-bearing age. Women who have ceased to menstruate in this way are infertile until their food intake improves. This is nature's way of preventing conception in undernourished individuals. Psychological consequences also result (see Chapter 24).

Numerous pregnancies and lactations, especially at short intervals, are likely to deplete the mother of nutrients unless she has an exceptionally good diet. Therefore, women with many children narrowly spaced are more likely to have poor nutritional status.

A woman whose diet is deficient during pregnancy, especially in terms of total food and energy, is likely to give birth to a baby that is smaller than it would have been if she were adequately nourished. Since mortality is more likely in underweight babies, a poor maternal diet is seen to increase the chances of death in the baby. Some studies, for example in Guatemala, have shown that when the diets of pregnant women were supplemented their infants had higher birth weights.

It has also been shown that a short interval between successive children may increase their risk of malnutrition and even of dying, particularly for fifth and subsequent children. Pregnancies that are too numerous and too narrowly spaced may be harmful to both the mother and the child. A mother practising family planning simply to space her children more widely benefits also in nutrition and health.

Family planning is intimately related to health and nutritional status. Small family size, long intervals between pregnancies and gradual termination of breastfeeding are all associated with good health, positive nutritional status and even decreased mortality rates in the mother and family.

The right to choose

Family planning is a concern of the family rather than the nation. People outside the family should become involved not in trying to limit the total number of children a couple should bear, but in giving the couple the means of determining themselves how many children they will have and at what intervals.

Family planning is also a right. Families, but women in particular, should be able to choose whether and when to have children. This choice used to be a luxury enjoyed only by those who had the knowledge to practise contraception and the funds to purchase contraceptive devices. Now education and services for family planning are available to more couples, providing them with the knowledge and means to prevent unwanted pregnancies. It has been said that every child born should be a wanted child; this is indeed a goal worthy of being pursued.

Breastfeeding, fertility and family planning

For many years the idea that lactation prevented pregnancy was considered an old wives' tale. Now it is known as a scientific fact that women who are intensively breastfeeding their babies do experience a longer interval before menstruation begins again, and they are therefore less likely to have an early successive pregnancy than those who do not breastfeed. Breastfeeding is likely to lengthen birth intervals by an average of five to eight months. In this way the prolongation of full breastfeeding in developing countries is having a major effect in reducing fertility, in population control and in child spacing. Breastfeeding is nature's way of helping to space children. If bottle-feeding were to replace breastfeeding without the availability of contraceptives, the result would be major increases in the number of children born.

Contraceptive pills, especially high-oestrogen pills, may reduce a woman's ability to produce breastmilk. Therefore care must be taken in advising women to take contraceptive pills soon after childbirth. In contrast, it has been suggested that the intra-uterine device (IUD) may enhance or improve lactation.

Some contraceptives may have an effect on nutritional status. Certain contraceptive pills are believed to cause anaemia because they affect folate utilization. The IUD may cause increased bleeding, which can lead to iron deficiency anaemia.

It seems likely that a decrease in infant and child mortality is a prerequisite to the wide acceptance of family planning in those societies in which childhood deaths are common. Parents need to have confidence that their children will survive before they will risk limiting their family size. As malnutrition is one of the leading causes or contributory causes of death in children, it follows that improved nutrition will expedite the acceptance of family planning.

Improved nutrition is part and parcel of a better quality of life. Having fewer children in a family means more food, more room and less poverty; these also contribute to an improved quality of life. Wider spacing of children results in improvements in the health and nutritional status of children and their mothers. There is thus a circular effect.

There is much sense in linking nutrition and family planning activities, and even in integrating them into one programme. Both are related to maternal and child health and to total family health care. It may be advantageous for the same health personnel to deal with nutrition, family planning and maternal and child health. Some countries, such as Indonesia, where family planning is having a significant impact in reducing the rate of population increase and where families are smaller than they were 20 years ago, have combined family planning activities with nutrition and health programmes; it appears to have worked well.

The nutritionist's role in population and family planning

Nutritionists may be concerned about the alarming rate of increase of the world's population. Kenya, for example, had a population of 26 million in 1994 and will have over 50 million people in 2020; nutritionists may be alarmed by all the implications of this population growth in terms of land shortage and mushrooming urban slums. In their work, however, nutritionists usually deal with problems of families or communities. It is important then to help people, especially women and their partners, understand the benefits of smaller families and the fact that more children require more resources: more food, more care, more time, more school fees, more money and so on. The appropriate strategy may be to persuade them that children today have a better chance of surviving than children had in 1955, and that quality of life is more important than numbers of children.

It is of particular importance in many developing countries first to empower women to control their own fertility and to be in a position to have the numbers of children they desire, and second to influence men to respect these rights of their female partners. The onus of having more children falls on the whole family, but in most countries by far the greatest additional burden of work falls on the mother. It is she who must endure pregnancy for another nine months, breast-feed the infant, drain her own health and perhaps impair her own nutritional status.

The education of girls and the empowerment of women to earn money, control resources and have more independence are all achievements that generally lead women to control their own fertility and have fewer babies. Women's support groups, sex education in schools, involvement of men in discussions, later marriage and more intensive breastfeeding are all likely to reduce the mean number of babies produced per mother.

Nutrition workers, be they in the field of health, agriculture, education or social services, should make themselves conversant with modern methods of family planning. They should be able to discuss these methods with people either individually or in groups, and they should know how to advise people to use local family planning services. If these services are inadequate or cause problems for women or families, nutrition workers should be advocates for improved family planning services. The more the choices available to women and men, the more likely it is that the babies born will be wanted babies. Of course workers must respect national laws and cultural norms. If abortion is illegal, the law will need to be respected. Communities have been most successful in limiting unwanted births where several family planning methods are available: contraceptive pills, condoms, IUDs, male and female surgical sterilization and, if legal, well-conducted abortions. In some countries newer methods such as hormone-releasing implants (Norplant) or the so-called abortion pill may be expected to help in family planning in the next five years. The use of breastfeeding as a family planning method is discussed in Chapter 7.

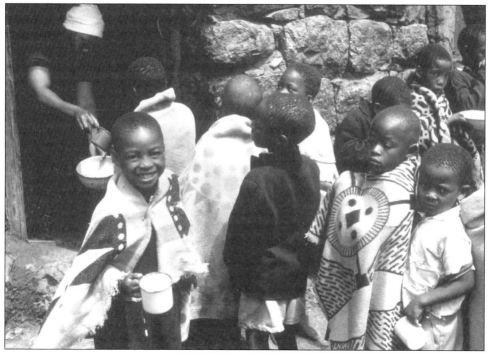

PHOTO 3
Child feeding in Lesotho: population increase causes food shortages

Chapter 6

Nutrition during particular times in the life cycle: pregnancy, lactation, infancy, childhood and old age

Nutrient requirements differ to some extent at different periods in the life cycle. Females of reproductive age have extra needs because of menstruation and, of course, during pregnancy and lactation. Infants and children have greater requirements on a unit weight basis than adults, mainly because they are growing. Older people are also a vulnerable group; they are at greater risk of malnutrition than younger adults.

Certain deficiency diseases are more prevalent in particular groups of the population. (The diseases are described and discussed in Part III.) In this chapter the emphasis is on the differing energy requirements of people at different stages of the life cycle.

Humans get energy from the foods and liquids they consume. The nutrient requirements of women of reproductive age (especially during pregnancy and lactation), of young children and adolescents and of older people are different from those of men between the ages of 15 and 60; therefore all people do not need the same amounts of food.

Figure 2 provides general guidance about the amounts of basic cooked foods needed each day by different categories of people.

WOMEN OF REPRODUCTIVE AGE

Women of child-bearing age have certain nutritional needs above those of adult males. One reason is that the loss of blood during menstruation leads to a regular loss of iron and other nutrients and makes women more prone than men to anaemia (see Chapter 13). In addition, however, in many developing countries women work much harder than men. In rural areas they are often heavily involved in agriculture, and in urban areas they may work long hours in factories and elsewhere; yet when they return home from the field or the factory they still have much work to do in the household, including food preparation and child care. Frequently the heavy burden of collecting water and fuel falls on women. All of this labour increases women's needs for nutritional energy and other nutrients.

The nutritional status of women before, during and after pregnancy contributes a good deal to their own general well-being, but also to that of their children and other members of the family. The field of maternal nutrition focuses attention on females as mothers. It has often concentrated on their nutritional status mainly as it is related to the well-being of the infants that they produce and their ability to breastfeed, nurture and raise their children. The health and well-being of the mother herself has been relatively neglected. Similarly, the field of maternal and child health has put major emphasis on the child and on providing services and help to women mainly so that they can have successful pregnancies and lactations; this is also in the interests of the infant,

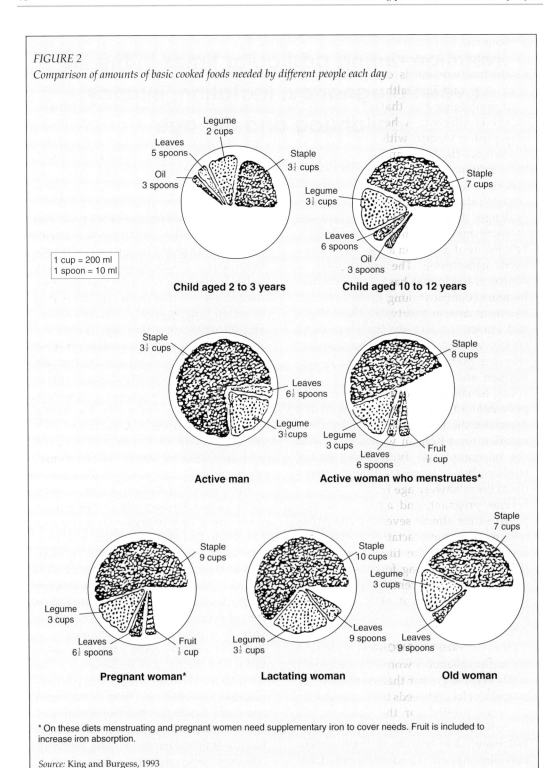

FIGURE 2

Comparison of amounts of basic cooked foods needed by different people each day

1 cup = 200 ml
1 spoon = 10 ml

Child aged 2 to 3 years

Legume 2 cups
Leaves 5 spoons
Oil 3 spoons
Staple 3½ cups

Child aged 10 to 12 years

Staple 7 cups
Legume 3½ cups
Leaves 6 spoons
Oil 3 spoons

Active man

Staple 3½ cups
Leaves 6½ spoons
Legume 3½ cups

Active woman who menstruates*

Staple 8 cups
Legume 3 cups
Leaves 6 spoons
Fruit ½ cup

Pregnant woman*

Staple 9 cups
Legume 3 cups
Leaves 6½ spoons
Fruit ½ cup

Lactating woman

Staple 10 cups
Legume 3½ cups
Leaves 9 spoons

Old woman

Staple 7 cups
Legume 3 cups
Leaves 9 spoons

* On these diets menstruating and pregnant women need supplementary iron to cover needs. Fruit is included to increase iron absorption.

Source: King and Burgess, 1993

without much concern for the mother. The dual role of women as mothers and productive workers is compromised by poor diets and ill health; not only their own well-being but that of the whole family is affected. A heavy work load may push a woman with marginal food intake over the brink and into a state of malnutrition.

A poor diet, frequent acute and some chronic infections, repeated pregnancies, prolonged lactation and a heavy burden of work may all contribute to serious physiological depletion and sometimes to overt malnutrition. The term "maternal depletion syndrome" has been suggested. In many countries young women in their late teens appear hearty, happy, healthy and attractive, but only ten or 15 years later, as young women in their late thirties, they are prematurely old, tired, down-trodden and unhealthy. Too often, the young female does not even live out her teens before her first pregnancy. Figure 3 illustrates the months of pregnancy and lactation for a Kenyan woman. She may not be completely typical of African mothers, but she is not atypical. During the 25 years between age 18, when she first became pregnant, and age 43, she was pregnant for almost seven years, or 27.7 percent of the time; lactating for 16 years, or 65 percent of the time; and neither pregnant nor lactating for less than two years, or only 7 percent of the time. She hardly menstruated at all during these 25 years.

PREGNANT WOMEN

During pregnancy a woman's nutritional needs become greater than at other times in her life. Her diet needs to provide all the elements needed for the growth of a fertilized ovum or egg into a viable foetus and baby (see Table 4). As the woman nourishes herself she also nourishes the growing foetus as well as the placenta to

which the foetus in her uterus is attached by its umbilical cord. At the same time her breast tissue prepares for lactation.

During the first half of pregnancy extra food is needed for the mother's uterus, breasts and blood – all of which increase in size or amount – as well as for the growth of the placenta. The increased need for food continues in the last half of the pregnancy, but during the last trimester the extra nutrients are required mainly for the rapidly growing foetus, which also needs to develop nutrient stores, particularly of vitamin A, iron and other micronutrients, and energy stores of fat. An adequate diet during pregnancy assists the mother to gain the extra weight that is physiologically desirable and helps ensure that the baby's birth weight is normal.

Healthy women gain weight during pregnancy if they are not overworked. Just as a heavy person needs more energy to perform the same amount of physical work as a lighter person, a pregnant woman also needs more energy. In industrialized countries many women have an easy life during pregnancy; they rest frequently, thus reducing their energy needs. However, in much of Africa and some other regions, pregnant women remain active, even during their last few months of pregnancy (Photo 4). The Basal metabolic rate (BMR) usually increases during pregnancy, which also raises energy requirements. Thus most women need more energy when they are pregnant, even if they are not overworked. For the overburdened woman of the developing world, who gets little rest and not much food, weight loss is a real and dangerous prospect.

There is little doubt that abortions, miscarriages and stillbirths are more common in women who are poorly nourished than in those who are adequately nourished. Dietary deficiencies probably also increase the risk of producing a malformed foetus. Severe malnutrition reduces

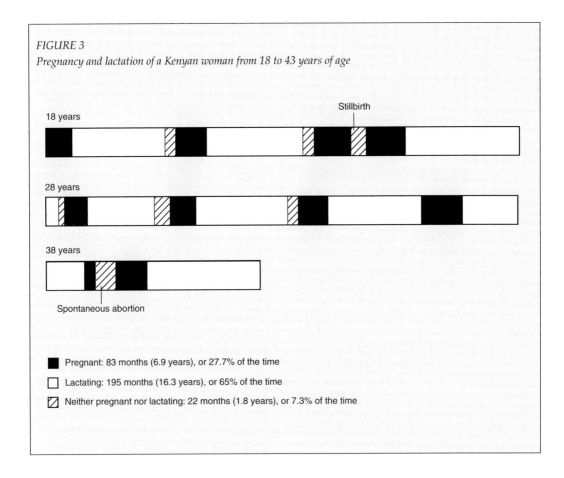

FIGURE 3
Pregnancy and lactation of a Kenyan woman from 18 to 43 years of age

■ Pregnant: 83 months (6.9 years), or 27.7% of the time

□ Lactating: 195 months (16.3 years), or 65% of the time

▨ Neither pregnant nor lactating: 22 months (1.8 years), or 7.3% of the time

fertility and therefore the likelihood of conception. A severely malnourished woman ceases to menstruate. This is clearly a natural device to stop the loss of nutrients in the menstrual flow and to protect the woman from the rigours of pregnancy and childbirth. Nevertheless, there is little evidence of lack of fertility among the less severely malnourished, and mildly malnourished women are the majority in Asia and parts of Africa.

The weight of the infant at birth is influenced by maternal nutrition. Low birth weights can be expected of infants born to malnourished mothers. Even a modest increase in energy intake during pregnancy tends to increase the birth weight of the infant.

In many developing countries 50 to 75 percent of pregnant women have anaemia (see Chapter 13). Anaemia often contributes to high maternal mortality rates. All pregnant women should attend a clinic at regular intervals for antenatal examination which should include checking of haemoglobin levels. Practical advice should be given regarding diet, taking into account what foods are locally available and what the mother can afford. It is accepted policy in many countries that pregnant women be advised to take medicinal supplements of iron, or sometimes iron-folate.

In areas where vitamin A deficiency is known to be a public health problem, infants of mothers who have poor vitamin A status are born with low vitamin A stores.

TABLE 4
Safe levels of intake of selected nutrients for active women of reproductive age

Condition	Weight (kg)	Energy (kcal)	Protein (g)	Iron (mg)	Vitamin A (µg retinol)	Vitamin C (mg)	Folate (µg)
Not pregnant or lactating	55	2 210	49	24-48	500	30	170
Pregnant	55	2 410	56	38-76	600	30	420
Lactating	55	2 710	69	13-26	850	30	270

A diet with adequate amounts of vitamin A is clearly important during pregnancy, both for the mother and the baby. However, high medicinal doses of vitamin A, as are given to young children, are not recommended during pregnancy. The recommended safe levels of intake of iron and folate, and also of vitamins A and C, are shown in Table 4. In the case of many other nutrients, however, the child is truly parasitic and takes all the nutrients it requires irrespective of whether the mother has a deficiency or not.

In some cultures there is a fear that extra food given during pregnancy will make the baby too large and thus cause a more difficult or complicated delivery. This is not true for healthy women of normal size. Women of short stature or with a contracted pelvis may have difficulty in delivering babies and may require special care before and during delivery.

At the time of birth the mother loses blood, not infrequently 500 to 1 000 ml, and she needs nutrients to regenerate that blood.

LACTATING MOTHERS

In most developing countries the majority of women breastfeed their newborn infants for a period of weeks or months after delivery (see Chapter 7). The nutritional stores of a lactating woman may already be more or less depleted as a result of the pregnancy and the loss of blood during childbirth. Lactation raises nutrient needs, mainly because of the loss of nutrients first through colostrum and then through breastmilk.

Breastmilk volume varies widely, but for fully breastfed babies around four months of age, it is often 700 to 800 ml per day. It may rise later to as much as 1 000 ml or more. The nutrients present in this milk come from the diet of the mother or from her nutrient reserves. It is recommended that mothers exclusively breastfeed their infants for six months and then begin to introduce other food while continuing to breastfeed for as long as they wish, often into the second year or beyond.

During the period of exclusive or full breastfeeding the woman usually will not menstruate. The duration of amenorrhoea varies from as little as four months to as long as 18 months or more. During that time the lactating woman will not be losing the iron normally lost with each menstrual period.

The conversion of nutrients in food to nutrients in breastmilk is not entire. In the case of energy, it is about 80 percent, so for every 800 kcal in breastmilk the mother needs to consume 1 000 kcal in her food. To have good nutritional status the breastfeeding woman has to raise nutrient intake (see Table 4).

There is a widely held belief that the composition of breastmilk varies enormously. This is not so. Human breastmilk has a fairly constant composition, and is only selectively affected by the diet of the mother. One litre of milk provides about 750 calories and contains approximately the following:

- 70 g carbohydrate,
- 46 g fat,
- 13 g protein,
- 300 mg calcium,
- 2 mg iron,
- 480 µg vitamin A,
- 0.2 mg thiamine,
- 0.4 mg riboflavin,
- 2 mg niacin,
- 40 mg vitamin C.

The fat content of breastmilk varies somewhat. The carbohydrate, protein, fat, calcium and iron contents do not change much even if the mother is short of these in her diet. A mother whose diet is deficient in thiamine and vitamins A and C, however, produces less of these in her milk. Thiamine deficiency in the lactating mother can lead to infantile beriberi in the baby (see Chapter 16). In general the effect of very poor nutrition on a lactating woman is to reduce the quantity rather than the quality of breastmilk.

Lactating mothers should be encouraged to attend a clinic with their babies during the months after delivery. At the clinic both mother and baby should be examined. The mother should have her haemoglobin level checked and also her weight. Medicinal iron in the same quantities as recommended during pregnancy should be given. The mother should be given advice on consuming a mixed diet. This is also a good time to discuss the mother's desire for further pregnancies and her view of the ideal spacing between pregnancies and to provide information and help regarding family planning. Relatively wide spacing between births is usually to the nutritional advantage of the mother, the infant and even the next foetus. Narrow spacing between births prevents the

mother from restoring her nutrient reserves before the next pregnancy, provides her with more work and a shorter time to care for her infant exclusively, and may influence her to breastfeed for a shorter period than is desirable.

At each postnatal visit both the mother and the baby should be examined, and advice on the diets of both mother and infant should be provided. A satisfactory gain in the infant's weight is the best way to judge the adequacy of the diet of the infant. In the first few months when there is exclusive breastfeeding the infant's adequate weight gain is a clear indication that the mother is producing sufficient breastmilk. Almost all mothers can successfully breastfeed their infants (Photo 5).

INFANTS AND PRESCHOOL-AGE CHILDREN

Provided that the mother has adequate breastmilk, breastfeeding alone with no added food or medicinal supplementation is all that is needed for the normal infant during the first six months of life. The advantages of exclusive breastfeeding during that period are discussed in the next chapter. Exclusive breastfeeding means that not even water, juice or other fluids are provided; none of these are needed. The infant should be examined regularly at the clinic, where weight gain is seen to indicate adequate nutrition. At the clinic a schedule for immunization will be set up, and this needs to be followed. Infants born with low weight (because of prematurity, for example) or twins may need special attention, and possibly iron or other supplements should be given. Up to six months of age many breastfed infants have considerable natural immunity to many infections.

As the children get older they gain weight and length. The increased energy requirements are based more on the weight of the child than on the age. Because healthy, well-nourished children follow a growth pattern, however, there is a close correlation between recommendations based on age and those based on weight. Table 5 shows the energy requirements of infants. A baby 2.5 months of age weighing 5 kg requires 5×120 kcal = 600 kcal, whereas a baby eight months of age weighing 8 kg requires 8×110 kcal = 880 kcal.

At six months of age complementary feeding should be introduced gradually while the infant continues to be breastfed intensively and to receive most of his or her energy and other nutrients from breast-milk and not from complementary foods. From six to 12 months, it is highly desirable that breastfeeding should continue and that the child should get as much milk as possible from the mother, while other foods, first semi-solid and then solid, should be introduced to the diet of the infant for normal growth and health.

Breastmilk is relatively deficient in iron, and the infant's store of iron is sufficient only until about six months of age. From six to 12 months, the normal infant may be expected to gain between 2 and 3 kg. The infant, while continuing to receive breast-milk, will now need foods to provide extra energy, protein, iron, vitamin C and other nutrients for growth.

The needed energy can usually be obtained from a gruel of whatever is the local staple food. The quantity and bulk can profitably be reduced if some edible oil or fat-containing food is also eaten. If the staple is a cereal such as maize, wheat, millet or rice, it will also provide a useful quantity of protein, but if it is plantain or a root such as cassava or yam, it will supply very little protein. In this case, once relatively little breastmilk is being consumed it is important to provide extra protein-rich foods from those available to the family.

In the 1950s and 1960s it was thought to be very important that complementary

TABLE 5
Energy requirements of infants during the first year

Age (*months*)	Energy requirement (*kcal/kg*)
0-3	120
3-6	115
6-9	110
9-12	105
Average	**112**

foods and then foods given after termination of breastfeeding should include animal protein in large amounts. This has been shown to be unnecessary. In developing countries these foods are often too expensive for poor families or are unavailable. More important is the need to feed the young child frequently, with foods that are not too bulky and are both nutritious and of high energy density.

Legumes such as beans, peas, lentils, cowpeas and groundnuts are good sources of protein and should be added to the diet of the child. They can be ground or crushed before or after cooking.

The above foods, as well as providing energy and protein, will also provide some iron. Additional iron can be obtained from edible green leaves, which also contain carotene and vitamin C. Carotene and vitamin C can also be obtained from fruit. Ripe papayas and mangoes are excellent sources and are usually most acceptable to young children. Vitamin C can alternatively be provided by citrus fruits (e.g. oranges) or other fruits (e.g. guavas). Gradually, as more teeth erupt, the child can be put on a more solid diet. By the age of two years, the child may have stopped breastfeeding and may be completely weaned.

The term "weaning" has been used to describe the introduction of foods and fluids other than breastmilk and the transition to a solid diet without breastmilk. However, people in Northern countries also talk of "weaning from the bottle". The word is therefore often misunderstood, and it may be better not to use it because of the confusion it causes. Rather, the transition can be described as four stages:

- the first four to six months when all the infant's nutrients come from breastmilk;
- the next few months when just as much (or more) breastmilk is provided but other appropriate, often soft, nutritious foods are introduced in increasing amounts, with efforts to prevent these from causing a decline in breastmilk consumption;
- the next stage, perhaps starting at about 12 to 15 months, when the baby is still breastfeeding but is getting considerably more of his or her nutrients from nutritious foods – most of them ordinary village or family foods – than from breastmilk;
- the end of breastfeeding, the stage termed "sevrage" (a good French term literally meaning "severance from the breast"), which can occur as late as the mother wants, sometimes when the infant is over two years of age.

After sevrage appropriate family foods are provided. These need to be nutritious, suitable for the child, energy dense and given frequently, perhaps four to six times per day, not just in two or three meals per day as may be the family practice. The young child should be fed between family mealtimes if these are limited to two or three per day.

The mother responsible for feeding a toddler who is no longer breastfeeding must keep in mind that the child, whether boy or girl, has special needs.

Special needs of a young girl in the months following sevrage

- She needs a variety of foods, as great as or greater than that given to any other member of the family.
- She is growing rapidly and needs energy-dense foods and extra protein-rich foods.
- She has few teeth, and requires soft food.
- She has a relatively small appetite and intake capacity and needs more frequent meals than older persons.
- She requires clean food and clean utensils to avoid infection.
- She must as far as possible be protected from communicable diseases.
- She should have the love, affection and personal attention of her mother for her mental and, indirectly, her physical well-being.
- Attention from the father and other members of the family will also contribute to her development and well-being.

The proper feeding of a toddler requires time and patience. Special utensils or equipment are not necessary, but a sieve or strainer is useful. Adult foods can be chopped up and forced through a strainer into a cup or on to a plateful of gruel for the child. A strainer can readily be made if none is available. Otherwise, various foods can be crushed before cooking using a pestle and mortar, which are found in most households.

In some societies gruel or porridge made from the local staple is made sour or partially fermented. This is a good practice. Small amounts of germinated cereal seeds, often millet or sorghum, are crushed and added to maize or other porridge. The amylase present breaks down some of the starch, causing the porridge to become thinner (more liquid), so it is easier for the young child to consume, and making it more energy dense. The food is also safer, because the growth of disease-causing organisms is inhibited in sour or fermented gruel. Some societies sour children's foods by addition of lime or lemon juice. This also is advantageous, and enhances the absorption of iron.

The period from six to 36 months of age is of paramount importance nutritionally. The mother should take the child regularly to a clinic if one is available. The happiness, general appearance and weight of the child are the best general indicators of adequate nutrition. The use of a weight chart to help the mother follow the growth of the child is described in Chapter 34. Many children of this age in developing countries do not grow at the rate they should, and some develop protein-energy malnutrition (see Chapter 12).

The first three years of life are also those when the important micronutrient deficiencies of vitamin A and iron are most likely to occur in children. From three years of age the risks are reduced, but in many parts of the world growth continues to lag, incidence of intestinal worms and other parasitic diseases may increase and other nutrition and health risks arise.

From three years of age onwards the child has usually stopped breastfeeding and is consuming family foods. The child can now obtain adequate nutrients in three meals per day, but until the child reaches the age of five years, parents should make certain that the child is eating adequately and getting his or her fair share of the most desirable foods, which may well be those that are most tasty and in shortest supply. Special attention may need to be given when children have a poor appetite or when they are ill and their appetite is reduced. For the whole family, but especially for children, care must be taken that food, water and other fluids are safe and not contaminated. Good personal and

---

Kimea or power flour: an approach to providing more energy-dense foods

Traditional ways of thinning porridge, using products which are termed "malted" (from the process used in beer production), are now being recommended for societies that do not customarily use them. Malted flour, termed *"kimea"* in the United Republic of Tanzania, is usually made by germinating cereal seeds or grains by moistening them, drying them for a few days and then pulverizing the dried grains into a powder. When added even in tiny amounts to stiff maize porridge (called *"ugali"* in Tanzania, Kenya and elsewhere in Africa), *kimea* thins the porridge into a more liquid gruel (termed *"uji"*). This remarkable property has led to its being called "power flour". The power lies in the enzyme amylase which is in the germinated flour. Amylase digests starch, the complex carbohydrate in cereal grains, into simple carbohydrates, thereby thinning the porridge. This makes the food easier for the young child to eat, safer because it harbours fewer disease-causing bacteria, and perhaps easier to digest. Above all it is more energy dense.

---

household hygiene are of the greatest importance. Washing hands with soap and water before meals or food handling is a good family rule.

Parents should understand the needs of the child and see that the right foods are available in adequate quantities and prepared in palatable ways.

The nutrient requirements of children of different ages and weights are provided in Annex 1. It is clear that as children increase in weight and age they need more food to provide them with more energy and more of the other nutrients essential for growth and health. Thus a child aged six to 12 months and weighing 8.5 kg requires

950 kcal per day, whereas a child aged five to seven years weighing 19 kg requires 1 820 kcal (almost twice as much) and a boy aged 17 years weighing about 60 kg requires 2 770 kcal (almost three times as much).

Mothers need to understand that as children grow beyond infancy, they increase in weight and require more food to eat. Table 6 indicates that as young boys and girls get older, heavier, taller and more active, they need to eat more food, especially a greater quantity of staple foods including cereals (e.g. rice, maize, wheat) and legumes (e.g. beans, cowpeas).

SCHOOL-AGE CHILDREN

The vast majority of schoolchildren in developing countries attend primary schools. Most are at day schools, few of which provide a midday meal. In rural areas the school is often some kilometres from the parents' home. The child frequently has to leave home early and walk a considerable distance to school. Often the child has little or no breakfast at home before he or she sets out; there is no meal at school; and the first, and sometimes only, meal of the day is late in the afternoon.

The nutritional needs of a schoolchild are high. The adolescent child has proportionately higher requirements for most nutrients than the average adult. It is practically impossible for an adolescent to obtain adequate quantities of the right foods from one or even two meals a day. It is highly desirable that school-age children eat some food before going to school and some food at school, or during the middle of the day outside the school grounds, as well as the food eaten at home.

Food before going to school

It is not practical for many mothers to rise before dawn to spend the considerable time necessary to light a fire and prepare a hot meal for children before school-time. Therefore, if no hot breakfast is available, some fruit, cold cooked potatoes, rice, cassava or even cold porridge should be left over from the previous day for the schoolchild to eat before leaving home in the morning. In some areas cold chapattis, tortillas or wheat products such as bread may be available.

Food eaten at school

This may consist of a midday school meal or a snack taken to school.

A midday school meal is the ideal. It should provide reasonable amounts of the nutrients most likely to be missing or short in the home diet. A whole-grain cereal as the basis and a side dish of legumes with vegetables or green leaves make an excellent school meal. There are many possibilities, depending on what foods are locally available. The meal might include some protein-rich food and some food containing vitamins A and C.

School meals are beneficial because they often supply much-needed nutrients; they can form the basis for nutrition education; they are a good way of introducing new foods; and they prevent hunger and malnutrition. School meals, in addition to improving nutritional status, may increase enrolment, especially for girls, and may reduce absenteeism. However, in many developing countries, for many reasons, school meals are unavailable. Parents' organizations can sometimes work with teachers to organize community school feeding or food supplementation or nutritious snacks. School meals can provide a good environment for nutrition education. Further nutrition education can be carried out as an extracurricular project (Photo 6). A school vegetable garden or orchard can provide foods with valuable extra nutrients for the midday meal. Poultry keeping, small animal production (rabbits, guinea-pigs, pigeons, etc.) and fish

TABLE 6
Amount of uncooked foods to satisfy the nutrient needs of children (g)

Age (years)	Cereal grains	Legumes	Vegetables	Fruit	Oils or fat
2-3	150-250	100-125	75-100	50-100	20
4-5	200-350	125-175	100-150	100-150	30
6-9	300-400	150-200	100-150	100-150	30
10-13	400-500	200-250	100-150	100-150	30

pond construction, in areas where they are suitable, are educative projects and can provide food for a school meal.

A midday school meal might be provided by the government or local authority as part of the education system and could be paid for from the normal school fees. Alternatively, a midday meal system might be started and paid for from special fees collected from the pupils daily, weekly or per term. Local organizations might provide certain food items free or at low prices for school feeding, thus reducing the overall cost.

The cost of school feeding can be reduced by local self-help efforts on the part of villagers, parents' committees and pupils. These efforts may fit in well with self-help community projects. For example, a small kitchen shelter can be built on a self-help basis. Instead of a paid cook, a rota of parents can take turns doing the cooking. Pupils can collect fuelwood at weekends. However, it must be stressed that the provision of a midday school meal must not detract from the parents' responsibilities to provide a good diet for schoolchildren at home.

In the absence of a school lunch, parents should send their children to school with some food to be eaten at midday. However, they may have real difficulty in finding suitable foods. The various foods suggested for a cold breakfast can equally provide the solution for a midday snack. The sort of food taken will vary according to what is available locally. Possibilities include a few bananas, cooked whole cassava, sweet or ordinary potatoes roasted in their skins, fruit, tomatoes, roasted maize on the cob, roasted groundnuts, coconuts, cold grilled fish, smoked cooked meat, hard-boiled eggs, a calabash of sour milk or some bread, a chapatti or tortillas.

Some schools above primary level are boarding schools. These usually provide three meals a day, and the menu should be based on recommendations made to the school by someone with dietetics training. Occasionally schools plead lack of money as an excuse for an inadequate diet. School meals need not be luxurious, but they should be balanced and should provide all the nutrients necessary for growth and health. The child with an inadequate diet will not only fail to grow properly, but may also develop anaemia and other signs of malnutrition and will not be able to concentrate on or benefit fully from the education provided.

Increasingly in urban areas, and even to some extent in more heavily populated rural districts, entrepreneurs set up stalls and the like near schools so they can prepare and sell foods to schoolchildren (see Chapter 40). These "street foods" often have the advantage of providing access to cooked foods at relatively low cost, but the disadvantages include poor hygiene, poor-quality food and high prices. Where the main source of a midday snack or meal for primary or secondary schoolchildren is a vendor, the food is available only to children who have money to purchase it. Often the wealthier children participate and the children from the poorest families, or those whose parents will not provide money, do not.

Other concerns

The health of schoolchildren also needs consideration. In many countries school health services are non-existent or very poor. Examination for sight and hearing defects is important. Routine deworming might be initiated. Attention to micro-nutrient deficiencies may be needed in areas where children are at risk of iron, vitamin A or iodine deficiency. Iodine is especially important when girls reach puberty and before they have their first pregnancy.

Unfortunately, in some countries a large percentage of school-age children do not attend school. In some countries far more boys than girls attend school. Out-of-school children have the same nutritional and health needs as children attending school, but they do not benefit from school meals and other services. They are an often forgotten and relatively neglected group of the population, including children from the poorest families as well as children with disabilities, either physical or psychological.

OLDER PERSONS

Older people, like all others, need a good diet that provides for all their nutrient needs. In more affluent societies, older adults are often plagued with chronic diseases that have nutritional origins or associations. These conditions include, among others, arteriosclerotic heart disease,

sometimes leading to coronary thrombosis; hypertension, which may lead to stroke or other manifestations; diabetes, with its serious complications; osteoporosis, which frequently leads to hip fracture or collapse of vertebrae; and loss of teeth because of dental caries and periodontal disease. As discussed in Chapter 23, these diseases are rapidly becoming more prevalent in developing countries.

Many older people, especially if unfit, take less exercise and so may need less energy (see Annex 1). They may, therefore, eat less food and as a result get fewer micronutrients, but their needs for micro-nutrients are unchanged (see Figure 2). Consequently, conditions such as anaemia are common. Older people who have lost many or all of their teeth or who have gingivitis or other gum problems may find it difficult to chew many ordinary foods and may need softer foods. Fed on a normal family diet, they may eat too little and become malnourished. They may also suffer from illnesses which reduce their appetite or desire for food, which may also lead to malnutrition.

In many rural traditional societies old people are cared for at home by relatives and others in the community. By contrast, many older people in the richer, industrialized countries of the North live lonely lives and are relegated to old people's nursing homes and other unpleasant institutions. In some developing countries the traditional support systems and extended families are breaking down, especially with urbanization and migration, and old people there may end up lonely, living in poverty, with chronic illnesses, poor hearing and vision and perhaps psychological problems. Compounding these problems, they will face difficulties in producing food, purchasing it and preparing it.

Many of the older people are poor women, who are especially vulnerable. They are members of society in special need of both good care and a good diet, just as children are in their early years.

In some countries special services are established to help older or poor people obtain food in soup kitchens or in their homes. These services can be helpful. Preferable, however, would be community and family efforts to care for older people who cannot care for themselves and who are at risk of malnutrition and disease.

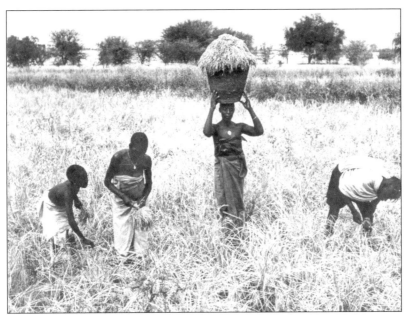

PHOTO 4
African women
remain active
during
pregnancy

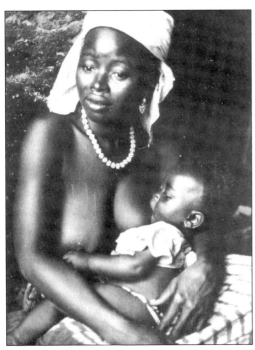

PHOTO 5
African women are usually good breastfeeders

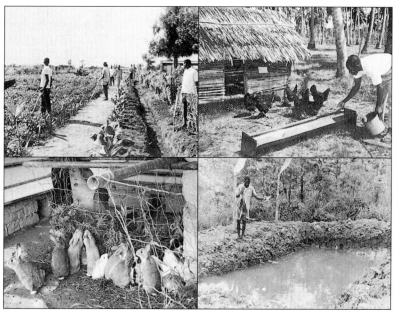

PHOTO 6
Examples of school food-production projects

Chapter 7
Breastfeeding

For most of human history nearly all mothers have fed their infants in the normal, natural, no-fuss way: breastfeeding. Most traditional societies in Africa, Asia and Latin America have had good local knowledge about breastfeeding, although practices have varied from culture to culture.

The famous paediatrician Paul Gyorgy said, "Cows' milk is best for baby cows and human breastmilk is best for human babies". No one can deny the truth of that statement. It is increasingly acknowledged, therefore, that every mother has the right to breastfeed her baby and every infant has the right to be breastfed. Any obstacles placed in the way of breastfeeding are an infringement of these rights; yet in almost all countries there are many babies who are not breastfed or are breastfed for a relatively short time.

In recent years interest in breastfeeding has grown. Part of the reason is the much-publicized controversy over the replacement of breastfeeding by bottle-feeding and the related aggressive promotion of manufactured breastmilk substitutes by multinational corporations. The womanly art of breastfeeding has in recent years been rediscovered in Europe and to a lesser extent in North America. Unfortunately, however, use of bottle-feeding continues to increase in many non-industrialized countries of the South. The most serious consequences of this shift from breast to bottle are seen among poor families in Africa, Asia and Latin America.

ADVANTAGES OF BREASTFEEDING
Extensive studies comparing the composition and relative benefits of human milk and its substitutes have been published over the past 50 years and especially in the last decade. Most of the new research has supported the many advantages of breastfeeding over other methods of infant feeding. A vast body of research from all over the world sustains the recommendation that only breastmilk be fed to infants for the first six months of life. Certainly in developing countries where the risks of complementary feeding usually outweigh any possible advantages, breastfeeding alone up to six months of age is advised.

The advantages of breastfeeding over bottle-feeding and the reasons why it is so strongly recommended are summarized as follows.

- Breastfeeding is convenient; the food is readily available for the infant, and no special preparation or equipment is needed.
- Breastmilk provides a proper balance and quantity of nutrients ideal for the human infant.
- Both colostrum and breastmilk have anti-infective constituents that help limit infections.
- Bottle-feeding enhances the risk of infections from contamination with pathogenic organisms in the milk, the formula and the water used in preparation, as well as in bottles, teats and other items used for infant feeding.
- Breastfeeding is more economical than bottle-feeding, which involves costs for infant formula or cows' milk, the bottles and teats and the fuel necessary for sterilization.
- Breastfeeding prolongs the duration of

post-partum anovulation, helping mothers to space their children.

- Breastfeeding fosters enhanced bonding and relationship between mother and infant.
- An apparent lowered risk of allergies, obesity and certain other health problems is seen in breastfed infants compared with those who are artificially fed.

There is now overwhelming evidence of the health advantages of breastfeeding as indicated by lower infant morbidity and mortality than for bottle-fed infants. The advantages accrue mainly to the two-thirds of the world's population who live in poverty, although some studies have shown lower rates of diarrhoea and other infections and less hospitalization among breastfed infants even in affluent communities. There is now evidence that women who breastfeed their infants have a reduced risk of breast cancer, and perhaps of uterine cancer, than women who do not.

PROBLEMS WITH BOTTLE-FEEDING OR FEEDING BREASTMILK SUBSTITUTES

An infant who is not breastfed, or even one who is not exclusively breastfed for the first four to six months of life, loses many or all of the advantages of breastfeeding mentioned above. The most common alternative to breastfeeding is bottle-feeding, usually with a manufactured infant formula, but not infrequently with cows' milk or other liquids. Less commonly an infant in the first four to six months of life is fed solid foods in place of breastmilk. Some mothers do use a cup and spoon rather than a bottle to provide cows' milk, infant formula or gruel to young babies. Spoon-feeding has some advantages over bottle-feeding but is much less satisfactory than breastfeeding.

Infection

Whereas breastmilk is protective, alternative infant feeding methods increase the risk of infection, mainly because contamination leads to the increased intake of pathogenic organisms. Poor hygiene, particularly with bottle-feeding, is a major cause of childhood gastro-enteritis and diarrhoea. Infant formula and cows' milk are good vehicles and culture media for pathogenic organisms. It is incredibly difficult to provide a clean, let alone sterile, feed to an infant from the bottle under the following circumstances:

- when the family water supply is a ditch or a well contaminated with human excrement (relatively few households in developing countries have their own safe supply of running water);
- when household hygiene is poor and the home environment is contaminated by flies and faeces;
- when there is no refrigerator or other safe storage space for reconstituted formula or for cows' milk;
- when there is no turn-on stove and on each occasion someone has to gather fuel and light a fire to boil water to sterilize a bottle;
- when there is no suitable equipment for cleaning the bottle between feeds and when the bottle used may be of cracked plastic or an almost uncleanable soda bottle;
- when the mother is relatively uneducated and has little or no knowledge of the role of germs in disease.

Malnutrition

Artificial feeding may contribute importantly in two ways to protein-energy malnutrition (PEM) including nutritional marasmus. First, as discussed earlier, formula-fed infants are more likely to get infections including diarrhoea, which then contribute to poor growth and PEM in infancy and early childhood. Second, mothers in poor families often overdilute infant formula. Because of the high cost of breastmilk substitutes, the family purchases too little and tries to stretch it by using less than the recommended amounts of powdered formula per feed. The infant may be given the correct number of feedings and the recommended volume of liquid, but if it is too dilute each feed may be too low in energy and other nutrients to sustain optimal growth. The result is first growth faltering and then perhaps the slow development of nutritional marasmus (Photos 7 and 8).

Economic problems

A very important disadvantage of formula feeding is the cost for the family and for the nation. Breastmilk is produced in all countries, but infant formula is not. Infant formula is a very expensive food, and if countries import it, then foreign exchange is unnecessarily spent. Choosing breastfeeding over bottle-feeding therefore confers significant economic advantages for families and for poor countries.

Infant formula is a better product for a one-month-old baby than fresh cows' milk or whole milk powder. Dried skimmed milk (DSM) and sweetened condensed milk are contraindicated. However, infant formula is extremely expensive relative to the incomes of poor families in developing countries. In India, Indonesia and Kenya it would cost a family 70 percent or more of the average labourer's wage to purchase adequate quantities of infant formula for a four-month-old baby. The purchase of formula as a substitute for breastmilk diverts scarce family monetary resources and increases poverty.

A baby three to four months of age needs about 800 ml of milk per day or perhaps 150 litres in the first six to seven months of life. In the first four months of life a baby of average weight would need about 22 kg or 44 half-kilogram cans of powdered formula. Health workers and those providing advice on infant feeding in any country should go to local shops, find the price of locally available breastmilk substitutes and estimate the cost of feeding that product in adequate amounts for a given period, say one or six months. This information should be publicized, made available to government officials and parents and used as far as possible to illustrate the economic implications for poor mothers who do not breastfeed.

For many countries that do not manufacture infant formula a decline in breastfeeding means an increase in the importation of manufactured breastmilk substitutes and the paraphernalia needed for bottle-feeding. These imports may lead to a worsening of the already horrendous foreign debt problems for many developing countries. Even where infant formula is locally made, the manufacture is frequently controlled by a multinational corporation, and profits are exported. Therefore, the preservation of breastfeeding or a reduction in artificial feeding is in the economic interests of most developing countries. Economists and politicians may be more inclined to support programmes to promote breastfeeding when they appreciate that such measures will save foreign exchange; the economic implications are often of more interest to them than arguments about the health advantages of breastfeeding.

PROPERTIES AND VALUE OF BREASTMILK

Immediately after giving birth to a baby, a mother produces colostrum from both breasts. Within a few days the milk "comes in", and it increases in quantity to match the needs of the baby. A mother's milk production is influenced mainly by the demands of her baby, whose sucking stimulates breastmilk secretion. The more the baby sucks, the more milk the mother will produce. The amount will often increase from about 100 to 200 ml on the third day after the baby's birth to 400 to 500 ml by the time the baby is ten days old.

Production can continue to increase to as much as 1 000 to 1 200 ml per day. A healthy, normally growing four-month-old infant of average weight will, if exclusively breastfed, receive 700 to 850 ml of breastmilk in 24 hours. Provided the babies can suckle as much as they want, they will always get enough milk. This is probably the only time in life when a person can eat as much of what he or she likes whenever he or she likes! Feeding on demand – any time, day or night – is the traditionally practised method of breastfeeding. It is best achieved by a mother who is happy, relaxed, confident and free to be with her baby all the time. In these circumstances, the mother and baby form what has been termed a dyad – a special twosome.

One litre of breastmilk produces about 750 kcal. Cows' milk provides about three times more protein and four times more calcium, but only about 60 percent of the carbohydrate present in human breastmilk (see Table 7).

Most studies now clearly indicate that the nutrients present in milk from a healthy, well-nourished mother satisfy all the nutritional needs of the infant if the infant is consuming enough milk. Even though the iron content of breastmilk is low, it is sufficient and well enough absorbed to prevent anaemia during the first four to six months of life. Cows' milk is even lower in its iron content and is not very well absorbed by the baby, so infants fed cows' milk are very likely to develop iron deficiency anaemia.

Breastmilk may vary somewhat between individuals, and probably to some minor extent in different parts of the world. It is also different at the beginning and end of each feed. The so-called foremilk is more watery and contains less fat in comparison with the milk of the latter part of the feed, which is somewhat thicker and whiter in appearance and more energy dense because it contains more fat.

Of particular importance is the presence in colostrum and breastmilk of anti-infective factors (which are not present in infant formula). These include:

- antibodies and immunoglobulins, some of which work in the baby's intestines and prevent disease-causing organisms from infecting the baby;
- living cells, mainly white blood cells, which may produce important substances such as interferon (which may fight viruses), immunoglobulin A, lactoferrin and lysosomes;
- other factors such as the bifidus factor which helps certain friendly bacteria such as lactobacilli to grow and proliferate in the infant's intestines, where they help ensure an acid environment (from lactic acid) which discourages the growth of harmful organisms.

In simple terms, breastmilk leads to an environment in the intestines of the baby that is harmful and unfriendly to disease-causing organisms. The stool of a breastfed infant differs in appearance from that of a formula-fed baby.

Science and industry have combined to produce breastmilk substitutes which are intended to mimic breastmilk in terms of quantities of known nutrients present in mothers' milk. These products, often called infant formulas, are the best alternative to breastmilk for those few babies who cannot receive breastmilk. All infant formulas are based on mammalian milk, usually cows' milk. Even though infant formulas may be the best alternative to human breastmilk, they are not the same. They do include the known nutrients that are needed by the infant, but they may not include those nutrients that have not yet been identified; in this case it is not possible to know what the bottle-fed infant is missing. Indeed, in some respects infant formulas are so different from human milk as to be at best unsuitable and at worst dangerous. The manufactured milks do not have the anti-

TABLE 7
Nutrient content of 100 g of human breastmilk and cows' milk compared

Type of milk	Energy (kcal)	Carbohydrate (g)	Protein (g)	Fat (g)	Calcium (mg)	Iron (mg)	Vitamin A (µg)	Folate (µg)	Vitamin C (mg)
Human milk	70	7.0	1.03	4.6	30	0.02	48	5	5
Cows' milk (whole)	61	5.4	3.3	3.3	119	0.05	31	5	1

infective properties and living cells that are present in human milk. The manufactured products may cause the infant to suffer health problems that would never be brought on by human milk.

Breastmilk, particularly because of the immunoglobulins it contains, seems to protect babies against allergies. In contrast, the non-human and cow proteins present in breastmilk substitutes, as well as other substances which enter infant formulas during manufacture, may provoke allergies. The important end result is a much higher rate of eczema, other allergies, colic and sudden infant death syndrome (SIDS) in formula-fed infants than in breastfed infants.

On top of everything else, the manufactured products are very expensive.

COLOSTRUM
Colostrum is the yellowish or straw-coloured fluid produced by the breasts for the first few days after the birth of the baby. Colostrum is highly nutritious and rich in anti-infective properties. It could be said that the living cells, immunoglobulins and antibodies in colostrum constitute the infant's first immunization.

In most societies, colostrum is recognized to differ from breastmilk because of its colour and its creamy consistency, but its enormous value to the baby is not universally acknowledged. In many parts of the world mothers do not feed colostrum to their babies; they wait until white milk

is secreted from the breast. Some mothers (and grandmothers) think that in the first days after birth the newborn infant should receive other fluids or foods, for example, tea in India, jamus (traditional medicinal potions) in Indonesia and sugar or glucose water in many Western hospitals. These foods are not needed and are in fact contraindicated. The baby at birth has adequate body water and fluids and enough nutrients, so the only feeding needed is colostrum and then breastmilk for the first four to six months of life.

HOW BREASTMILK IS MADE
The milk in the breasts is produced in large numbers of sac-like structures called the alveoli and is then carried in milk ducts to the nipple. The nipple has nerves and is sensitive to stimuli. Around the nipple is a roundish pigmented area called the areola, beneath which are glands which produce oil to keep the nipple and areola surface healthy. Milk production is influenced by hormones, particularly prolactin and oxytocin, and by reflexes.

The infant's sucking at the nipple stimulates the anterior pituitary gland in the brain to produce prolactin, which influences the alveoli to secrete milk. This mechanism is sometimes called the "milk secretion reflex".

Sucking also influences the posterior pituitary gland to release the hormone oxytocin into the blood. It travels to the breasts and causes contractions around the alveoli and the ducts to let down or eject the milk. This oxytocin effect is often termed the "let-down reflex". Oxytocin also has another action in that it stimulates the uterine muscles to contract; soon after the delivery of an infant, these uterine contractions reduce haemorrhage. They also help to return muscle tone, eliminating the pregnant look and giving back to the post-partum mother the shape that she hasn't seen for so long.

INFANT FEEDING TRENDS

The percentage of mothers who breastfeed their infants and the duration of breast-feeding varies among countries and within them. Exclusive or near exclusive breast-feeding for the first four to six months of life, followed by breastfeeding for many more months while other foods are introduced, is considered by scientists to provide optimum infant feeding. This ideal, however, does not exist in any country, North or South.

Most mothers in traditional societies, particularly in rural areas in developing countries, still breastfeed all their children for a long time. Few, however, practise exclusive breastfeeding, and many do not provide colostrum to their babies.

Many mothers in Europe and North America, by contrast, do not breastfeed their children. The trend away from breast-feeding was most marked in the 1950s and 1960s, when fewer than 15 percent of American babies two months of age were breastfed. During those years a marked decline in breastfeeding was reported from some Asian and Latin American countries. By the mid-1990s there was a modest resurgence of breastfeeding in the indus-trialized countries of the North, especially among better-educated mothers. In poor Asian, African and Latin American coun-tries breastfeeding rates are often lower in urban areas and higher in the rural areas where people have less education.

Breastmilk myths

Myth: Breastmilk varies from person to person.
There is a widely held belief that the composition of breastmilk varies enormously. This is not so. Human breastmilk has a fairly constant composition.
Myth: The milk in one breast is different from the milk in the other breast.
Contrary to some beliefs, the milk in both breasts has the same composition.
Myth: Breastmilk ferments in the breasts in the heat.
When the breastmilk is in the breasts it is perfectly safe.
Myth: Breastmilk can spoil in the breasts.
Just as it cannot ferment in the breasts, breast-milk does not spoil in other ways.

There are many reasons for a decline in breastfeeding or for the unnecessary use of breastmilk substitutes, and the reasons vary from country to country. Aggres-sive promotion by the manufacturers of breast-milk substitutes is one cause. Promotional practices have now been regulated in many countries, but the manufacturers continue to circumvent the accepted codes of conduct and to promote their products, even though such practices may contribute to infant morbidity.

Actions by the medical profession have also contributed to the reduction in breast-feeding. In general, health care systems in most countries have not adequately supported breastfeeding. Even in many developing countries doctors and other health care professionals have had a negative role and have contributed to reduced levels of breastfeeding. This situation is changing, but many health professionals are still relatively ignorant about breastfeeding.

Breastfeeding often declines when rural

women move to urban areas, where traditional practices may get replaced by modern ones or be influenced by urbanization. Women who take jobs in factories and offices may come to believe that they cannot combine their employment with breastfeeding, and labour conditions and labour laws may also make it difficult for women to hold a job and breastfeed.

The female breast is accentuated in books and magazines, by the media (especially television) and by manufacturers and advertisers of women's clothes. The breast may become regarded as a dominant sex symbol, and women may then not wish to breastfeed their babies in public, or they may falsely come to believe that breastfeeding will mar the appearance of the breasts. At the same time, a belief may develop that it is superior, chic and sophisticated to bottle-feed. Breastfeeding may be regarded as a primitive practice, and the feeding bottle may become a status symbol. As a result in many areas of the world breastfeeding is declining despite all recent efforts in its favour.

Traditional breastfeeding practices do not fit in with the demands of modern societies in which women have to be absent from their homes and their children for extended periods, usually for work. Although employment legislation in some countries provides for breastfeeding breaks for workers, distance from home and transport problems make it impractical for mothers to take advantage of the breaks. Thus, while it may well be possible for a mother to breastfeed her baby when they are together (usually at home), when they are apart the baby must be bottle-fed with infant formula. The mother could also express her own milk and leave it for someone else to feed to the baby using a bottle or a cup and spoon, but in practice few women do this. Some consider expressing milk a bother (although it is very easy once the technique is acquired) or

unpleasant, and many worry about storing the breastmilk safely.

Giving babies breastmilk substitutes at an early age is dangerous even where breastfeeding is continued. The unnecessary very early partial replacement of breastmilk with breastmilk substitutes from a bottle introduces risks and sometimes serious problems for the infant, the mother and the family.

MANAGEMENT OF BREASTFEEDING

If at all possible, breastfeeding should begin within minutes of delivery (or certainly within one hour). This early suckling has physiological advantages because it raises the levels of the hormone oxytocin secreted into the mother's blood. As described above, oxytocin causes uterine contractions which first help expel the placenta and then have an important role in reducing blood loss.

Soon after delivery the mother and her baby should be together in bed at home or in the hospital ward (Photo 9). In the past it was considered normal in modern hospitals to take the baby to a nursery ward and the mother to a maternity ward, but this practice is highly undesirable. Wherever "rooming-in" is not the current hospital practice, procedures need to be changed. It is absolutely safe for the baby to sleep in the same bed as the mother. There are very few contraindications (save serious illness in the mother or infant) for rooming-in or breastfeeding.

In the days after delivery, and as the baby gets older, breastfeeding should be done "on demand". That is, the baby should be breastfed when he or she wants to be fed and not, as used to be common in Western countries, on a scheduled basis, such as every three or four hours. The epic poem "Song of Lawino", by the Ugandan poet Okot p'Bitek, praises breastfeeding on demand, in sickness and in health, and satirizes the mostly Western practice of regulated feeding, now widely acknowledged as harmful:

> When the baby cries
> Let him suck
> From the breast.
> There is no fixed time
> For breastfeeding.
> When the baby cries
> It may be he is ill:
> The first medicine for a child
> Is the breast.
> Give him milk
> And he will stop crying.

Feeding on demand stimulates the nipple and boosts production of milk, and it helps prevent breast engorgement.

The duration of feedings will vary and in general should not be limited. Usually a baby feeds for 8 to 12 minutes, but there are fast and slow feeders, and both types usually get an adequate quantity of milk. Some mothers believe that the milk from the left breast is different from that from the right, but this is not so; the baby should feed from both breasts more or less equally.

Babies in the first few days after birth usually lose weight, so a baby with birth weight of 3 kg may weigh 2.75 kg at five days of age. A loss of up to about 10 percent is not unusual, but by seven to ten days the baby should have regained or overtaken the birth weight.

Almost all experts now agree that the infant should be exclusively breastfed for the first four to six months. An adequate gain in weight is the best way of judging the adequacy of the diet. No water, juices or other fluids are needed for a baby getting adequate breastmilk, even in hot humid or hot arid areas of the tropics; the baby will simply feed more often if thirsty. If the baby has diarrhoea breastfeeding should continue, but other fluids such as oral rehydration solutions or local preparations may be needed.

Experience from countries in East Africa, Asia and Latin America suggests that most mothers living in extended families in traditional societies are very successful, often very expert breastfeeders, and failure of lactation is uncommon. Traditional family life is undoubtedly of great importance to the beginning breastfeeder. Other women in the family provide the support and comfort – especially if there are difficulties – that people in Europe and North America have to seek from organizations such as La Leche League.

At clinics, time is often wasted on lessons on Western textbook ideas about breastfeeding, including insistence on burping, timing of feeds or frequent washing of the nipples. This emphasis on rules and strictures rather than on relaxation and pleasure is not good for anyone anywhere. It has been known to have grave psychological effects, often resulting in failure of lactation. The low rate of successful breastfeeders in North America and Western Europe is an indication of how inadequate Western-style breastfeeding has been, except in Scandinavia.

Breastfeeding should not be a complicated, difficult procedure. It should be enjoyable for both mother and child, and given the right circumstances of security, support and encouragement it can be. Some women in all societies do have problems with breastfeeding, but many of these are solvable or can be relieved. It is important that mothers have easy access to good advice and support. Many books dealing with lactation and related problems are available, and they should be consulted.

Common breastfeeding problems include:

- inverted or short nipples, or nipples that do not seem to be very protractile;
- nipples so long as to interfere with feeding, because some babies suck only the nipple and not the areola;
- refusal to feed, which needs to be checked in case the baby is ill or has a mouth problem such as a cleft palate;

- soreness of the breasts, which may be caused by cracked nipples, by mastitis or by a breast abscess requiring antibiotics and good medical care;
- so-called insufficient milk, which is discussed below;
- leakage from the breasts, which may cause embarrassment but is usually self-limiting and can be dealt with by expression of milk and by using an absorbent pad to prevent wetting of clothing.

BREASTFEEDING PROBLEMS
Complete lactation failure

Very few mothers – fewer than 3 percent – experience complete or nearly complete lactation failure. If the mother has serious difficulties, seeks help and really wants to breastfeed her very young baby, then some heroic methods may be necessary. The mother may need to be admitted to hospital and placed in a ward where other women are successfully breastfeeding. She and her infant should be examined for any physical reason for inability to breastfeed. The mother should be given plenty of fluids, including milk. These are mainly psychological inducements aimed to encourage lactation. In some societies local foods or potions are considered to be lactagogues, or substances that stimulate breastmilk production. There is no harm in trying these substances. A knowledgeable doctor or senior health worker may prescribe one of two drugs which are sometimes effective in improving or stimulating milk production: the tranquillizer chlorpromazine, 25 mg three times a day by mouth, or the newer drug metoclopramide, 10 mg three times a day.

In general, the important basis for treatment is to help the mother relax, to assist her in getting the baby to suck at the breast and to make certain that, while the breast is relied upon as much as possible, the baby is not losing weight. The dilemma is that the more the infant suckles at the breast, the greater the stimulation to production and let-down of milk; while the more the supplementary foods given, the less the infant will want to suckle.

If breastfeeding remains unsuccessful in an infant of up to three months of age, the mother should be taught to feed infant formula or milk to the baby either with a cup and spoon or with a feeding bowl. A cup and spoon are easier to keep clean than a bottle and teat. Some means should be found to provide the mother with adequate infant formula, fresh milk or full-cream milk powder if she cannot afford to buy it, which will often be the case. The infant should attend a clinic regularly.

This method of feeding also applies to the infant of a mother who dies in childbirth. It is then desirable to admit to hospital both the child and the female relative or care-giver who is to be responsible for the infant's feeding. An alternative is to find a lactating relative or friend to act as a wet nurse and to breastfeed the infant. Sometimes a friend or relative will be willing and able.

Failure of lactation or death of the mother after the infant is four months of age calls for a different regime. The child can be fed a thin gruel of whatever is the local staple food, to which should be added adequate quantities of milk or milk powder. It is advantageous to provide some extra fat in the infant's diet. A relatively small quantity of groundnut, sesame, cottonseed, red palm or other edible oil will markedly increase the baby's energy intake without adding too much bulk to the diet. If milk or milk powder is not available then any protein-rich food such as legumes, eggs, ground meat, fish or poultry may be used.

Insufficient milk production

Much more common than lactation failure is the belief by a mother that she is not producing enough breastmilk to satisfy her baby. Insufficient milk is very commonly reported by mothers in industrialized countries; perhaps the baby cries a lot or the mother feels that the baby is not growing adequately, or there may be any of a number of other reasons. In medicine this common condition is termed "insufficient milk syndrome". It is often at first a psychological concern rather than a serious condition, but it may rapidly lead to a real problem of milk production. Too often physicians, nurses and friends of the mother provide exactly the wrong advice to the mother concerned about her milk production.

In many studies, especially in industrialized countries, "insufficient milk" is cited as the most common reason given by mothers for their early termination of breastfeeding or for early supplementation with other foods, especially formula. It is all too easy to assume simply that many women are incapable of producing enough milk to feed their young infants. The busy practitioner's answer, when faced with a mother complaining of insufficient milk, is simply to advise her to supplement her breastmilk with bottle feeds. This may be exactly the wrong advice to give.

Suckling at the breast encourages the release of prolactin. The maintenance of lactation is dependent on adequate nipple stimulation by the suckling infant. It is now evident that diminishing breastmilk production results from reduced nipple stimulation. The cause of insufficient milk may therefore often be that alternative feeding has replaced breastfeeding to a variable degree. Therefore, advice to provide or increase supplementation is almost always going to contribute to a reduction in breastmilk production; supplementary bottle feeds are used as a cure for insufficient milk when in fact they are the cause.

The most appropriate treatment for insufficient milk syndrome in a mother who wishes to breastfeed is to advise her to try to increase milk production by putting the infant to the breast more frequently, in this way increasing stimulation of the nipples. The common medical advice, increasing bottle feeds, is likely to worsen the situation, leading to a further decline in milk production and eventual cessation of lactation. This is not to condemn supplementary feeding, especially after the infant is six months of age, but it should be clear that its use will almost inevitably contribute to a decline in milk production.

Maternal employment away from home is frequently cited as the most important reason for a decline in breastfeeding. Published surveys, however, seldom cite work as an important reason for not initiating breastfeeding or for early weaning from the breast. Clearly, employment out of the home for more than a few hours a day does place constraints on the opportunity to breastfeed and provides a reason for supplementary feeding. It may therefore contribute to the development of insufficient milk production.

Working mothers can continue to breastfeed successfully and can maintain good levels of lactation. Nipple stimulation from adequate suckling during the time they spend with their infants is particularly important for them. There is a need for labour laws and work conditions that recognize the special needs of lactating mothers in the labour force. If breastfeeding were accepted as necessary and usual practice by governments and employers, then arrangements would have to be made for a woman's baby to be near her for the first six months of life.

Past and present promotional practices by manufacturers of breastmilk substitutes may be an important factor contributing to the problem of insufficient milk. The companies find it advantageous to influence both the public and the medical profession to believe that supplementary bottle-feeding is the answer to insufficient milk.

The best and easiest way to judge whether or not a baby is getting enough breastmilk, when no other feeding is provided, is to weigh the baby regularly. Normal or near-normal weight gain provides the best evidence of adequate breastmilk production.

BREASTFEEDING, FERTILITY AND BIRTH SPACING

The traditional wisdom of many societies long included a belief that breastfeeding reduced the likelihood of an early pregnancy. Often this belief was regarded as an old wives' tale. Scientific evidence now proves beyond question that the intensity, frequency and duration of breastfeeding bears a positive relationship to the length of post-partum amenorrhoea, anovulation and reduced fertility. Mothers who breastfeed intensively find that there is a relatively long period after birth before menstruation resumes. In contrast, the interval between birth and the onset of monthly periods is short in women who do not breastfeed their babies. The physiology of this phenomenon is now reasonably clear; it is related to hormones produced as a result of sucking stimulation of the nipple.

This knowledge has important implications in terms of birth spacing and population dynamics. In many developing countries, breastfeeding now contributes more to child spacing and to prolonging intervals between births than does the combined use of contraceptive pills, intra-uterine devices (IUDs), condoms, diaphragms and other modern contraceptives. Therefore the fertility-controlling benefits of breastfeeding should now be added to its other advantages.

Recent data from Kenya and elsewhere suggest that women who continue to breastfeed for a long time but also introduce bottle-feeding in the first few months of the infant's life may have shorter post-partum amenorrhoea than women who practise breastfeeding exclusively. The use of breastmilk substitutes in the first few months of life reduces sucking at the breast, thus lowering prolactin levels and leading to an earlier return of ovulation and menstruation even in mothers who breastfeed for a year or more. Thus bottle-feeding of babies contributes to a narrower spacing between births.

The so-called lactational amenorrhoea method (LAM) of natural family planning is now being widely and successfully used. If a mother has an infant under six months of age, is amenorrhoeic (with no vaginal bleeding from 56 days post partum) and is exclusively or almost fully breastfeeding her infant, then she is said to be 98 percent protected against pregnancy. She does not need to use any artificial family planning method.

BREASTFEEDING AND AIDS

Human immunodeficiency virus (HIV) infection is now a major health challenge worldwide. Infection with HIV is followed, often some years later, by progressive disease and eventually by immunosuppression. The resulting syndrome, called acquired immunodeficiency syndrome (AIDS), is characterized by the development of various infections, often with diarrhoea and pneumonia, and malignancies such as Kaposi's sarcoma, leading eventually to death. In many developing countries HIV infection is almost as common in females as in males. Increasing numbers of infants and young children appear to be infected from their mothers. The exact mechanisms of transmission from the mother to the foetus or infant is not known. Transmission could occur *in utero* through passage of the virus across the placenta; around the time of delivery through exposure to vaginal secretions, ingestion of maternal blood or maternal-foetal transfusion during labour and delivery; and in infancy through ingestion of the virus in breastmilk. In many countries HIV infection has been reported in 25 to 45 percent of infants born to HIV-positive mothers.

Evidence suggests that HIV can be transmitted from infected mothers to their uninfected infants through breastmilk. The virus has been isolated from human breast-milk. It was thought that the fragile virus might be destroyed by gastric acid and enzymes in the infant's gut and that the stomach and intestines of infants might be relatively impervious to the virus. This is probably largely true; by far the majority of babies breastfed by HIV-infected mothers do not become infected through breastmilk. It has been difficult, however, to determine whether a particular infant was infected prior to delivery, at the time of delivery or through breastfeeding. This uncertainty is partly due to the fact that both infected and uninfected infants acquire HIV antibodies passively from their infected mothers, but the presence of antibodies in standard HIV tests cannot be interpreted to mean active infection.

A pregnant woman with poor vitamin A status is more likely than others to pass the HIV infection to the foetus. Transmission from mother to infant through breast-milk is currently thought to be relatively rare. Some apparent differences in rates of transmission among groups of women from different countries may be related to vitamin A intake and other factors.

A consultation of the World Health Organization (WHO) and the United Nations Children's Fund (UNICEF) was clear in its recommendation, despite the current evidence of HIV transmission through breastmilk (WHO/UNICEF, 1992):

Where infectious diseases and malnutrition are the main cause of infant deaths and the infant mortality rate is high, breast-feeding should be the usual advice to pregnant women, including those who are HIV-infected. This is because their baby's risk of HIV infection through breast milk is likely to be lower than the risk of death from other causes if it is not breast-fed.

Many infants in Africa, Asia and Latin America live in settings where gastro-intestinal infections are prevalent, hygiene is poor and water supplies are suspect. In these circumstances the many advantages of breastfeeding far outweigh the risk to the infant of AIDS infection through breast-milk from an HIV-positive mother. Only where the common causes of morbidity and mortality in infancy are not infectious diseases should public policy advise the use of bottle-feeding in place of breast-feeding to reduce the possibility of AIDS transmission. The individual mother should, of course, where feasible, be counselled by a doctor or trained health worker and cautioned about the relative risks to the infant of breastfeeding or alternative feeding methods in terms of disease and survival (Photo 10). This counselling will allow the mother to make an informed decision.

CONTROL OF INFANT FORMULA PROMOTION

Two factors stand out as the major reasons for a decline in breastfeeding: first, the promotion of breastmilk substitutes by their manufacturers, particularly the multinational corporations; and second, the failure of the health profession to advocate, protect and support breast-feeding. In the 1950s and 1960s a small group of physicians, paediatricians and nutritionists working in developing countries drew attention to the dangers of bottle-feeding and decried the role of industry in the decline of breastfeeding. In the 1970s public outrage arose over the aggressive promotion of infant formula using advertising, free supplies and other "hard sell" tactics. Most doctors and health workers in countries of both North and South were at best unsupportive of the growing public pressure to rein in the promotional activities of the corporations; at the worst, doctors sided with the manufacturers against the critics of the corporations.

In 1979, WHO and UNICEF organized a meeting in Geneva, Switzerland, at which a number of experts met with representatives of industry and of non-governmental organizations (NGOs) and delegates from selected countries to discuss possible regulations to control the promotion of breastmilk substitutes. At this conference participants took a decision to develop a code of conduct and agreed upon some of its main principles. Several meetings followed to develop wording for the code. On 21 May 1981 the World Health Assembly overwhelmingly adopted the International Code of Marketing of Breast-milk Substitutes. In 1994 the United States Government finally decided to support it. The code applies to the marketing of breastmilk substitutes, and its most important article states: "There should be no advertising or other form of promotion to the general public of products within the scope of this Code." Other details concern provision of samples at sales points; contact between marketing personnel and mothers; the use of health facilities for the promotion of infant formula; and the labelling and quality of products.

The code was a compromise between industry and those who believe that all promotion of infant formula should be barred, and it surely represents the minimum requirements. Its major provisions include:

- no advertising in health care facilities;
- no free samples;
- no promotion in health care facilities;
- no inducement or unscientific promotion to health workers;
- no free or low-cost supplies to maternity wards and hospitals;
- factual rather than promotion-oriented literature;
- non-promotional labels that state the superiority of breastfeeding and the hazards of bottle-feeding.

The international code is not binding on individual countries, but it suggests that governments should take action to give effect to its principles and aims. Many countries have introduced legislation based on the code. The use of samples has declined but has not been halted. Many ministries of health are now more supportive of breastfeeding than in the past. However, it is often forgotten that the code was a compromise agreement, that it is the very minimum needed to address a small part of a large problem and that all codes have loopholes.

Although advertising to the public has ceased, manufacturers continue to advertise to health professionals; and companies are increasingly advertising to the public the use of their manufactured weaning foods for consumption by very young babies. Free formula is still provided by many manufacturers to hospitals in many countries. In exchange, the hospitals hand out free formula together with company literature to new mothers as they leave the hospital. This offering gives the mother the impression of medical endorsement of formula feeding.

Passage of the International Code of Marketing of Breast-milk Substitutes and of some other resolutions that are very supportive of breastfeeding has led to some complacency and to a false belief that the problem has been solved. Those who worked for the code knew that it could at best solve only a part of the problem, yet support for actions to deal with other important causes of decreased breastfeeding is now more difficult to obtain. There is currently a need to strengthen and broaden the code, to make it applicable to manufactured weaning foods as well as breastmilk substitutes and to prevent advertising to health professionals as well as to the general public. More support is needed for NGOs involved in monitoring the code and for their work to protect, support and promote breastfeeding.

The attitude of health professionals with regard to breastfeeding has improved over the last two decades. However, there is still much ignorance, and as a result the medical and health profession often has a negative impact on breastfeeding. The first need then is to educate all future health workers about breastfeeding and to re-educate present professionals. It follows that training of doctors, nurses, midwives and other health professionals must be improved. In some countries major efforts are under way, in which seminars and refresher courses are used to educate active health workers about sound infant-feeding practices.

PROTECTION, SUPPORT AND PROMOTION OF BREASTFEEDING

A country's or community's strategy to empower women and to assist mothers and their infants regarding the right to breastfeed needs to include three levels or categories of activity:

- protection of breastfeeding through policies, programmes and activities that shield women who are already breastfeeding or plan to do so against forces that might influence them to do otherwise;
- support of breastfeeding through activities, both formal and informal, that may help women to have confidence in their ability to breastfeed, which is important for women who have a desire to breastfeed but have

anxieties or doubts about it, or for those who face conditions that make breastfeeding seem difficult;
- promotion of breastfeeding through activities that are designed mainly to influence groups of women to breastfeed their infants when they are disinclined to do so or have not done so with their previous babies.

Although all three categories of activity are important, the relative effort put into each should depend on the current situation in the particular country. Thus, where traditional breastfeeding practices are the norm but infant formula is just beginning to make inroads, protection activities deserve highest priority. In contrast, in a country where the majority of women do not breastfeed at all, the major efforts should concern promotion. To use a health analogy, it can be said that protection and support are preventive measures, and promotion is a curative approach.

Protection of breastfeeding is aimed at guarding women who normally would successfully breastfeed against those forces that might cause them to alter this practice. All actions that prevent or curtail promotion of breastmilk substitutes, baby bottles and teats will have this effect. A strong code, properly enforced and monitored, will help protect breastfeeding. Various forms of formula promotion need to be curtailed, including promotion aimed at health professionals; distribution of samples, calendars and promotional materials; and hospital visits by manufacturers' staff. Legislative measures to curb these practices may be needed. Papua New Guinea has placed infant formula on prescription as a means of protecting breastfeeding. New measures need to be adopted in some countries to reduce the promotion of manufactured weaning foods and items such as glucose for child feeding.

What needs to be done to support breast-feeding in a country depends on the factors or problems that make breastfeeding more difficult. In many urban areas paid employment away from home is one such factor. Actions to allow women both to work away from home and to breastfeed are needed. A second factor relates to maternal morbidity, including breast problems during lactation. Unless health workers are supportive of breastfeeding, it is often found that mothers unnecessarily resort to breastmilk substitutes when they face such problems. A third important issue involves current health facility practices. Doctors need to understand that very few health conditions are absolute contra-indications for breastfeeding. In many industrialized and non-industrialized countries, private voluntary agencies and NGOs have very useful roles in support of breastfeeding. La Leche League and other breastfeeding information groups have been important.

Promotion of breastfeeding includes motivation or re-education of mothers who otherwise might not be inclined to breast-feed their babies. In theory, promotion is the most difficult and certainly the most costly of the three options. In some societies, however, promotion is essential if breastfeeding is to become the preferred method of infant feeding. The usual approach involves mass media and edu-cation campaigns to make known the disadvantages of bottle-feeding and the advantages of breastfeeding (Photo 11). It is important to know the factors that have led to a decline in breastfeeding in an area and to understand how women regard breast- and bottle-feeding. A lack of such understanding has led to the failure of many promotional campaigns. Social marketing techniques, properly applied, have a greater chance of success. Pro-motion should address not only the health benefits, but also the economic and contra-ceptive advantages of breastfeeding. Often it is first necessary for politicians to be educated about these matters.

Both a strong political will and an ability to implement new policies are necessary for any plan to protect, support and promote breastfeeding.

The Baby Friendly Hospital Initiative (BFHI)

In 1992, UNICEF and WHO launched an initiative to help protect, support and promote breastfeeding by addressing problems in hospitals, such as practices that were not supportive of breastfeeding (for example, separation of mothers from their infants) and those that directly influenced mothers to formula-feed (for example, presentation of free formula packs to mothers). The two major objectives of BFHI were to end the distribution of free or low-cost supplies of breastmilk substitutes; and to ensure hospital practices supportive of breastfeeding.

BFHI may be less relevant for countries and communities where most babies are born outside the hospital setting. It may also be less influential in maternity hospitals in large cities in developing countries, where babies are discharged within 24 or 36 hours of delivery.

Breastfeeding and employment legislation

Some countries have made it easier for working women to breastfeed, and some employers of female labour have facilitated breastfeeding for mothers. These are exceptions, however, when they should be the rule. The FAO/WHO International Conference on Nutrition (ICN), held in Rome in 1992, acknowledged "the right of infants and mothers to exclusive breast-feeding". The Plan of Action for Nutrition adopted at the conference states that governments and others should "support and encourage mothers to breast-feed and adequately care for their children, whether formally or informally employed or doing

Ten steps to successful breastfeeding

The joint WHO/UNICEF statement *Protecting, promoting and supporting breast-feeding: the special role of maternity services* (WHO/UNICEF, 1989) spelled out the following practices, termed "Ten steps to successful breast-feeding", which hospitals and all facilities providing maternity services and care for newborn infants are expected to undertake in order to be considered baby friendly.

1. Have a written breastfeeding policy that is routinely communicated to all health care staff.
2. Train all health care staff in skills necessary to implement this policy.
3. Inform all pregnant women about the benefits and management of breastfeeding.
4. Help mothers initiate breastfeeding within a half-hour of birth.
5. Show mothers how to breastfeed, and how to maintain lactation even if they should be separated from their infants.
6. Give newborn infants no food or drink other than breastmilk, unless medically indicated.
7. Practise rooming-in – allow mothers and infants to remain together – 24 hours a day.
8. Encourage breastfeeding on demand.
9. Give no artificial teats or pacifiers (also called dummies or soothers) to breast-feeding infants.
10. Foster the establishment of breastfeeding support groups and refer mothers to them on discharge from the hospital or clinic.

many countries serious obstacles are placed in the way of mothers' rights to breastfeed. Among the common obstacles are very short maternity leave, or rejection of maternity leave for casual employees; job dismissal for those who do take maternity leave; lack of child care facilities which could be available in places where large numbers of women are employed; failure to provide breastfeeding breaks for women who could breastfeed during a long work shift; and open targeting of working women by formula companies to persuade them to formula-feed rather than breastfeed their infants.

What can be done? First, governments and the general public should ensure that at the very minimum the terms of the ILO Maternity Protection Convention are adhered to and never infringed. These terms include 12 weeks of maternity leave with cash benefits of at least 66 percent of previous earnings; two 30-minute breast-feeding breaks during each working day; and prohibition of dismissal during maternity leave. Other actions can be taken to:

• ensure that every country has legislation to protect working women's rights to breastfeed and that these laws are implemented;

• increase public awareness of the very great benefits – not only to infants, but to society as a whole – of combining work and breastfeeding;

• take concrete steps to make as many workplaces as possible mother friendly and baby friendly;

• use workers' associations, groups and trade unions to advocate and insist on a set of entitlements related to maternity leave and breastfeeding;

• encourage the establishment of child care facilities in or near the workplace where infants can be safely kept and where mothers can visit to breastfeed.

Figure 4, taken from an action folder produced by the World Alliance for Breast-

unpaid work. ILO conventions and regulations covering this subject may be used as a starting point...".

The Maternity Protection Convention adopted by the International Labour Organisation (ILO) recognizes that women have a right to maternity leave and a right to breastfeed their infants. However, in feeding Action (WABA) for World Breast-feeding Week in 1993, illustrates the requirements of time, space and support for mother-friendly workplaces.

International commitments in favour of breastfeeding

The nine years between 1981 and 1990 witnessed many international actions or pledges in support of breastfeeding. These include the adoption of the International Code of Marketing of Breast-milk Substitutes by the World Health Assembly in May 1981; the Innocenti Declaration on the Protection, Promotion and Support of Breastfeeding, adopted by the WHO/UNICEF policy-makers' meeting Breast-feeding in the 1990s: A Global Initiative, in Florence, Italy in 1990; and the World Declaration on Nutrition and Plan of Action for Nutrition approved at the ICN in 1992.

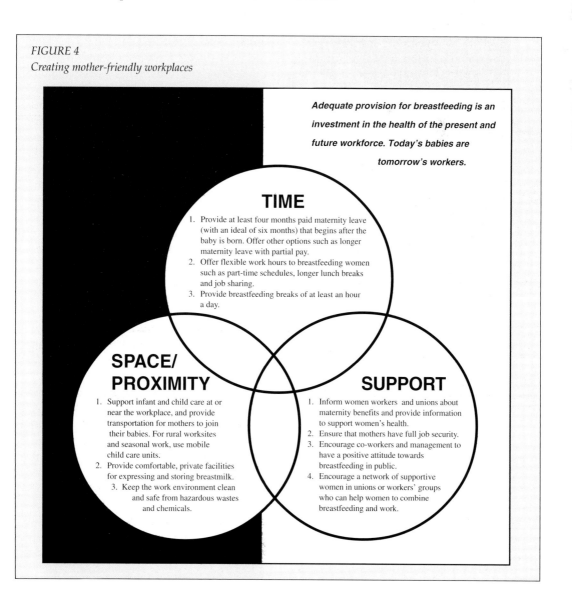

FIGURE 4
Creating mother-friendly workplaces

Adequate provision for breastfeeding is an investment in the health of the present and future workforce. Today's babies are tomorrow's workers.

TIME
1. Provide at least four months paid maternity leave (with an ideal of six months) that begins after the baby is born. Offer other options such as longer maternity leave with partial pay.
2. Offer flexible work hours to breastfeeding women such as part-time schedules, longer lunch breaks and job sharing.
3. Provide breastfeeding breaks of at least an hour a day.

SPACE/ PROXIMITY
1. Support infant and child care at or near the workplace, and provide transportation for mothers to join their babies. For rural worksites and seasonal work, use mobile child care units.
2. Provide comfortable, private facilities for expressing and storing breastmilk.
3. Keep the work environment clean and safe from hazardous wastes and chemicals.

SUPPORT
1. Inform women workers and unions about maternity benefits and provide information to support women's health.
2. Ensure that mothers have full job security.
3. Encourage co-workers and management to have a positive attitude towards breastfeeding in public.
4. Encourage a network of supportive women in unions or workers' groups who can help women to combine breastfeeding and work.

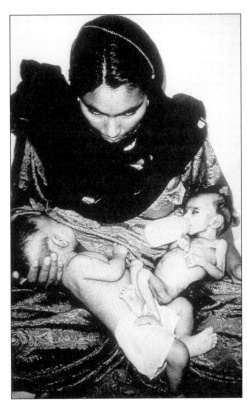

PHOTO 7
Asian mother with twins:
the baby on the left is male,
breastfed, well nourished
and healthy; the baby on the
right is female, bottle-fed
and seriously
undernourished (she died
the day after this photo was
taken)

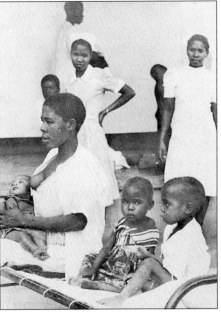
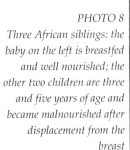

PHOTO 8
Three African siblings: the
baby on the left is breastfed
and well nourished; the
other two children are three
and five years of age and
became malnourished after
displacement from the
breast

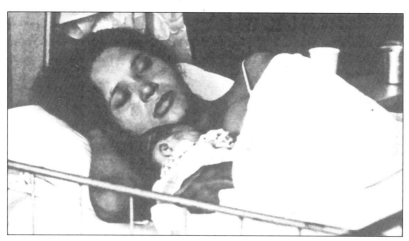

PHOTO 9
Rooming-in

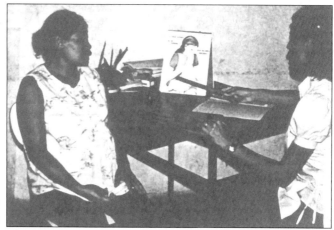

PHOTO 10
Advice during pregnancy

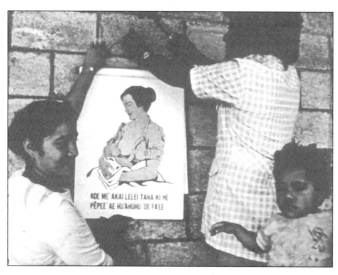

PHOTO 11
Promotion of breastfeeding

Part II
Basic nutrition

Chapter 8
Body composition, the functions of food, metabolism and energy

The phrase "we are what we eat" is frequently used to signify that the composition of our bodies is dependent in large measure on what we have consumed. The many chemical elements in the human body occur mainly in the form of water, protein, fats, mineral salts and carbohydrates, in the percentages shown in Table 8. Each human body is built up from food containing these five constituents, and vitamins as well.

Food serves mainly for growth, energy and body repair, maintenance and protection. Food also provides enjoyment and stimulation, since eating and drinking are among the pleasures of life everywhere. Truly food nourishes both the body and soul. Even if technology could produce a perfect diet in terms of content, such a diet could still lack, for example, the aroma and flavour of a curry, or the stimulating taste of hot coffee.

What controls appetite or the feeling of hunger is not fully understood. The hypothalamus in the brain has a role, as do other central nervous system sites. Other probable factors include blood sugar levels, body hormones, body fat, many diseases, emotions and of course food type and availability, personal likes and dislikes and the social setting where food is to be consumed.

DIETARY CONSTITUENTS AND THE FUNCTIONS OF FOOD

A simple classification of dietary constituents is given in Table 9.

Human beings eat food, and not individual nutrients. Most foods, including staples such as rice, maize and wheat, provide mainly carbohydrate for energy but also significant quantities of protein, a little fat or oil and useful micronutrients. Thus cereal grains provide some of the constituents needed for energy, growth and body repair and maintenance. Breastmilk provides all the macro- and micronutrients necessary to satisfy the total needs of a young infant up to six months of age including those for energy, growth and body repair and maintenance. Cows' milk has the balance of nutrients for all the requirements of a calf.

Water

Water can be considered the most important dietary constituent. A normal man or woman can live without food for 20 to 40 days, but without water humans die in four to seven days. Over 60 percent of human body weight is made up of water, of which approximately 61 percent is intracellular and the rest extracellular. Water intake, except under exceptional circumstances (e.g. intravenous feeding), comes from the food and fluids consumed. The amount consumed varies widely in individuals and may be influenced by climate, culture and other factors. Often as much as 1 litre is consumed in solid food, and 1 to 3 litres as fluids drunk. Water is also formed in the body as a result of oxidation of macronutrients, but the water thus obtained usually constitutes less than 10 percent of total water.

Water is excreted mainly by the kidneys

TABLE 8
Chemical composition of a human body weighing 65 kg

Component	Percentage of body weight
Water	61.6
Protein	17
Fats	13.8
Minerals	6.1
Carbohydrate	1.5

TABLE 9
Simple classification of dietary constituents

Constituent	Use
Water	To provide body fluid and to help regulate body temperature
Carbohydrates	As fuel for energy for body heat and work
Fats	As fuel for energy and essential fatty acids
Proteins	For growth and repair
Minerals	For developing body tissues and for metabolic processes and protection
Vitamins	For metabolic processes and protection
Indigestible and unabsorbable particles, including fibre	To form a vehicle for other nutrients, add bulk to the diet, provide a habitat for bacterial flora and assist proper elimination of refuse

as urine. The kidneys regulate the output of urine and maintain a balance; if smaller amounts of fluid are consumed, the kidneys excrete less water, and the urine is more concentrated. While most water is eliminated by the kidneys, in hot climates as much or more can be lost from the skin (through perspiration) and the lungs. Much smaller quantities are lost from the gut in the faeces (except in the presence of diarrhoea, when losses may be high).

Metabolism of sodium and potassium, which are known as electrolytes, is linked with body water. The sodium is mainly in the extracellular water and the potassium in the intracellular water. Most diets contain adequate amounts of both these minerals. In fluid loss caused, for example, by diarrhoea or haemorrhage, the balance of electrolytes in the blood may become disturbed. Water intake and electrolyte balance are particularly important in sick infants. In healthy infants, breastmilk alone from a healthy mother provides adequate quantities of fluids and electrolytes without additional water for the first six months of life even in hot climates. Infants with diarrhoea and disease, however, may require additional fluids.

While food intake is largely regulated by appetite and food availability, fluid intake is influenced by the sensation termed thirst. Thirst may arise for various reasons. In dehydration it may be caused by drying of the mouth but also by signals from the same satiety centre in the hypothalamus that controls hunger sensations. Dehydration, an important feature of diarrhoea, is discussed in Chapter 37.

The phenomenon of water accumulation in the body is manifested in the condition known as oedema, when disease causes an excess of extracellular fluid. Two important deficiency diseases in which generalized oedema is a feature are kwashiorkor (see Chapter 12) and wet beriberi (see Chapter 16). The excess fluid may result from electrolyte disturbances and accumulation of water in the extracellular compartment. A person can have oedema and still be dehydrated from diarrhoea; this condition is a form of heart failure. Water can also collect in the peritoneal cavity, in the condition known as ascites, which may be caused by liver disease.

BODY COMPOSITION

The human body is sometimes said to be divided into three compartments, accounting for the following shares of the total body weight of a well-nourished healthy adult male:

- body cell mass, 55 percent;
- extracellular supporting tissue, 30 percent;
- body fat, 15 percent.

The body cell mass is made up of cellular components such as muscle, body organs (viscera, liver, brain, etc.) and blood. It comprises the parts of the body that are involved in body metabolism, body functioning, body work and so on.

The extracellular supporting tissue consists of two parts: the extracellular fluid (for example, the blood plasma supporting the blood cells) and the skeleton and other supporting structures.

Body fat is nearly all present beneath the skin (subcutaneous fat) and around body organs such as the intestine and heart. It serves in part as an energy reserve. Small quantities are present in the walls of body cells or in nerves.

Physiologists and those interested in metabolism have developed various ways to estimate body composition, including the amount of fluids in the body and body density. A common determination is to estimate lean body mass (LBM) or the fat-free mass of the body. These measures vary from the very simple to the very difficult. The simpler ones are of course less precise. Anthropometry using weight, height, skinfold thickness and body circumferences is relatively easy and very cheap to undertake, and does provide some estimate of LBM and body composition. In contrast, methods using, for example, bioelectrical impedance, computerized axial tomography (CAT scans) and nuclear magnetic resonance require expensive apparatus and highly trained staff.

The fluid in the cells (intracellular fluid) has mainly potassium ions, and the extracellular fluid is mainly a solution of sodium chloride. Both also have other ions. Total body water can be estimated using different methods including dilution techniques to measure, for example, plasma volume.

Body fat is estimated using different methods. Because a large portion of adipose tissue is present beneath the skin, it can be estimated by using a skinfold calliper to measure skinfold thickness in different sites (see Chapter 33). Another method is to weigh the person both in air and under water using a special apparatus and tank. This method really provides an estimate of body density.

The various methods of determining body composition are described in detail in textbooks of physiology or nutrition (see Bibliography).

Body composition is much influenced by nutrition. The two extremes are the wasting of nutritional marasmus (see Chapter 12) and starvation (see Chapter 24) and the overweight of obesity (see Chapter 23). Body composition differs between the genders and, perhaps only slightly, among races. African Americans have been shown to have heavier skeletons than whites of the same body build in the United States. In females pregnancy and lactation influence body composition.

The body composition of children is influenced by their age and growth. Disturbances of growth resulting from nutritional deficiencies influence body composition, including the eventual size of the body and of body organs.

METABOLISM AND ENERGY

The general term for all the chemical processes carried out by the cells of the body is "metabolism". Chief among these processes is the oxidation (combustion, or burning) of food which produces energy. This process is analogous to a car engine burning petrol to produce the energy that makes it run. In most forms of combustion, be it in the car or in the human, heat is produced as well as energy.

Classical physics taught that energy can be neither created nor destroyed. Although this law of nature is not completely correct (as the conversion of matter to energy in a nuclear reactor shows), it is still true in most instances. All three macronutrients in food – carbohydrate, protein and fat – provide energy. Energy for the body comes mainly from food, and in the absence of food it can be produced only by the breakdown of body tissues.

All forms of energy can be converted into heat energy. It is possible to measure the heat produced by burning a litre of petrol, for example. Food energy can also be and is expressed as heat energy. The unit of measurement used has been the large calorie (Cal) or kilocalorie (kcal) (which is 1 000 times the small calorie used in physics), but this measure is increasingly being replaced by the joule (J) or kilojoule (kJ). The kilocalorie is defined as the heat necessary to raise the temperature of 1 litre of water from 14.5° to 15.5°C. Whereas the kilocalorie is a unit of heat, the joule is truly a unit of energy. The joule is defined as the amount of energy used when 1 kg is moved 1 m by 1 newton (N) of force. In nutrition the kilojoule (1 000 J) is used. The equivalent of 1 kcal is 4.184 kJ. These are units of measurement in the same way that litres and pints are measures of quantity, and metres and feet are measures of length. In many scientific journals the joule is being introduced in place of the kilocalorie (see conversion tables, Annex 5), but the general public and most health workers still prefer to express food energy in kilocalories rather than joules. Kilocalories are therefore used in this book.

The human body requires energy for all bodily functions, including work, the maintenance of body temperature and the continuous action of the heart and lungs. In children energy is essential for growth. Energy is also needed for breakdown, repair and building of tissues. These are metabolic processes. The rate at which these functions are carried out while the body is at rest is the Basal metabolic rate (BMR).

Basal metabolic rate

BMR for an individual person is usually defined as the amount of energy [expressed in kilocalories or megajoules (MJ) per day] expended when the person is at complete rest, both physical (i.e. lying down) and psychological. It can also be expressed as kilocalories per hour or per kilogram of weight. BMR provides the energy required by the body for maintenance of body temperature; for the work of body organs such as the beating heart and the muscles working for normal, at rest, breathing; and for the functioning of other organs such as the liver, kidneys and brain.

BMR varies from individual to individual. Important general factors influencing BMR are the person's weight, gender, age and state of health. BMR is also influenced by the person's body composition, for example the amounts of muscle and adipose tissue and therefore the amounts of protein and fat in the body. In broad terms, bigger people with more muscle and larger body organs have higher BMR than smaller people. Elderly people tend to have lower BMR than they had when they were young, and females tend to have lower BMR than males even on a per kilogram body weight basis. There are exceptions, however, to all these generalizations.

BMR is important as a component of energy requirements. Table 10 shows BMR of adult men and women according to height and weight, both per kilogram body weight and as total energy per day. The

TABLE 10

Basal metabolic rate in adult men and women in relation to height and median acceptable weight for height

Height (m)	Weight[a] (kg)	18-30 years		30-60 years		Over 60	
		kcal(kJ)[b]/kg/day	kcal(kJ)/day	kcal(kJ)/kg/day	kcal(kJ)/day	kcal(kJ)/kg/day	kcal(kJ)/day
Men							
1.5	49.5	29.0 (121)	1 440 (6.03)	29.4 (123)	1 450 (6.07)	23.3 (98)	1 150 (4.81)
1.6	56.5	27.4 (115)	1 540 (6.44)	27.2 (114)	1 530 (6.40)	22.2 (93)	1 250 (5.23)
1.7	63.5	26.0 (109)	1 650 (6.90)	25.4 (106)	1 620 (6.78)	21.2 (89)	1 350 (5.65)
1.8	71.5	24.8 (104)	1 770 (7.41)	23.9 (99)	1 710 (7.15)	20.3 (85)	1 450 (6.07)
1.9	79.5	23.9 (100)	1 890 (7.91)	22.7 (95)	1 800 (7.53)	19.6 (82)	1 560 (6.53)
2.0	88.0	23.0 (96)	2 030 (8.49)	21.6 (90)	1 900 (7.95)	19.0 (80)	1 670 (6.99)
Women							
1.4	41	26.7 (112)	1 100 (4.60)	28.8 (120)	1 190 (4.98)	25.0 (105)	1 030 (4.31)
1.5	47	25.2 (105)	1 190 (4.98)	26.3 (110)	1 240 (5.19)	23.1 (97)	1 090 (4.56)
1.6	54	23.9 (100)	1 290 (5.40)	24.1 (101)	1 300 (5.44)	21.6 (90)	1 160 (4.85)
1.7	61	22.9 (96)	1 390 (5.82)	22.4 (94)	1 360 (5.69)	20.3 (85)	1 230 (5.15)
1.8	68	22.0 (92)	1 500 (6.28)	20.9 (87)	1 420 (5.94)	19.3 (81)	1 310 (5.48)

Source: WHO, 1985.
[a] Median acceptable weight for height; body mass index (BMI = wt/ht^2) = 22 in men, 21 in women (see Chapter 23).
[b] Kilojoules are given in parentheses.

table shows, for example, that in females aged 30 to 60 years BMR ranges from 1 190 to 1 420 kcal per day. This is the amount of energy required by a woman at complete rest for 24 hours. Of course many adult females in developing countries are smaller than 1.4 m in height and 41 kg in weight; their BMR might then be a little lower than 1 190 kcal per day.

Energy requirements

The mean daily energy requirements of adult men and women doing work classified as light, moderate and heavy are given in Table 11, expressed as multiples of BMR. The table shows, for example, that a woman doing heavy work requires energy equal to 1.82 times her BMR. If the woman is aged 25 years, is 1.4 m tall and weighs 41 kg, according to Table 10 her BMR would be 1 100 kcal per day. Thus her daily requirements are: 1 100 kcal × 1.82 = 2 002 kcal.

It is often useful to estimate energy needs for various activities that a person may do for particular lengths of time. The energy expenditure is usually calculated by multiplying an activity factor or metabolic constant, which varies according to the activity, by the individual's BMR. Table 12 gives the activity factors for calculating gross energy expenditure of various activities for adult males and females.

The average human burns energy at his or her BMR only when at complete rest. All ordinary movements require additional energy, and physical work, of course, requires more still. For a healthy male with

TABLE 11
Average daily energy requirements of adults by category of occupational work, expressed as a multiple of BMR

Classification of work	Men	Women
Light	1.55	1.56
Moderate	1.78	1.64
Heavy	2.10	1.82

Source: WHO, 1985.

TABLE 12
Activity factors for calculating gross energy expenditure (multiply by BMR)

Activity	Adult males	Adult females
Sleeping	1.0	1.0
Lying	1.2	1.2
Sitting quietly	1.2	1.2
Standing quietly	1.5	1.5
Walking slowly	2.8	2.8
Walking at normal pace	3.2	3.3
Walking fast uphill	7.5	6.6
Cooking	1.8	1.8
Office work (moving around)	1.6	1.7
Driving lorry	1.4	1.4
Labouring	5.2	4.4
Cutting sugar cane	6.5	–
Pulling loaded cart	5.9	–
Playing soccer	6.6	6.3
Fetching water from well	–	4.1
Pounding grain	–	4.6

Source: WHO, 1985.
Note: These values apply only as approximate mean values for the time actually spent on the activity. They do not allow for rests. In heavy work individuals usually take frequent pauses or rests.

BMR of 1 kcal/min, an average day may involve the energy expenditure shown in Table 13.

If the person in this example did – instead of eight hours of light work – five hours of herding and three hours of heavy work, hoeing hard ground at 8 kcal/min, then his output of energy would be as shown in Table 14.

If the individual undertaking the activities in the first example gets exactly 2 640 kcal in his food, his weight will be steady, and he will be functioning normally. However, if he then undertakes the activities in the second example and eats no extra food, his weight will gradually drop, because he will have to burn up his fuel reserve, which forms part of his own body. He would fairly soon, however, begin to limit his activities in order to stop this process. He would therefore probably work much less hard at hoeing, so that instead of burning 8 kcal/min he might use only, say, 3.2 kcal/min; he would also tend to be tired at the end of the day, and might well increase his period of complete rest (at 1 kcal/min) by reducing the period of minor activities. He would therefore have reduced his energy requirements to 2 646 kcal, as shown in Table 15.

This is just an example. In most instances, when people increase their output of energy, including work, they feel more hungry and increase their consumption of their staple food, be it rice, millet, maize, wheat, cassava or anything else.

The energy requirements of a human being are affected by several factors. The important ones are:

- *Body size.* A small person needs less energy than a large person.
- *Basal metabolic rate.* BMR varies and can be affected by factors such as disease of the thyroid gland.
- *Activity.* The more physical work or recreation performed, the more energy is required.

TABLE 13
Energy expenditure of an average day for a healthy male

Activity	Time *(hours)*	Energy expenditure *(kcal/min)*	Calculation	Total energy expenditure *(kcal)*
Sleep	8	1 (=BMR)	$8 \times 60 \times 1$	480
Light work: herding animals	8	2.5	$8 \times 60 \times 2.5$	1 200
Other: sitting and minor activities	8	2	$8 \times 60 \times 2$	960
Total				**2 640**

TABLE 14
Energy expenditure when the person in Table 13 performs three hours of hard work

Activity	Time *(hours)*	Energy expenditure *(kcal/min)*	Total energy expenditure *(kcal)*
Sleep	8	1	480
Light work: herding	5	2.5	750
Hard work: hoeing	3	8	1 440
Other: sitting and minor activities	8	2	960
Total			**3 630**

TABLE 15
Energy expenditure when the person in Table 14 adjusts his work to a less adequate diet

Activity	Time *(hours)*	Energy expenditure *(kcal/min)*	Total energy expenditure *(kcal)*
Sleep	10	1	600
Light work	5	2.5	750
Less hard work: hoeing	3	3.2	576
Other: sitting and minor activities	6	2	720
Total			**2 646**

- *Pregnancy.* A woman requires extra energy to develop the foetus and to carry its additional weight.
- *Lactation.* The lactating mother needs additional energy to produce energy-containing milk for the suckling baby. The relatively long duration of breast-feeding among most Asians and Africans results in a large proportion of women requiring extra energy.
- *Age.* Infants and children need more energy, for growth and activity, than adults. In older persons, the need for energy is sometimes reduced because there is a decline in activity and because their BMR is usually lower.
- *Climate.* In warm climates, i.e. in most of the tropics and subtropics, less energy is necessary to keep the body at its normal temperature than in cold climates.

Chapter 9
Macronutrients: carbohydrates, fats and proteins

CARBOHYDRATES

The main source of energy for most Asians, Africans and Latin Americans is carbohydrates in the food they eat. Carbohydrates constitute by far the greatest portion of their diet, as much as 80 percent in some cases. In contrast, carbohydrates make up only 45 to 50 percent of the diet of many people in industrialized countries.

Carbohydrates are compounds containing carbon, hydrogen and oxygen in the proportions 6:12:6. They are burned during metabolism to produce energy, liberating carbon dioxide (CO_2) and water (H_2O). The carbohydrates in the human diet are mainly in the form of starches and various sugars. Carbohydrates can be divided into three groups:

• monosaccharides, e.g. glucose, fructose, galactose;
• disaccharides, e.g. sucrose (table sugar), lactose, maltose;
• polysaccharides, e.g. starch, glycogen (animal starch), cellulose.

Monosaccharides

The simplest carbohydrates are the monosaccharides, or simple sugars. These sugars can pass through the wall of the alimentary tract without being changed by the digestive enzymes. The three most common are glucose, fructose and galactose.

Glucose, sometimes also called dextrose, is present in fruit, sweet potatoes, onions and other plant substances. It is the substance into which many other carbohydrates, such as the disaccharides and starches, are converted by the digestive

enzymes. Glucose is oxidized to produce energy, heat and carbon dioxide, which is exhaled in breathing.

Because glucose is the sugar in blood, it is most often used as an energy-producing substance for persons fed intravenously. Glucose dissolved in sterile water, usually in concentrations of 5 or 10 percent, is frequently used for this purpose.

Fructose is present in honey and some fruit juices. Galactose is a monosaccharide that is formed, along with glucose, when the milk sugar lactose is broken down by the digestive enzymes.

Disaccharides

The disaccharides, composed of simple sugars, need to be converted by the body into monosaccharides before they can be absorbed from the alimentary tract. Examples of disaccharides are sucrose, lactose and maltose. Sucrose is the scientific name for table sugar (the kind that is used, for example, to sweeten tea). It is most commonly produced from sugar cane but is also produced from beets. Sucrose is also present in carrots and pineapple. Lactose is the disaccharide present in human and animal milk. It is much less sweet than sucrose. Maltose is found in germinating seeds.

Polysaccharides

The polysaccharides are chemically the most complicated carbohydrates. They tend to be insoluble in water, and only some can be used by human beings to produce energy. Examples of polysaccharides are starch, glycogen and cellulose.

Starch is an important source of energy for humans. It occurs in cereal grains as well as in root foods such as potatoes and cassava. Starch is liberated during cooking when the starch granules rupture because of heating.

Glycogen is made in the human body and is sometimes known as animal starch. It is formed from monosaccharides produced by the digestion of dietary starch. Starch from rice or cassava is broken down in the intestines to form monosaccharide molecules, which pass into the bloodstream. Those surplus monosaccharides that are not used to produce energy (and carbon dioxide and water) are fused together to form a new polysaccharide, glycogen. Glycogen is usually present in muscle and in the liver, but not in large amounts.

Any of the digestible carbohydrates when consumed in excess of body needs are converted by the body into fat which is laid down as adipose tissue beneath the skin and at other sites in the body.

Cellulose, hemicellulose, lignin, pectin and gums are sometimes called unavailable carbohydrates because humans cannot digest them. Cellulose and hemicellulose are plant polymers that are the main components of cell walls. They are fibrous substances. Cellulose, which is a polymer of glucose, is one of the fibres of green plants. Hemicellulose is a polymer of other sugars, usually hexose and pentose. Lignin is the main component of wood. Pectins are present in plant tissue and sap and are colloidal polysaccharides. Gums are also viscous carbohydrates extracted from plants. Pectins and gums are both used by the food industry. The human alimentary tract cannot break down these carbohydrates or utilize them to produce energy. Some animals, such as cattle, have microorganisms in their intestines that break down cellulose and make it available as an energy-producing food. In humans, any of the unavailable carbohydrates present in food pass through the intestinal tract. They form much of the bulk and roughage evacuated in human faeces, and are often termed "dietary fibre".

There is increasing interest in fibre in diets, because high-fibre diets are now considered healthful. A clear advantage of a high-fibre diet is a lower incidence of constipation than among people who consume a low-fibre diet. The bulk in high-fibre diets may contribute a feeling of fullness or satiety which may lead to less consumption of energy, and this may help reduce the likelihood of obesity. A high-fibre diet results in more rapid transit of food through the intestinal tract and is thus believed to assist normal and healthy intestinal and bowel functioning. Dietary fibre has also been found to bind bile in the intestines.

It is now recognized that the high fibre content of most traditional diets may be an important factor in the prevention of certain diseases which appear to be much more prevalent in people consuming the low-fibre diets common in industrialized countries. Because it facilitates the rapid passage of materials through the intestine, fibre may be a factor in the control of diverticulitis, appendicitis, haemorrhoids and also possibly arteriosclerosis, which leads to coronary heart disease and some cancers.

Frequent consumption of any sticky fermentable carbohydrates, either starch or sugar, can contribute to dental caries, particularly when coupled with poor oral hygiene. Adequate intake of fluoride and/or a topical application is the best protection against caries (see Chapter 21).

FATS

In many developing countries dietary fats make up a smaller part of total energy intake (often only 8 or 10 percent) than carbohydrates. In most industrialized countries the proportion of fat intake is much higher. In the United States, for example, an average of 36 percent of total energy is derived from fat.

Fats, like carbohydrates, contain carbon, hydrogen and oxygen. They are insoluble in water but soluble in such chemical solvents as ether, chloroform and benzene. The term "fat" is used here to include all fats and oils that are edible and occur in human diets, ranging from those that are solid at cool room temperatures, such as butter, to those that are liquid at similar temperatures, such as groundnut or cottonseed oils. (In some terminologies the word "oil" is used to refer to those materials that are liquid at room temperature, while those that are solid are called fats.)

Fats (also referred to as lipids) in the body are divided into two groups: storage fat and structural fat. Storage fat provides a reserve storehouse of fuel for the body, while the structural fats are part of the essential structure of the cells, occurring in cell membranes, mitochondria and intracellular organelles.

Cholesterol is a lipid present in all cell membranes. It has an important role in fat transport and is the precursor from which bile salts and adrenal and sex hormones are made.

Dietary fats consist mainly of triglycerides, which can be split into glycerol and chains of carbon, hydrogen and oxygen called fatty acids. This action, the digestion or breakdown of fats, is achieved in the human intestine by enzymes known as lipases, which are present primarily in the pancreatic and intestinal secretions. Bile salts from the liver emulsify the fatty acids to make them more soluble in water and hence more easily absorbed.

The many fatty acids in human diets are divided into two main groups: saturated and unsaturated. The latter group includes both polyunsaturated and monounsaturated fatty acids. Saturated fatty acids have the maximum number of hydrogen atoms that their chemical structure will permit. All fats and oils eaten by humans are mixtures of saturated and unsaturated fatty acids. Broadly speaking, fats from land animals (i.e. meat fat, butter and ghee) contain more saturated fatty acids than do those of vegetable origin. Fats from plant products and to some extent those from fish have more unsaturated fatty acids, particularly polyunsaturated fatty acids (PUFAs). There are exceptions, however. For example, coconut oil has a large amount of saturated fatty acids.

These groupings of fats have important health implications because excess intake of saturated fats is one of the risk factors associated with arteriosclerosis and coronary heart disease (see Chapter 23). In contrast, PUFAs are believed to be protective.

PUFAs also include two unsaturated fatty acids, linoleic acid and linolenic acid, which have been termed "essential fatty acids" (EFAs) as they are necessary for good health. EFAs are important in the synthesis of many cell structures and several biologically important compounds. Recent studies have also shown the benefits of other longer-chain fatty acids in the growth and development of young children, and arachidonic acid and docosahexaenoic acid (DHA) should conditionally be considered essential during early development. Experiments with animals and studies in humans have shown definite skin and growth changes and abnormal vascular and neural function in the absence of these fatty acids, and there is no doubt that they are essential for the nutrition of individual cells and tissues of the body.

Fat is desirable to make the diet more palatable. It also yields about 9 kcal/g, which is more than twice the energy yielded by carbohydrates and proteins (about 4 kcal/g); fat can therefore reduce the bulk of the diet. A person doing very heavy work, especially in a cold climate, may require as many as 4 000 kcal a day. In such a case it is highly desirable that a good proportion of the energy should come from fat; otherwise the diet would be very bulky. Bulky diets can be a particularly serious problem in young children as well. A reasonable increase in the fat or oil content of the diets of young children raises the energy density of predominantly bulky carbohydrate diets and is highly desirable.

Fat also functions as a vehicle that assists the absorption of fat-soluble vitamins (see Chapter 11).

Thus fats, and even specific types of fat, are essential to health. However, practically all diets provide the small amount required.

Fat deposited in the human body serves as a reserve fuel. It is an economic way of storing energy, because, as mentioned above, fat yields about twice as much energy, weight for weight, as does carbohydrate or protein. Fat is present beneath the skin as an insulation against cold, and it forms a supporting tissue for many organs such as the heart and intestines.

All fat in the body is not necessarily derived from fat that has been eaten. However, excess calories from the carbohydrate and protein in, for example, maize, cassava, rice or wheat can be converted into fat in the human body.

PROTEINS

Like carbohydrates and fats, proteins contain carbon, hydrogen and oxygen, but they also contain nitrogen and often sulphur. They are particularly important as nitrogenous substances, and are necessary for growth and repair of the body. Proteins are the main structural constituents of the cells and tissues of the body, and they make up the greater portion of the substance of the muscles and organs (apart from water). The proteins in different body tissues are not all exactly the same. The proteins in liver, in blood and in specific hormones, for example, are all different.

Proteins are necessary

- for growth and development of the body;
- for body maintenance and the repair and replacement of worn out or damaged tissues;
- to produce metabolic and digestive enzymes;
- as an essential constituent of certain hormones, such as thyroxine and insulin.

Although proteins can yield energy, their main importance is rather as an essential constituent of all cells. All cells may need replacement from time to time, and their replacement requires protein.

Any protein eaten in excess of the amount needed for growth, cell and fluid replacement and various other metabolic functions is used to provide energy, which the body obtains by changing the protein into carbohydrate. If the carbohydrate and fat in the diet do not provide adequate energy, then protein is used to provide energy; as a result less protein is available for growth, cell replacement and other metabolic needs. This point is especially important for children, who need extra protein for growth. If they get too little food for their energy requirements, then the protein will be diverted for daily energy needs and will not be used for growth.

Amino acids

All proteins consist of large molecules which are made of amino acids. The amino acids in any protein are linked together in chains, called peptide linkages. The various proteins are made of different amino acids linked together in different chains. Because there are many different amino acids, there are many different possible configurations, so there are many different proteins.

During digestion proteins break down to form amino acids much as complex carbohydrates such as starches break down into simple monosaccharides and fats break down into fatty acids. In the stomach and intestines various proteolytic enzymes hydrolyse the protein, releasing amino acids and peptides.

Plants are able to synthesize amino acids from simple inorganic chemical substances. Animals do not have this ability; they derive all the amino acids necessary for building their protein from consumption of plants or animals. As the animals eaten by humans initially derived their protein from plants, all amino acids in human diets have originated from this source.

Animals have differing abilities to convert one amino acid into another. In the human this ability is limited. Conversion occurs mainly in the liver. If the ability to convert one amino acid into another were unlimited, then the question of the protein content of diets and the prevention of protein deficiency would be simple. It would be enough merely to supply sufficient protein, irrespective of the quality or amino acid content of the protein supplied.

Of the large number of amino acids, 20 are common in plants and animals. Of these, eight have been found to be essential for the adult human and have thus been termed "essential amino acids" or "indispensable amino acids", namely: phenylalanine, tryptophan, methionine, lysine, leucine, isoleucine, valine and threonine. A ninth amino acid, histidine, is required for growth and is essential for infants and children; it may also be necessary for tissue repair. Other amino acids include glycine, alanine, serine, cystine, tyrosine, aspartic acid, glutamic acid, proline, hydroxy-proline, citrulline and arginine. Each protein in a food is composed of a particular mixture of amino acids which might or might not contain all eight of the essential ones.

Protein quality and quantity

To assess the protein value of any food it is useful to know how much total protein it contains, which amino acids it has and how many essential amino acids are present and in what proportion. Much is now known about the individual proteins present in various foods, their amino acid content and therefore their quality and quantity. Some have a better mixture of amino acids than others, and these are said to have a higher biological value. The proteins albumin in egg and casein in milk, for example, contain all the essential amino acids in good proportions and are nutritionally superior to such proteins as zein in maize, which contains little tryptophan or lysine, and the protein in wheat, which contains only small quantities of lysine. It is not true, however, to say that the proteins in maize and wheat are not valuable. Although they contain less of certain amino acids, they do contain some amount of all the essential amino acids as well as many of the other important ones. The relative deficiency of maize and wheat proteins can be overcome by providing other foodstuffs containing more of the limited amino acids. It is therefore possible for two foods with low-value protein to complement each other to form a good protein mixture when eaten together.

Humans, especially children on diets deficient in animal protein, require a variety of foods of vegetable origin, not just one staple food. In many diets, pulses or legumes such as groundnuts, beans and cowpeas, though short of sulphur-containing amino acids, supplement the cereal proteins, which are often short of lysine. A mixture of foods of vegetable origin, especially if taken at the same meal, can serve as a substitute for animal protein (Photo 12).

FAO has produced tables showing the content of essential amino acids in different foodstuffs, from which it can be seen which foods best complement each other. It is also necessary, of course, to ascertain the total quantity of protein and amino acids in any food.

The quality of the protein depends largely on its amino acid composition and its digestibility. If a protein is deficient in one or more essential amino acids, its quality is lower. The most deficient of the essential amino acids in a protein is called the "limiting amino acid". The limiting amino acid determines the efficiency of utilization of the protein present in a food or combination of foods. Human beings usually eat food in meals which contain many proteins; they seldom consume just one protein. Therefore nutritionists are interested in the protein quality of a person's diet or meals, rather than just one food. If one essential amino acid is in short supply in the diet, it limits the use of the other amino acids for building protein.

Readers who wish to become familiar with the methods used for determining protein quality are advised to consult comprehensive textbooks on nutrition, which describe them in detail (see Bibliography). One method uses experiments on growth and nitrogen retention in young rats. Another involves determination of the amino acid or chemical score, usually by examining the efficiency of utilization of proteins in the foods consumed by comparing their amino acid composition with that of protein known to be of high quality, such as that in whole eggs.

The chemical score may thus be defined as the efficiency of utilization of food protein in comparison with whole egg protein. Net protein utilization (NPU) is a measure of the amount or percentage of protein retained in relation to that consumed. As an example, Table 16 gives the chemical score and NPU of the protein in five foods.

It is not usual or easy to obtain NPU values in people, and in most studies rats are used. Table 16 suggests that there is a good correlation between the values in rats and in children, and that chemical score provides a reasonable estimate of protein quality.

For the professional involved in nutritional activities to help people – be it a dietitian in a health facility, an agricultural extension worker or a nutrition educator – what is important is that the protein value differs among foods and that mixing foods improves the protein quality of the meal or the diet. Table 17 gives the protein content and the limiting amino acid score of some commonly eaten plant-based foods. Because lysine is most commonly the limiting amino acid in many foods of plant origin, the lysine score is also given.

Protein digestion and absorption

Proteins consumed in the diet undergo a series of chemical changes in the gastrointestinal tract. The physiology of protein digestion is complicated; pepsin and rennin from the stomach, trypsin from the pancreas and erepsin from the intestines hydrolyse proteins into their component amino acids. Most of the amino acids are absorbed into the bloodstream from the small intestine and thus travel to the liver and from there all over the body. Any surplus amino acids are stripped of the amino (NH_2) group, which goes to form urea in the urine, leaving the rest of the molecule to be transformed into glucose. There is now some evidence that a little intact protein is taken up into certain cells lining the intestines. Some of this protein in the infant may have a role in the passive immunity conveyed from the mother to her newborn child.

A little of the protein and amino acids

TABLE 16
Chemical score and net protein utilization in selected foods

Food	Chemical score	NPU determined in children	NPU determined in rats
Eggs (whole)	100	87	94
Milk (human)	100	94	87
Rice	67	63	59
Maize	49	36	52
Wheat	53	49	48

Source: Adapted from FAO/WHO, 1973.

TABLE 17
Protein content, limiting amino acid score and lysine score of selected plant foods

Food	Protein content (%)	Limiting amino acid score	Lysine score
Cereals			
Maize	9.4	49 (Lys)	49
Rice (white)	7.1	62 (Lys)	62
Wheat flour	10.3	38 (Lys)	38
Millet	11.0	33 (Lys)	33
Legumes			
Kidney beans	23.6	100	118
Cowpea	23.5	100	117
Groundnut	25.8	62 (Lys)	62
Vegetables			
Tomato	0.9	56 (Leu)	64
Squash	1.2	70 (Thr)	95
Pepper, sweet	0.9	77 (Lys Leu)	77
Cassava	1.3	44 (Leu)	56
Potato	2.1	91 (Leu)	105

Source: Adapted from Young and Pellett, 1994.

released in the intestines is not absorbed. The unabsorbed amino acids, plus cells shed from the intestinal villi and acted upon by bacteria, together with gut organisms, contribute to the nitrogen found in faeces.

Much of the protein in the human body is present in muscle. There is no true storage of protein in the body as there is with fat and to a small extent glycogen. However, there is now little doubt that a well-nourished individual has sufficient protein accumulated to be able to last several days without replenishment and to remain still in good health.

Protein requirements

Children need more protein than adults because they need to grow. Infants in the first few months of life require about 2.5 g of protein per kilogram of body weight. This requirement drops to about 1.5 g/kg at nine to 12 months of age. Unless energy intakes are adequate, however, the protein will not all be used for growth. A pregnant woman needs an additional supply of protein to build up the foetus inside her. Similarly, a lactating woman needs extra protein, because the milk she secretes contains protein. In some societies it is common for women to breastfeed their babies for as long as two years. Thus some women need extra protein for two years and nine months for every infant they bear.

Protein requirements and recommended allowances have been the subject of much research, debate and disagreement over the past 50 years. FAO and the World Health Organization (WHO) periodically assemble experts to review current knowledge and to provide guidelines. The most recent guidelines were the outcome of an Expert Consultation held jointly by FAO, WHO and United Nations University (UNU) in Rome in 1981 (WHO, 1985). The safe level of intake for a one-year-old child was put at 1.5 g per kilogram of body weight. The amount then falls to 1 g/kg at age six years. The United States recommended dietary allowance (RDA) is a little higher, namely 1.75 g/kg at age one year and 1.2 g/kg at age six years. In adults the FAO/WHO/UNU safe intake of protein is 0.8 g/kg for females and 0.85 g/kg for males.

The safe levels of intake of protein by age and gender, including those for pregnant and lactating women, are given in Annex 1. Values are provided both for a diet high in fibre, comprising mainly cereals, roots and legumes with little food of animal origin, and for a mixed balanced diet with less fibre and plenty of complete protein. As an example, a non-pregnant adult woman weighing 55 kg requires 49 g of protein per day for the first diet and 41 g per day for the second. Fibre reduces protein utilization.

Inadequate protein intake jeopardizes growth and repair in the body. Protein deficiency is especially dangerous for children because they are growing and also because the risk of infection is greater during childhood than at almost any other time of life. In children inadequate energy intake also has an impact on protein. As stated above, in the absence of adequate energy some protein needs to be diverted and therefore will not be used for growth.

In many developing countries (though not all), the intake of protein is relatively low and of predominantly vegetable origin. The paucity of foods of animal origin in the diet is not always a matter of choice. For example, many low-income Africans and Latin Americans like animal products but find them less freely available, more difficult to produce and store and more expensive than most vegetable products. Diets low in meat, fish and dairy products are very common in countries where most people are poor.

Infections lead to an increased loss of nitrogen from the body, which has to be replaced by proteins in the diet. Therefore children and others who have frequent infections will have greater protein needs than healthy persons. This fact must constantly be borne in mind, for in developing countries many children suffer an almost continual series of infectious diseases; they may frequently get diarrhoea, and they may harbour intestinal parasites.

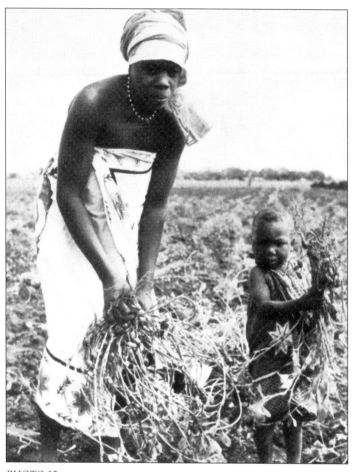

PHOTO 12
A woman and child harvesting groundnuts, a food rich in fat, protein and B vitamins: a dietary addition of a handful of groundnuts per person per day could rid Africa of most existing malnutrition

Chapter 10
Minerals

Minerals have a number of functions in the body. Sodium, potassium and chlorine are present as salts in body fluids, where they have a physiological role in maintaining osmotic pressure. Minerals form part of the constitution of many tissues. For example, calcium and phosphorus in bones combine to give rigidity to the whole body. Minerals are present in body acids and alkalis; for example, chlorine occurs in hydrochloric acid in the stomach. They are also essential constituents of certain hormones, e.g. iodine in the thyroxine produced by the thyroid gland.

The principal minerals in the human body are calcium, phosphorus, potassium, sodium, chlorine, sulphur, copper, magnesium, manganese, iron, iodine, fluorine, zinc, cobalt and selenium. Phosphorus is so widely available in plants that a shortage of this element is unlikely in any diet. Potassium, sodium and chlorine are easily absorbed and are physiologically more important than phosphorus. Sulphur is consumed by humans mainly in the form of sulphur-containing amino acids; thus sulphur deficiency, when it occurs, is linked with protein deficiency. Copper, manganese and magnesium deficiencies are not believed to be common. The minerals that are of most importance in human nutrition are thus calcium, iron, iodine, fluorine and zinc, and only these are discussed in some detail here. Some mineral elements are required in very tiny amounts in human diets but are still vital for metabolic purposes; these are termed "essential trace elements".

The table giving the nutrient content of selected foods in Annex 3 shows the relative content of some important minerals in different foods.

CALCIUM

The body of an average-sized adult contains about 1 250 g of calcium. Over 99 percent of the calcium is in the bones and teeth, where it is combined with phosphorus as calcium phosphate, a hard substance that gives the body rigidity. However, although hard and rigid, the skeleton of the body is not the unchanging structure it appears to be. In fact, the bones are a cellular matrix, and the calcium is continuously taken up by the bones and given back to the body. The bones, therefore, serve as a reserve supply of this mineral.

Calcium is present in the serum of the blood in small but important quantities, usually about 10 mg per 100 ml of serum. There are also about 10 g of calcium in the extracellular fluids and soft tissues of the adult body.

Properties and functions

In humans and other mammals, calcium and phosphorus together have an important role as major components of the skeleton. They are also important, however, in metabolic functions such as muscular function, nervous stimuli, enzymatic and hormonal activities and transport of oxygen. These functions are described in detail in textbooks of physiology and nutrition.

The skeleton of a living person is physiologically different from the dry skeleton in a grave or museum. The bones are living tissues, consisting mainly of a mineralized protein collagen substance. In the living body there is continuous turnover of calcium. Bone is laid down and resorbed all the time, in people of all ages. Bone cells called osteoclasts take up or resorb bone, while others, termed osteoblasts, lay down or form new bone. The bone cells in the mineralized collagen are called osteocytes.

Up to full growth or maturity (which has usually taken place by age 18 to 22 years), new bone is formed as the skeleton enlarges to its adult size. In young adults, despite bone remodelling, the skeleton generally maintains its size. However, as persons get older there is some loss of bone mass.

A complex physiological system maintains proper calcium and phosphorus levels. The control involves hormones from the parathyroid gland, calcitonin and the active form of vitamin D (1,25-dihydroxy-cholecalciferol).

Small but highly important amounts of calcium are present in extracellular fluids, particularly blood plasma, as well as in various body cells. In serum most of the calcium is in two forms, ionized and protein bound. Laboratories usually measure only total plasma calcium; the normal range is 8.5 to 10.5 mg/dl (2.1 to 2.6 mmol/litre). A drop in the level of calcium to below 2.1 mmol/litre is termed hypocalcaemia and can lead to various symptoms. Tetany (not to be confused with tetanus resulting from the tetanus bacillus), characterized by spasms and sometimes fits, results from low levels of ionized calcium in the blood.

Dietary sources

All the calcium in the body, except that inherited from the mother, comes from food and water consumed. It is especially necessary to have adequate quantities of calcium during growth, for it is at this stage that the bones develop.

The foetus in the mother's uterus has most of its nutritional requirements satisfied, for in terms of nutrition the unborn child is almost parasitic. If the mother's diet is poor in calcium, she draws extra supplies of this mineral from her bones.

An entirely breastfed infant will obtain adequate calcium from breastmilk as long as the volume of milk is sufficient. Contrary to popular belief, the calcium content of human milk varies rather little; 100 ml of breastmilk, even from an undernourished mother on a diet very low in calcium, provides approximately 30 mg of calcium (Table 18). A lactating mother secreting 1 litre will thus lose 300 mg of calcium per day.

Cows' milk is a very rich source of calcium, richer than human milk. Whereas a litre of human milk contains 300 mg of calcium, a litre of cows' milk contains 1 200 mg. The difference arises because a cow has to provide for her calf, which grows much more rapidly than a human infant and needs extra calcium for the hardening of its fast-growing skeleton. Similarly, the milk of most other domestic animals has a higher calcium content than human milk. This does not mean, however, that a child would be better off drinking cows' milk rather than human milk. Cows' milk yields more calcium than a child needs. A child (or even a baby) who drinks large quantities of cows' milk excretes any excess calcium, so it is of no benefit; it does not increase the child's growth rate beyond what is optimal.

Milk products such as cheese and yoghurt are also rich sources of calcium. Small saltwater and freshwater fish such as sardines and sprats supply good quantities of calcium since they are usually eaten whole, bones and all. Small dried fish known as *dagaa* in the United Republic of Tanzania, *kapenta* in Zambia and *chela* in India add useful calcium to the diet (Photo 13). Vegetables and pulses provide some calcium. Although cereals and roots

TABLE 18

Calcium content of various milks commonly used in developing countries

Source of milk	Calcium content (mg/100 ml)
Human	32
Cow	119
Camel	120
Goat	134
Water buffalo	169
Sheep	193

are relatively poor sources of calcium, they often supply the major portion of the mineral in tropical diets by virtue of the quantities consumed.

The calcium content of drinking-water varies from place to place. Hard water usually contains high levels of calcium.

Absorption and utilization

The absorption of calcium is variable and generally rather low. It is related to the absorption of phosphorus and the other important mineral constituents of the bones. Vitamin D is essential for the proper absorption of calcium. Thus a person seriously deficient in vitamin D absorbs too little calcium, even if the intake of calcium is more than adequate, and could have a negative calcium balance. Phytates, phosphates and oxalates in food reduce calcium absorption.

Persons customarily consuming diets low in calcium appear to have better absorption of calcium than those on high-calcium diets. Unabsorbed calcium is excreted in the faeces. Excess calcium is excreted in the urine and in sweat.

Requirements

It is not easy to state categorically the human requirements for calcium, because there are several factors influencing absorption and considerable variations in calcium losses among individuals.

Needs for calcium are increased during pregnancy and lactation, and children require more calcium because of growth. Those on high-protein diets require more calcium in the diet.

The following are recommended levels of daily calcium intake:

- adults, 400 to 500 mg;
- children, 400 to 700 mg;
- pregnant and lactating women, 800 to 1 000 mg.

Deficiency states

Disease or malformation caused primarily by dietary deficiency of calcium is rare. There is little convincing evidence to show that the many diets of adults in developing countries supplying perhaps only 250 to 300 mg of calcium daily are harmful to health. It is assumed that adults achieve some sort of balance when intakes of calcium are low. Females who go through a series of pregnancies and long lactations may lose calcium and be at risk of osteomalacia. However, vitamin D deficiency, not calcium deficiency, is more often implicated in this condition.

In children the development of rickets results from vitamin D deficiency, not from dietary lack of calcium, in spite of increased calcium requirements in childhood. Calcium balance in childhood is generally positive, and calcium deficiency has not been shown to have an adverse influence on growth.

Osteoporosis is a common disease of ageing, especially in women (see Chapter 23). The skeleton becomes demineralized, which leads to fragility of bones and commonly to fractures of the hip, vertebrae and other bones, particularly in older women. High calcium intake is often recommended but has not been proved effective in prevention or treatment.

Exercise appears to reduce the loss of calcium from bones; this may explain, in part, why osteoporosis is less prevalent in many developing countries, where women work hard and are very active. There is now clear evidence that providing the female hormone oestrogen to women after menopause reduces bone loss and osteoporosis.

IRON

Iron deficiency is a very common cause of ill health in all parts of the world, both South and North. The average iron content in a healthy adult is only about 3 to 4 g, yet this relatively small quantity is vital.

Properties and functions

Most of the iron in the body is present in the red blood cells, mainly as a component of haemoglobin. Much of the rest is present in myoglobin, a compound occurring mainly in muscles, and as storage iron or ferritin, mainly in the liver, spleen and bone marrow. Additional tiny quantities are found binding protein in the blood plasma and in respiratory enzymes.

The main, vital function of iron is in the transfer of oxygen at various sites in the body. Haemoglobin is the pigment in the erythrocytes that carries oxygen from the lungs to the tissues. Myoglobin in skeletal and heart muscle accepts the oxygen from the haemoglobin. Iron is also present in peroxidase, catalase and the cytochromes.

Iron is an element that is neither used up nor destroyed in the properly functioning body. Unlike some minerals, it is not required for excretion, and only very small amounts appear in urine and sweat. Minute quantities are lost in desquamated cells from the skin and intestine, in shed hair and nails and in the bile and other body secretions. The body is, however, efficient, economical and conservative in the use of iron. Iron released when the erythrocytes are old and broken down is

taken up and used again and again for the manufacture of new erythrocytes. This economy of iron is important. In normal circumstances, only about 1 mg of iron is lost from the body daily by excretion into the intestines, in urine, in sweat or through loss of hair or surface epithelial cells.

Because iron is conserved, the nutritional needs of healthy males and post-menopausal females are very small. Women of child-bearing age, however, must replace the iron lost during menstruation and childbirth and must meet the additional requirements of pregnancy and lactation. Children have relatively high needs because of their rapid growth, which involves increases not only in body size but also in blood volume.

Dietary sources

Iron is present in a variety of foods of both plant and animal origin. Rich food sources include meat (especially liver), fish, eggs, legumes (including a variety of beans, peas and other pulses) and green leafy vegetables. Cereal grains such as maize, rice and wheat contain moderate amounts of iron, but because these are often staple foods and eaten in large quantities, they provide most of the iron for many people in developing countries. Iron cooking pots may be a source of iron.

Milk, contrary to the notion that it is the "perfect food", is a poor source of iron. Human milk contains about 2 mg of iron per litre and cows' milk only half this amount.

Absorption and utilization

Absorption of iron takes place mainly in the upper portion of the small intestine. Most of the iron enters the bloodstream directly and not through the lymphatic system. Evidence indicates that absorption is regulated to some extent by physiological demand. Persons who are iron deficient tend to absorb iron more efficiently and in greater quantities than do normal subjects.

Several other factors affect iron absorption. For example, tannins, phosphates and phytates in food reduce iron absorption, whereas ascorbic acid increases it. Studies have indicated that egg yolk, despite its relatively high iron content, inhibits absorption of iron – not only the iron from the egg yolk itself, but also that from other foods.

Healthy subjects normally absorb only 5 to 10 percent of the iron in their foods, whereas iron-deficient subjects may absorb twice that amount. Therefore, on a diet that supplies 15 mg of iron, the normal person would absorb 0.75 to 1.5 mg of iron, but the iron-deficient person would absorb as much as 3 mg. Iron absorption generally increases during growth and pregnancy, after bleeding and in other conditions in which the demand for iron is enhanced.

Of greatest importance is the fact that the availability of iron from foods varies widely. Absorption of the haem iron in foods of animal origin (meat, fish and poultry) is usually very high, whereas the non-haem iron in foods such as cereals, vegetables, roots and fruits is poorly absorbed.

However, people usually eat meals, not single individual foods, and a small amount of haem iron consumed with a meal where most of the iron is non-haem iron will enhance the absorption of all the iron. Thus the addition of a quite small amount of haem iron from perhaps fish or meat to a large helping of rice or maize containing non-haem iron will result in much greater absorption of iron from the cereal staple. If this meal also includes fruits or vegetables, the vitamin C in them will also enhance iron absorption. However, if tea is consumed with this meal, the tannin present in the tea will reduce the absorption of iron.

Requirements

The dietary requirements for iron are approximately ten times the body's physiological requirements. If a normally healthy man or post-menopausal woman requires 1 mg of iron daily because of iron losses, then the dietary requirements are about 10 mg per day. This recommendation allows a fair margin of safety, as absorption is increased with need.

Menstrual loss of iron has been estimated to average a little less than 1 mg per day during an entire year. It is recommended that women of child-bearing age have a dietary intake of 18 mg per day.

During pregnancy, the body requires on average about 1.5 mg of iron daily to develop the foetus and supportive tissues and to expand the maternal blood supply. Most of this additional iron is required in the second and third trimesters of pregnancy.

Breastfeeding women use iron to provide the approximately 2 mg of iron per litre of breastmilk. However, during the first six to 15 months of intensive breastfeeding they may not menstruate, so they do not lose iron in menstrual blood.

Newborn infants are born with very high haemoglobin levels (a high red blood cell count), termed polycythaemia, which provides an extra store of iron. This iron, together with that present in breastmilk, is usually sufficient for the first four to six months of life, after which iron from other foods becomes necessary.

Premature and other low-birth-weight infants may have lower iron stores and be at greater risk than other infants.

An excess intake of iron over long periods can lead to the disease siderosis or haemachromatosis. This disease is reported to occur most commonly where beer or other alcoholic beverages are brewed in iron cooking pots, particularly in South Africa. In alcoholics siderosis leading to iron deposits in the liver may be associated with cirrhosis.

Average safe levels of iron intake are provided in Annex 1.

Deficiency states

Consideration of the iron requirements and the iron content of commonly eaten foods might suggest that iron deficiency is rare, but this is not the case. Food iron is poorly absorbed. Iron is not readily excreted into the urine or the gastro-intestinal tract; thus severe iron deficiency is usually associated with an increased need for iron resulting from conditions such as pregnancy, blood loss or expansion of the total body mass during growth. Iron deficiency is most common in young children, in women of child-bearing age and in persons with chronic blood loss.

The end result of iron deficiency is anaemia. Anaemia is described in detail in Chapter 13, and its control is discussed in Chapter 39.

Hookworm infections, which are extremely prevalent in many countries, result in loss of blood which may cause iron deficiency anaemia. In some parts of the tropics schistosomiasis is also common, and this disease also causes blood loss.

IODINE

The body of an average adult contains about 20 to 50 mg of iodine, much of it in the thyroid gland. Iodine is essential for the formation of thyroid hormones secreted by this gland.

Properties and functions

In humans iodine functions as an essential component of the hormones of the thyroid gland, an endocrine gland situated in the lower neck. Thyroid hormones, of which the most important is thyroxine (T4), are important for regulating metabolism. In children they support normal growth and development, including mental development.

Iodine is absorbed from the gut as iodide, and excess is excreted in the urine. The adult thyroid gland, in a person consuming adequate iodine, traps about 60 µg of iodine per day to make normal amounts of thyroid hormones. If there is insufficient iodine, the thyroid works harder to trap more; the gland enlarges in size (a condition known as goitre), and its iodine content might become markedly reduced.

Thyroid stimulating hormone (TSH) from the pituitary gland influences thyroxine secretion and iodine trapping. In severe iodine deficiency, TSH levels are raised and thyroxine levels are low.

Dietary sources

Iodine is widely present in rocks and soils. The quantity in different plants varies according to the soil in which they are grown. It is not meaningful to list the iodine content of foodstuffs because of the large variations in iodine content from place to place, depending on the iodine content of the soil. Iodine tends to get washed out of the soil, and throughout the ages a considerable quantity has flowed into the sea. Sea fish, seaweed and most vegetables grown near the sea are useful sources of iodine. Drinking-water provides some iodine but very seldom enough to satisfy human requirements.

In many countries where goitre is prevalent the authorities have added iodine to salt, a strategy which has successfully controlled iodine deficiency disorders (IDD). Iodine has usually been added to salt in the form of potassium iodide, but another form, potassium iodate, is more stable and is better in hot, humid climates. Iodated salt is an important dietary source of iodine.

Deficiency states

A lack of iodine in the diet results in several health problems, one of which is goitre, or enlargement of the thyroid gland. Goitre is extremely prevalent in many countries. There are other contributing causes of goitre, but iodine deficiency is by far the most common. Iodine deficiency during pregnancy may lead to cretinism, mental retardation and other problems, which may be permanent, in the child. It is now known that endemic goitre and cretinism are not the only problems caused by iodine deficiency. The decrease in mental capacity associated with iodine deficiency is of particular concern (see Chapter 14).

IDD, although previously prevalent in Europe, North America and Australia, is now seen predominantly in developing countries. The greatest prevalence tends to be in mountainous areas such as the Andes and the Himalayas and in plateau areas far from the sea. For example, an investigation carried out by the author in the Ukinga Highlands of Tanzania revealed that 75 percent of the population had some enlargement of the thyroid.

FLUORINE

Fluorine is a mineral element found mainly in the teeth and skeleton. Traces of fluorine in the teeth help to protect them against decay. Fluorides consumed during childhood become a part of the dental enamel and make it more resistant to the weak organic acids formed from foods that adhere to or get stuck between the teeth. This strengthening greatly reduces the chances of decay or caries developing in the teeth. Some studies have suggested that fluoride may also help strengthen bone, particularly later in life, and may thus inhibit the development of osteoporosis.

Dietary sources

The main source of fluorine for most human beings is the water they drink. If the water has a fluorine content of about one part per million (1 ppm), then it will supply adequate fluorine for the teeth. However, many water supplies contain much less than this amount. Fluorine is present in bone; consequently small fish that are consumed whole are a good source. Tea has a high fluorine content. Few other foods contain much fluorine.

Deficiency

If the fluoride content of drinking-water in any locality is below 0.5 ppm, dental caries will probably be much more prevalent than where the concentration is higher.

The recommended level of fluoride in water is between 0.8 and 1.2 ppm. In some countries or localities where the content of fluorine in the water is less than 1 ppm, it has now become the practice to add fluoride to the water supply. This practice is strongly recommended, but it is only practicable for large piped-water supplies; in some developing countries where most people do not have piped water, it is not feasible. The addition of fluoride to toothpaste also helps reduce dental caries. Fluorine does not totally prevent dental caries, but it can reduce the incidence by 60 to 70 percent.

Excess

An excessively high intake of fluoride causes a condition known as dental fluorosis, in which the teeth become mottled. It is usually caused by consuming excessive fluoride in water supplies that have high fluoride levels. In some parts of Africa and Asia, natural waters contain over 4 ppm of fluoride. Very high fluorine intakes also cause bone changes with sclerosis (added bone density), calcification of muscle insertions and exostoses. A survey carried out by the author in Tanzania revealed a high incidence of fluorotic bone changes (as shown by X-ray) in older subjects who normally drank water containing over 6 ppm of fluoride. Similar findings have been well described in India. Skeletal fluorosis can cause severe pain and serious bone abnormalities.

ZINC

Zinc is an essential element in human nutrition, and its importance to human health has received much recent attention. Zinc is present in many important enzymes essential for metabolism. The body of a healthy human adult contains 2 to 3 g of zinc and requires around 15 mg of dietary zinc per day. Most of the zinc in the body is in the skeleton, but other tissues (such as the skin and hair) and some organs (particularly the prostate) have relatively high concentrations.

Dietary sources

Zinc is present in most foods both of vegetable and of animal origin, but the richest sources tend to be protein-rich foods such as meat, seafoods and eggs. In developing countries, however, where most people consume relatively small amounts of these foods, most zinc comes from cereal grains and legumes.

Absorption and utilization

As with iron, absorption of zinc from the diet is inhibited by food constituents such as phytates, oxalate and tannins. No simple tests of human zinc status are known, however. Indicators used include evidence of low dietary intake, low blood serum zinc levels and low quantities of zinc in hair specimens.

Much research on this mineral has been undertaken in the last two decades, and a great deal of knowledge concerning zinc metabolism and zinc deficiency in animals and humans has been gathered. Nonetheless, there is little evidence to suggest that zinc deficiency is an important public health problem for large numbers of people in any country, industrialized or developing. However, research now under way may show that poor zinc status is responsible for poor growth, reduced appetite and other conditions; in this way zinc deficiency may contribute especially to what is now called protein-energy malnutrition (PEM).

Zinc deficiency is responsible for a very rare congenital disease known as acrodermatitis enteropathica. It responds to zinc therapy. Some patients receiving all of their nutrients intravenously have developed skin lesions which also respond to zinc treatment. In the Near East, particularly in the Islamic Republic of Iran and Egypt, a condition has been described in which adolescent or near-adolescent boys are dwarfed and have poorly developed genitalia and delayed onset of puberty; this condition has been said to respond to zinc treatment.

Zinc deficiency has also been reported as secondary to, or as a part of, other conditions such as PEM, various malabsorption conditions, alcoholism including cirrhosis of the liver, renal disease and metabolic disorders.

OTHER TRACE ELEMENTS

Numerous minerals are present in the human body. For most of the trace elements, besides those discussed above, there is no evidence that deficiency is responsible for major public health problems anywhere. Some of these minerals are very important in metabolism or as constituents of body tissues. Many of them have been studied, and their chemistry and biochemistry have been described. Experimental deficiencies have been produced in laboratory animals, but most human diets, even poor diets, do not appear to lead to important deficiencies. These minerals therefore are not of public health importance. Other trace elements are present in the body but do not have any known essential role. Some minerals, for example lead and mercury, are of great interest to health workers because excess intake has commonly resulted in toxic manifestations.

Cobalt, copper, magnesium, manganese

and selenium deserve mention because of their important nutritional role, and lead and mercury because of their toxicity. These minerals are considered in detail in large comprehensive textbooks of nutrition.

Cobalt

Cobalt is of interest to nutritionists because it is an essential part of vitamin B_{12} (cyanocobalamin). When isolated as a crystalline substance, the vitamin was found to contain about 4 percent cobalt. However, cobalt deficiency does not play a part in the anaemia that results from vitamin B_{12} deficiency.

Copper

Copper deficiency is known to cause anaemia in cattle, but no such risk is known in adult humans. Some evidence suggests that copper deficiency leads to anaemia in premature infants, in people with severe PEM and in those maintained on parenteral nutrition. An extremely rare congenital condition known as Menkes' disease is caused by failure of copper absorption.

Magnesium

Magnesium is an essential mineral present mainly in the bones but also in most human tissues. Most diets contain adequate dietary magnesium, but under some circumstances, such as diarrhoea, severe PEM and other conditions, excessive body losses of magnesium occur. Such losses may lead to weakness and mental changes and occasionally to convulsions.

Selenium

Both deficiency and excess of selenium have been well described in livestock. In areas of China where the soil selenium, and therefore the food selenium, is low, a heart condition has been described; termed Keshan's disease, it is a serious condition affecting heart muscle. Chinese researchers believe it can be prevented by providing dietary selenium. Selenium deficiency has also been associated with certain cancers.

Lead

Lead is of great public health importance because it commonly causes toxicity. Human lead deficiency is not known. Lead poisoning is especially an urban problem and is most important in children. It may lead to neurological and mental problems and to anaemia. Excess lead intake may result from consumption of lead in the household (from lead-based paint or water pipes containing lead) and from intake of atmospheric lead (from motor vehicle emissions).

Mercury

Mercury deficiency is not known in humans. The concern is with excessively high intakes of mercury and the risks of toxicity. Fish in waters contaminated with mercury concentrate the mineral. There is a danger of toxicity in those who consume fish with high mercury content. Mercury poisoning resulting from consumption of seeds coated with a mercury-containing fungicide has been described in Asia, Latin America and the Near East. The effects include severe neurological symptoms and paralysis.

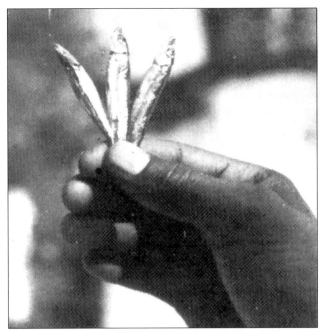

PHOTO 13
Small fish consumed whole are a rich source of calcium

Chapter 11

Vitamins

Vitamins are organic substances present in minute amounts in foodstuffs and necessary for metabolism. They are grouped together not because they are chemically related or have similar physiological functions, but because, as their name implies, they are vital factors in the diet and because they were all discovered in connection with the diseases resulting from their deficiency. Moreover, they do not fit into the other nutrient categories (carbohydrates, fats, protein and minerals or trace metals).

When vitamins were first being classified, each was named after a letter of the alphabet. Subsequently, there has been a tendency to drop the letters in favour of chemical names. The use of the chemical name is justified when the vitamin has a known chemical formula, as with the main vitamins of the B group. Nevertheless, it is advantageous to include certain vitamins under group headings, even if they are not chemically related, since they do tend to occur in the same foodstuffs.

In this book only vitamin A, five of the B vitamins (thiamine, riboflavin, niacin, vitamin B_{12} and folic acid), vitamin C and vitamin D are described in detail. Other vitamins known to be vital to health include pantothenic acid (of which a deficiency may cause the burning feet syndrome mentioned below), biotin (vitamin H), *para*-aminobenzoic acid, choline, vitamin E and vitamin K (antihaemorrhagic vitamin). These vitamins are not described in detail here for one or more of the following reasons:

- deficiency is not known to occur under natural conditions in humans;
- deficiency is extremely rare even in grossly abnormal diets;
- lack of the vitamin results in disease only if it follows some other disease process that is adequately described in textbooks of general medicine;
- the role of the vitamin in human nutrition has not yet been elucidated.

None of the vitamins omitted from discussion is important from the point of view of workers studying nutrition as community health problems in most developing countries. Those wishing to learn more about these vitamins are referred to textbooks of general medicine or more detailed textbooks of nutrition. A summary of the conditions associated with vitamin Deficiencies is given in Chapter 33, Table 37.

VITAMIN A (RETINOL)

Vitamin A was discovered in 1913 when research workers found that certain laboratory animals stopped growing when lard (made from pork fat) was the only form of fat present in their diet, whereas when butter was supplied instead of lard (with the diet remaining otherwise the same) the animals grew and thrived. Further animal experiments showed that egg yolk and cod-liver oil contained the same vital food factor, which was named vitamin A.

It was later established that many vegetable products had the same nutritional properties as the vitamin A in butter; they were found to contain a yellow pigment called carotene, some of which can be converted to vitamin A in the human body.

Properties

Retinol is the main form of vitamin A in human diets. (Retinol is the chemical name of the alcohol derivative, and it is used as the reference standard.) In its pure crystalline form, retinol is a very pale yellow-green substance. It is soluble in fat but insoluble in water, and it is found only in animal products. Other forms of vitamin A exist, but they have somewhat different molecular configurations and less biological activity than retinol, and they are not important in human diets.

Carotenes, which act as provitamins or precursors of vitamin A, are yellow substances that occur widely in plant substances. In some foodstuffs their colour may be masked by the green plant pigment chlorophyll, which often occurs in close association with carotenes. There are several different carotenes. One of these, beta-carotene, is the most important source of vitamin A in the diets of most people living in non-industrialized countries. The other carotenes, or carotenoids, have little or no nutritional importance for humans. In the past, food analyses have often failed to distinguish beta-carotene from other carotenes.

Vitamin A is an important component of the visual purple of the retina of the eye, and if vitamin A is deficient, the ability to see in dim light is reduced. This condition is called night blindness. The biochemical basis for the other lesions of vitamin A deficiency has not been fully explained. The main change, in pathological terms, is a keratinizing metaplasia which is seen on various epithelial surfaces. Vitamin A appears to be necessary for the protection of surface tissue.

Several studies have shown that adequate vitamin A status reduces infant and child mortality in certain populations. Vitamin A supplementation reduces case fatality rates from measles. In other illnesses such as diarrhoea and respiratory infections, however, there is not strong evidence that the prevalence or duration of morbidity is reduced by vitamin A dosing.

Calculating vitamin A content in foods

1 IU retinol = 0.3 µg retinol = 0.3 RE
1 RE = 3.33 IU retinol
1 RE = 6 µg beta-carotene

Since pure crystalline vitamin A, which is termed retinol alcohol, is now available, the vitamin A activity in foods is now widely expressed and measured using retinol equivalents (RE) rather than the international units (IU) previously used. One IU of vitamin A is equivalent to 0.3 µg retinol.

Humans obtain vitamin A in food either as preformed vitamin A (retinol) or as carotenes which can be converted to retinol in the body. Beta-carotene is the most important in human diets and is better converted to retinol than other carotenes. It has been determined that six molecules of beta-carotene are needed to produce one molecule of retinol; thus it takes 6 µg of carotene to make 1 µg of retinol, or 1 RE.

Dietary sources

Vitamin A itself is found only in animal products; the main sources are butter, eggs, milk, meat (especially liver) and some fish. However, most people in developing countries rely mainly on beta-carotene for their supply of vitamin A. Carotene is contained in many plant foods. Dark green leaves such as those of amaranth, spinach, sweet potato and cassava are much richer sources than paler leaves such as those of cabbage and lettuce. Various pigmented fruits and vegetables, such as mangoes, papayas and tomatoes, contain useful quantities. Carotene is also present in yellow varieties of sweet potatoes and in yellow vegetables such as pumpkins. Carrots are rich sources. Yellow maize is the only cereal that contains carotene. In West Africa much carotene is obtained from red palm oil, which is widely used in cooking. The cultivation of the very valuable oil palm has spread to other tropical regions. In Malaysia it is widely cultivated as a cash crop, but its products are mainly exported rather than consumed locally.

Both carotene and vitamin A withstand ordinary cooking temperatures fairly well. However, a considerable amount of carotene is lost when green leaves and other foods are dried in the sun. Sun-drying is a traditional method of preserving wild leaves and vegetables often used in arid regions. Since serious disease from vitamin A deficiency is common in these areas, it is important that other methods of preservation be established.

Absorption and utilization

The conversion of beta-carotene into vitamin A takes place in the walls of the intestines. Even the most efficient intestine can absorb and convert only a portion of the beta-carotene in the diet; therefore 6 mg of beta-carotene in food is equivalent to about 1 mg of retinol. If no animal products are consumed and the body must rely entirely on carotene for its vitamin A, consumption of carotene must be great enough to achieve the required vitamin A level.

Carotene is poorly utilized when the diet has a low fat content, and diets deficient in vitamin A are often deficient in fat. Intestinal diseases such as dysentery, coeliac disease and sprue limit the absorption of vitamin A and the conversion of carotene. Malabsorption syndromes and infections with common intestinal parasites such as roundworm, which are prevalent in the tropics, may also reduce the ability of the body to convert carotene into vitamin A. Bile salts are essential for the absorption of vitamin A and carotene, so persons with obstruction of the bile duct are likely to become deficient in vitamin A. Even in ideal circumstances, infants and young children do not convert carotene to vitamin A as readily as adults do.

The liver acts as the main store of vitamin A in the human and most other vertebrates, which is why fish-liver oils have a high content of this vitamin. Retinol is transported from the liver to other sites in the body by a specific carrier protein called retinol binding protein (RBP). Protein deficiency may influence vitamin A status by reducing the synthesis of RBP.

Storage in the body

The storage of vitamin A in the liver is important, for in many tropical diets foods containing vitamin A and carotene are available seasonally. If these foods are eaten in fairly large quantities when available (usually during the wet season), a store can be built up which will help tide the person over the dry season, or at least part of it. The short mango season provides an excellent opportunity for youngsters, who may happily spend their leisure hours foraging for this fruit, to replenish the vitamin A stored in the liver.

Toxicity

If taken in excess, vitamin A has undesirable toxic effects. The most marked toxic effect is an irregular thickening of some long bones, usually accompanied by headache, vomiting, liver enlargement, skin changes and hair loss. Cases of vitamin A toxicity from dietary sources are rare, but toxicity can be a serious problem with supplemental doses of vitamin A. A high risk of birth defects is associated with supplements given before or during pregnancy.

Human requirements

The intake recommended by FAO and the World Health Organization (WHO) is 750 µg of retinol per day for adults; lactating mothers need 50 percent more, and children and infants less. It should be noted that these figures are based upon mixed diets containing both vitamin A and carotene. When the diet is entirely of vegetable origin, larger amounts of carotene are suggested, because the conversion from carotene to retinol is not very efficient.

Deficiency

Deficiency results in pathological drying of the eye, leading to xerophthalmia and sometimes keratomalacia and blindness. Other epithelial tissues may be affected; in the skin, follicular keratosis may be the result. These conditions are described in detail in Chapter 15.

THIAMINE (VITAMIN B₁)

During the 1890s in Java, Indonesia, Christiaan Eijkman of the Netherlands noticed that when his chickens were fed on the same diet as that normally consumed by his beriberi patients, they developed weakness in their legs and other signs somewhat similar to those of beriberi. The diet of the beriberi patients consisted mainly of highly milled and refined rice (known as polished rice). When Eijkman changed the diet of the chickens to whole-grain rice, they began to recover. He showed that there was a substance in the outer layers and germ of the rice grain that protected the chickens from the disease.

Researchers continued to work on isolating the cause of the different effects of diets of polished and whole-grain rice, but despite many attempts it was not until 1926 that vitamin B₁ was finally isolated in crystalline form. It was synthesized ten years later, and now the term thiamine is used, rather than vitamin B₁.

Properties

Thiamine is one of the most unstable vitamins. It has a rather loosely bound structure and decomposes readily in an alkaline medium. Thiamine is highly soluble in water. It resists temperatures of up to 100°C, but it tends to be destroyed if heated further (e.g. if fried in a hot pan or cooked under pressure).

Much research has been carried out on the physiological effects and biochemical properties of thiamine. It has been shown that thiamine has a very important role in carbohydrate metabolism in humans. It is utilized in the complicated mechanism of the breakdown, or oxidation, of carbohydrate and the metabolism of pyruvic acid.

The energy used by the nervous system is derived entirely from carbohydrate, and a deficiency of thiamine blocks the final utilization of carbohydrate, leading to a shortage of energy and lesions of the nervous tissues and brain. Because thiamine is involved in carbohydrate metabolism, a person whose main supply of energy comes from carbohydrates is more likely to develop signs of thiamine deficiency if his or her food intake is decreased. For this reason, thiamine requirements are sometimes expressed in relation to intake of carbohydrate.

Thiamine has been synthesized in pure form and is now measured in milligrams.

Dietary sources

Thiamine is widely distributed in foods of both vegetable and animal origin. The richest sources are cereal grains and pulses. Green vegetables, fish, meat, fruit and milk all contain useful quantities. In seeds such as cereals, the thiamine is present mainly in the germ and in the outer coats; thus much can be lost during milling (see Chapter 32). Bran of rice, wheat and other cereals tends to be naturally rich in thiamine. Yeasts are also rich sources. Root crops are poor sources. Cassava, for example, contains only about the same low quantity as polished, highly milled rice. It is surprising that beriberi is not common among the many people in Africa, Asia and Latin America whose staple food is cassava.

Because it is very soluble in water, thiamine is liable to be lost from food that is washed too thoroughly or cooked in excess water that is afterwards discarded. For people on a rice diet, it is especially important to prepare rice with just the amount of water that will be absorbed in cooking, or to use water that is left over in soups or stews, for this water will contain thiamine and other nutrients.

Cereals and pulses maintain their thiamine for a year or more if they are stored well, but if they are attacked by bacteria, insects or moulds the content of thiamine gradually diminishes.

Absorption and storage in the body

Thiamine is easily absorbed from the intestinal tract, but little is stored in the body. Experimental evidence indicates that humans can store only enough for about six weeks. The liver, heart and brain have a higher concentration than the muscles and other organs. A person with a high intake of thiamine soon begins to excrete increased quantities in the urine. The total amount in the body is about 25 mg.

Human requirements

A daily intake of 1 mg of thiamine is sufficient for a moderately active man and 0.8 mg for a moderately active woman. Pregnant and lactating women may need more (see Annex 1). FAO and WHO recommend an intake of 0.4 mg per 1 000 kcal for most persons.

Deficiency

Deficiency of thiamine leads to the disease beriberi, which in advanced forms pro-duces paralysis of the limbs. In alcoholics thiamine deficiency leads to a condition termed Wernicke-Korsakoff syndrome. These disorders are described in Chapter 16.

RIBOFLAVIN (VITAMIN B$_2$)

Early work on the properties of vitamins in yeast and other foodstuffs showed that antineuritic factors were destroyed by excessive heat, but that a growth-promoting factor was not destroyed in this way. This factor, riboflavin, was later isolated from the heat-resistant portion. It was synthesized in 1935.

Properties

Riboflavin is a yellow crystalline substance. It is much less soluble in water and more heat resistant than thiamine. The vitamin is sensitive to sunlight, so milk, for example, if left exposed may lose considerable quantities of riboflavin. Riboflavin acts as a coenzyme involved with tissue oxidation. It is measured in milligrams.

Dietary sources

The richest sources of riboflavin are milk and its non-fat products. Green vegetables, meat (especially liver), fish and eggs contain useful quantities. However, the main sources in most Asian, African and Latin American diets, which do not contain much of the above products, are usually cereal grains and pulses. As with thiamine, the quantity of riboflavin present is much reduced by milling. Starchy foods such as cassava, plantains, yams and sweet potatoes are poor sources.

Human requirements

Approximately 1.5 mg of riboflavin per day is an ample amount for an average adult, but rather more may be desirable during pregnancy and lactation. The FAO/WHO requirement is 0.55 mg per 1 000 kcal in the diet.

Deficiency

In humans a deficiency of riboflavin is termed ariboflavinosis. It may be characterized by painful cracking of the lips (cheilosis) and at the corners of the mouth (angular stomatitis). The clinical manifestations are described in Chapter 22. Ariboflavinosis is common in most countries but is not life threatening.

NIACIN (NICOTINIC ACID, NICOTINAMIDE, VITAMIN PP)

As the history of thiamine is linked with the disease beriberi, so the history of niacin is closely linked with the disease pellagra. beriberi is associated with the East and a rice diet, and pellagra with the West and a maize diet. Pellagra was first attributed to a poor diet over 200 years ago by the Spanish physician Gaspar Casal. At first, it was believed that pellagra might be caused by a protein deficiency, because the disease could be cured by some diets rich in protein. Later it was shown that a liver extract almost devoid of protein could cure pellagra. In 1926 J. Goldberger, in the United States, demonstrated that yeast extract contained a pellagra-preventing (PP) non-protein substance. In 1937 niacinamide or nicotinamide (nicotinic acid amide) was isolated, and this was found to cure a pellagra-like disease of dogs known as black tongue.

Because pellagra was found mainly in those whose staple diet was maize, it was assumed that maize was particularly poor in niacin. It has since been shown that white bread contains much less niacin than maize. However, the niacin in maize is not fully available because it is in a bound form.

The discovery that the amino acid tryptophan prevents pellagra in experimental animals, just as niacin does, complicated the picture until it was shown that tryptophan is converted to niacin in the human body. This work vindicated and explained the early theories that protein could prevent pellagra. The fact that zein, the main protein in maize, is very deficient in the amino acid tryptophan further explains the relationship between maize and pellagra. It has also been shown that a high intake of leucine, as occurs with diets based on sorghum, interferes with tryptophan and niacin metabolism and may cause pellagra.

Properties

Niacin, a derivative of pyridine, is a white crystalline substance, soluble in water and extremely stable. It has been synthesized. The main role of niacin in the body is in tissue oxidation. The vitamin occurs in two forms, nicotinic acid and nicotinamide (niacinamide). Niacin is measured in milligrams.

Dietary sources

Niacin is widely distributed in foods of both animal and vegetable origin. Particularly good sources are meat (especially liver), groundnuts and cereal bran or germ. As for other B vitamins, the main source of supply tends to be the staple food. Wholegrain or lightly milled cereals, although not rich in niacin, contain much more than highly milled cereal grains. Starchy roots, plantains and milk are poor sources. Beans, peas and other pulses contain amounts similar to those in most cereals.

Although the niacin in maize does not seem to be fully utilizable, treatment of maize with alkalis such as lime water, which is a traditional method of processing in Mexico and elsewhere, makes the niacin much more available.

Cooking, preservation and storage of food cause little loss of niacin.

Human requirements

An adequate quantity for any person is 20 mg per day. Niacin requirements are affected by the amount of tryptophan-containing protein consumed and also by the staple diet (i.e. whether it is maize-based or not). The FAO/WHO requirement is 6.6 mg per 1 000 kcal in the diet.

Deficiency

A deficiency of niacin leads to pellagra (see Chapter 17), the "disease of the three Ds": dermatitis, diarrhoea and dementia. Initially manifested as skin trouble, pellagra, if untreated, can continue for many years, growing steadily worse.

VITAMIN B$_{12}$ (CYANOCOBALAMIN)

Pernicious anaemia, so named because it invariably used to be fatal, was known for many years before its cause was determined. In 1926 it was found that patients improved if they ate raw liver. This finding led to the preparation of liver extracts, which controlled the disease when given by injection. In 1948 scientists isolated from liver a substance they called vitamin B$_{12}$. When given in very small quantities by injection, this substance was effective in the treatment of pernicious anaemia.

Properties

Vitamin B$_{12}$ is a red crystalline substance containing the metal cobalt. It is necessary for the production of healthy red blood cells. A small addition of vitamin B$_{12}$ or of foods rich in this substance to the diet of experimental animals results in increased growth. It is measured in micrograms.

Dietary sources

Vitamin B$_{12}$ is present only in foods of animal origin. It can also be synthesized by many bacteria. Herbivorous animals such as cattle get their vitamin B$_{12}$ from the action of bacteria on vegetable matter in their rumen. Humans apparently do not obtain vitamin B$_{12}$ by bacterial action in their digestive tracts. However, fermented vegetable products may provide vitamin B$_{12}$ in human diets.

Human requirements

The human daily requirement of this vitamin is quite small, probably around 3 µg for adults. Diets containing smaller amounts do not seem to lead to disease.

Deficiency

Pernicious anaemia is not caused by a dietary deficiency of vitamin B$_{12}$, but by an inability of the subject to utilize the vitamin B$_{12}$ in the diet because of a lack of an intrinsic factor in gastric secretions. It may be that an autoimmune reaction limits absorption of vitamin B$_{12}$. In pernicious anaemia the red blood cells are macrocytic (larger than normal) and the bone marrow contains many abnormal cells called megaloblasts. This macrocytic or megaloblastic anaemia is accompanied by a lack of hydrochloric acid in the stomach (achlorhydria). Later, serious changes take place in the spinal cord, leading to progressive neurological symptoms. If left untreated, the patient dies.

Treatment consists of injection of large doses of vitamin B$_{12}$. When the blood characteristics have returned to normal, the patient can usually be maintained in good health if given one injection of 250 mg of vitamin B$_{12}$ every two to four weeks.

Vitamin B$_{12}$ will also cure the anaemia accompanying the disease sprue. This is a tropical condition in which the absorption of vitamin B$_{12}$, folic acid and other nutrients is impaired.

The tapeworm *Diphyllobothrium latum*, acquired from eating raw or undercooked fish, lives in the intestines and has a propensity for removing vitamin B$_{12}$ from the food of its host. This results in the development in humans of a megaloblastic anaemia which can be cured by injection of vitamin B$_{12}$ and treatment to rid the patient of the tapeworm.

Some medicines interfere with absorption of vitamin B$_{12}$.

Except in the above conditions deficiency

of vitamin B$_{12}$ is likely to occur only in those on a vegetarian diet. Deficiency causes macrocytic anaemia and may produce neurological symptoms; however, even though strict vegetarians get very little vitamin B$_{12}$ in their diet, it appears that macrocytic anaemia due to vitamin B$_{12}$ deficiency is not prevalent and is not a major public health problem.

FOLIC ACID OR FOLATES

In 1929 Lucy Wills first described a macrocytic anaemia (an anaemia in which the red cells are abnormally large) commonly found among pregnant women in India. This condition responded to certain yeast preparations even though it did not respond to iron or any known vitamin. The substance present in the yeast extract that cured the macrocytic anaemia was at first called "Wills' factor". In 1946 a substance called folic acid, which had been isolated from spinach leaves, was found to have the same effect.

Properties

Folic acid is the group name (also termed folates or folacin) given to a number of yellow crystalline compounds related to pteroglutamic acid. Folic acid is involved in amino acid metabolism. The folic acid in foodstuffs is easily destroyed by cooking. It is measured in milligrams.

Dietary sources

The richest sources are dark green leaves, liver and kidney. Other vegetables and meats contain smaller amounts.

Human requirements

The recommended daily intake for adults has been set at 400 µg in the United States.

Deficiency

Folate deficiency is most commonly due to poor diets, but it may result from malabsorption. It can be induced by

medicines such as those used in treatment of epilepsy. A deficiency leads to the development of macrocytic anaemia. Anaemia resulting from folate deficiency is the second most common type of nutritional anaemia, after iron deficiency.

Folic acid deficiency during pregnancy has been found to cause neural tube defects in newborn babies. The role of folic acid in prevention of ischaemic heart disease has also recently received increased attention.

The main therapeutic use of folic acid is in the treatment of nutritional macrocytic or megaloblastic anaemias of pregnancy and infancy and for the prevention of neural tube defects. A dose of 5 to 10 mg daily is recommended for an adult.

Although administration of folic acid will improve the blood picture of persons with pernicious anaemia, the nervous system symptoms will neither be prevented nor improved by it. For this reason, folic acid should never be used in the treatment of pernicious anaemia, except in conjunction with vitamin B$_{12}$.

VITAMIN C (ASCORBIC ACID)

The discovery of vitamin C is associated with scurvy, which was first recorded by seafarers who made prolonged journeys. In 1497 Vasco da Gama described scurvy among the crew of his historical voyage from Europe around the southern tip of Africa to India; more than half the crew died of the disease. It gradually became apparent that scurvy occurred only in persons who ate no fresh food. It was not until 1747, however, that James Lind of Scotland demonstrated that scurvy could be prevented or cured by the consumption of citrus fruit. This finding led to the introduction of fresh food, especially citrus products, to the rations of seafarers. Subsequently scurvy became much less common.

In the nineteenth century, however, scurvy began to occur among infants receiving the newly introduced preserved milk instead of breastmilk or fresh cows' milk. The preserved milk contained adequate carbohydrate, fat, protein and minerals, but the heat used in its processing destroyed the vitamin C, so the infants got scurvy.

Later vitamin C was found to be ascorbic acid, which had already been identified.

Properties

Ascorbic acid is a white crystalline substance that is highly soluble in water. It tends to be easily oxidized. It is not affected by light, but it is destroyed by excessive heat, especially when in an alkaline solution. It is a powerful reducing agent and antioxidant and can therefore reduce the harmful action of free radicals. It is also important in enhancing the absorption of the non-haem iron in foods of vegetable origin.

Ascorbic acid is necessary for the proper formation and maintenance of intercellular material, particularly collagen. In simple terms, it is essential for producing part of the substance that binds cells together, as cement binds bricks together. In a person suffering from ascorbic acid deficiency, the endothelial cells of the capillaries lack normal solidification. They are therefore fragile, and haemorrhages take place. Similarly, the dentine of the teeth and the osteoid tissue of the bone are improperly formed. This cell-binding property also explains the poor scar formation and slow healing of wounds manifest in persons deficient in ascorbic acid.

It is a common belief, claimed also by some scientists, that very large doses of vitamin C both prevent and reduce symptoms of the common cold (coryza). This claim has not been verified. One large study did suggest a modest reduction in the severity of cold symptoms in those taking vitamin C medicinally, but the vitamin Did not prevent colds from occurring. It is not advisable to take very large doses of medicinal vitamin C for long periods of time.

Dietary sources

The main sources of vitamin C in most diets are fruits, vegetables and various leaves (Photo 14). In pastoral tribes milk is often the main source. Plantains and bananas are the only common staple foods containing fair quantities of vitamin C. Dark green leaves such as amaranth and spinach contain far more than pale leaves such as cabbage and lettuce. Root vegetables and potatoes contain small but useful quantities. Young maize provides some ascorbic acid, as do sprouted cereals and pulses. Animal products such as meat, fish, milk and eggs contain small quantities.

As vitamin C is easily destroyed by heat, prolonged cooking of any food may destroy much of the vitamin C present.

Ascorbic acid is measured in milligrams of the pure vitamin.

Human requirements

Opinions regarding human requirements differ widely. It seems clear that as much as 75 mg per day is necessary if the body is to remain fully saturated with vitamin C. However, individuals appear to remain healthy on intakes as low as 10 mg per day. A recommendation of 25 mg for an adult, 30 mg for adolescents, 35 mg during pregnancy and 45 mg during lactation seems to be a reasonable compromise.

Deficiency

Scurvy and the other clinical manifestations of vitamin C deficiency are described in Chapter 19. Scurvy is not now a prevalent disease. Outbreaks have occurred in famine areas and recently in several refugee camps in Africa.

In its early stages vitamin C deficiency may lead to bleeding gums and slow healing of wounds.

VITAMIN D

Vitamin D is associated with prevention of the disease rickets and its adult counterpart osteomalacia (softening of the bones). Rickets was for many years suspected to be a nutritional deficiency disease, and in certain parts of the world cod-liver oil was used in its treatment. However, it was not until 1919 that Sir Edward Mellanby, using puppies, demonstrated conclusively that the disease was indeed of nutritional origin and that it responded to vitamin D in cod-liver oil. Later it was proved that action of sunlight on the skin leads to the production of the vitamin D used by humans.

Properties

A number of compounds, all sterols closely related to cholesterol, possess antirachitic properties. It was found that certain sterols that did not have these properties became antirachitic when acted upon by ultraviolet light. The two important activated sterols are vitamin D_2 (ergocalciferol) and vitamin D_3 (cholecalciferol).

In human beings, when the skin is exposed to the ultraviolet rays of sunlight, a sterol compound is activated to form vitamin D, which is then available to the body and which has exactly the same function as vitamin D taken in the diet. Dietary vitamin D is only absorbed from the gut in the presence of bile.

The function of vitamin D in the body is to allow the proper absorption of calcium. Vitamin D formed in the skin or absorbed from food acts like a hormone in influencing calcium metabolism. Rickets and osteomalacia, though diseases in which calcium is deficient in certain tissues, are caused not by calcium deficiency in the diet but by a lack of vitamin D which would allow proper utilization of the calcium in the diet.

Vitamin D is often expressed in international units; 1 IU is equivalent to 0.025 µg of vitamin D_3.

Dietary sources

Vitamin D occurs naturally only in the fat in certain animal products. Eggs, cheese, milk and butter are good sources in normal diets. Meat and fish contribute small quantities. Fish-liver oils are very rich. Cereals, vegetables and fruit contain no vitamin D.

Storage in the body

The body has a considerable capacity to store vitamin D in fatty tissue and in the liver. An adequate store is important in a pregnant woman, to avoid predisposition to rickets in the child.

Human requirements

It is not possible to define human dietary requirements, because the vitamin is obtained both by eating foods containing vitamin D and by the action of sunlight on the skin. There is no need for adults to have any vitamin D in their diets, provided they are adequately exposed to sunlight, and many children in Asia, Latin America and Africa survive in good health on a diet almost completely devoid of vitamin D. It has been shown that fish-liver oil containing 400 IU (10 µg) of vitamin D will prevent the occurrence of rickets in infants or children not exposed to sunlight. This amount seems to be a safe allowance.

Deficiency

Rickets and osteomalacia, two diseases resulting from a deficiency of vitamin D, are described in Chapter 18. As vitamin D is produced in humans by the action of the sun on the skin, deficiency is not common in tropical countries, although synthesis of vitamin D may possibly be reduced in darkly pigmented skin. Rickets and osteomalacia are seen sporadically but are more common in areas where tradition or religion keeps women and children indoors. Many cases have been reported from Yemen and Ethiopia. The conditions are manifested mainly by skeletal changes.

Toxicity

Like other fat-soluble vitamins, vitamin D taken in excess in the diet is not well excreted. Consumption of large doses, which has most commonly resulted from overdosing of children with fish-liver oil preparations, can lead to toxicity. Overdosing may lead to hypercalcaemia, diagnosed from high levels of calcium in the blood. Toxicity usually begins with loss of appetite and weight, which may be followed by mental disorientation and finally by kidney failure. Fatalities have been recorded.

OTHER VITAMINS

The two fat-soluble vitamins (A and D) and the six water-soluble vitamins (thiamine, riboflavin, niacin, vitamin B_{12}, folates and vitamin C) have been described in some detail because these are the vitamins most likely to be deficient and to be of public health importance in non-industrialized countries. Five other vitamins, although vital to human health, are not very commonly deficient in human diets and so are of less public health importance. These are vitamin B_6, biotin, pantothenic acid, vitamin E and vitamin K.

Vitamin B₆ (pyridoxine)

Vitamin B_6 is a water-soluble vitamin widely present in foods of both animal and vegetable origin. It is important as a coenzyme in many metabolic processes. Primary dietary deficiency is extremely rare, but vitamin B_6 deficiency became common in tuberculosis patients treated with the drug isoniazid. The patients developed neurological signs and sometimes also anaemia and dermatosis. Now it is common to provide 10 mg of vitamin B_6 by mouth daily to those receiving large doses of isoniazid. Vitamin B_6 is

relatively expensive, however, and the routine administration of vitamin B_6 to patients receiving isoniazid increases the cost of treatment of tuberculosis.

Biotin

Biotin is another water-soluble vitamin of the B complex group. It is found widely in food, and deficiency in humans is extremely rare. The vitamin is very important, however, in physiological and biochemical metabolic processes. Avidin in uncooked egg white prevents absorption of biotin in animals and humans. Rats fed egg white as their only source of protein become thin and wasted and develop neuropathies and dermatitis. Biotin deficiency has been reported in a very few cases, in people consuming mainly egg white and in a few intravenously-fed patients with some special forms of malabsorption.

Pantothenic acid

Pantothenic acid, a water-soluble vitamin, is present in adequate amounts in almost all human diets. It has important biochemical functions in various enzyme reactions, but deficiency in humans is very rare. A neurological condition described as burning feet syndrome, reported in prisoners of war held by the Japanese between 1942 and 1945, was ascribed to a deficiency of this vitamin.

Vitamin E (tocopherol)

Vitamin E, a fat-soluble vitamin, is obtained by humans mainly from vegetable oils and whole-grain cereals. It has been termed the "anti-sterility vitamin" or even the "sex vitamin" because rats fed on tocopherol-deficient diets cannot reproduce: males develop abnormalities in the testicles and females abort spontaneously.

Because of its relationship to fertility and to many conditions in animals, vitamin E is widely self-prescribed and is not uncommonly recommended by physicians for a variety of human ills. However, true deficiency is probably rare; it occurs mainly in association with severe malabsorption states (when fat is poorly absorbed), in genetic anaemias [including glucose-6-phosphatase dehydrogenase (G-6PD) deficiency] and occasionally in very low-weight babies.

Vitamin E (like vitamin C) is an antioxidant, and because of its ability to limit oxidation and to deal with damaging free radicals it is sometimes recommended as a possible preventive for both arteriosclerosis and cancer. Its presence in oils helps prevent the oxidation of unsaturated fatty acids.

Vitamin K

Vitamin K has been termed the "coagulation vitamin" because of its relationship to prothrombin and blood coagulation, and because it is successfully used to treat a bleeding condition of newborn infants (haemorrhagic disease of the newborn). Humans obtain some vitamin K from food, and some is also made by bacteria in the intestines. Newborn infants have a gut free of organisms, so they do not get vitamin K from bacterial synthesis. It is now believed that intravenously-fed or starved patients receiving broad-spectrum antibiotics that kill gut bacteria may bleed because of vitamin K deficiency. In many hospitals vitamin K is given routinely to newborn infants to prevent haemorrhagic disease.

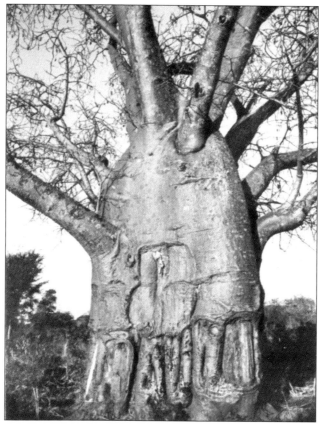

PHOTO 14
*Among the variety of wild fruits eaten, that of the baobab
is particularly rich in vitamin C*

Part III
Disorders of malnutrition

Chapter 12

Protein-energy malnutrition

Protein-energy malnutrition (PEM) in young children is currently the most important nutritional problem in most countries in Asia, Latin America, the Near East and Africa. Energy deficiency is the major cause. No accurate figures exist on the world prevalence of PEM, but World Health Organization (WHO) estimates suggest that the prevalence of PEM in children under five years of age in developing countries has fallen progressively, from 42.6 percent in 1975 to 34.6 percent in 1995. However, in some regions this fall in percentage has not been as rapid as the rise in population; thus in some regions, such as Africa and South Asia, the number of malnourished children has in fact risen. In fact the number of underweight children worldwide has risen from 195 million in 1975 to an estimated 200 million at the end of 1994, which means that more than one-third of the world's under-five population is still malnourished.

Failure to grow adequately is the first and most important manifestation of PEM. It often results from consuming too little food, especially energy, and is frequently aggravated by infections. A child who manifests growth failure may be shorter in length or height or lighter in weight than expected for a child of his or her age, or may be thinner than expected for height.

The conceptual framework described in Chapter 1 suggests that there are three necessary conditions to prevent malnutrition or growth failure: adequate food availability and consumption; good health and access to medical care; and adequate care and feeding practices. If any one of these is absent, PEM is a likely outcome.

The term protein-energy malnutrition entered the medical literature fairly recently, but the condition has been known for many years. In earlier literature it was called by other names, including protein-calorie malnutrition (PCM) and protein-energy deficiency.

The term PEM is used to describe a broad array of clinical conditions ranging from the mild to the serious. At one end of the spectrum, mild PEM manifests itself mainly as poor physical growth in children; at the other end of the spectrum, kwashiorkor (characterized by the presence of oedema) and nutritional marasmus (characterized by severe wasting) have high case fatality rates.

It has been known for centuries that grossly inadequate food intake during famine and food shortages leads to weight loss and wasting and eventually to death from starvation. However, it was not until the 1930s that Cicely Williams, working in Ghana, described in detail the condition she termed "kwashiorkor" (using the local Ga word meaning "the disease of the displaced child"). In the 1950s kwashiorkor began to get a great deal of attention. It was often described as the most important form of malnutrition, and it was believed to be caused mainly by protein deficiency. The solution seemed to be to make more protein-rich foods available to children at risk. This stress on kwashiorkor and on protein led to a relative neglect of nutritional marasmus and adequate food and energy intakes for children.

The current view is that most PEM is the

result of inadequate intake or poor utilization of food and energy, not a deficiency of one nutrient and not usually simply a lack of dietary protein. It has also been increasingly realized that infections contribute importantly to PEM. Nutritional marasmus is now recognized to be often more prevalent than kwashiorkor. It is unknown why a given child may develop one syndrome as opposed to the other, and it is now seen that these two serious clinical forms of PEM constitute only the small tip of the iceberg. In most populations studied in poor countries, the point prevalence rate for kwashiorkor and nutritional marasmus combined is 1 to 5 percent, whereas 30 to 70 percent of children up to five years of age manifest what is now termed mild or moderate PEM, diagnosed mainly on the basis of anthropometric measurements.

CAUSES AND EPIDEMIOLOGY

PEM, unlike the other important nutritional deficiency diseases, is a macronutrient deficiency, not a micronutrient deficiency. Although termed PEM, it is now generally accepted to stem in most cases from energy deficiency, often caused by insufficient food intake. Energy deficiency is more important and more common than protein deficiency. It is very often associated with infections and with micronutrient deficiencies. Inadequate care, for example infrequent feeding, may play a part.

The cause of PEM (and of some other deficiency diseases prevalent in developing countries) should not, however, be viewed simply in terms of inadequate intake of nutrients. For satisfactory nutrition, foods and the nutrients they contain must be available to the family in adequate quantity; the correct balance of foods and nutrients must be fed at the right intervals; the individual must have an appetite to consume the food; there

must be proper digestion and absorption of the nutrients in the food; the metabolism of the person must be reasonably normal; and there should be no conditions that prevent body cells from utilizing the nutrients or that result in abnormal losses of nutrients. Factors that adversely influence any of these requisites can be causes of malnutrition, particularly PEM. The aetiology, therefore, can be complex. Certain factors that contribute to PEM, particularly in the young child, are related to the host, the agent (the diet) and the environment. The underlying causes could also be categorized as those related to the child's food security, health (including protection from infections and appropriate treatment of illness) and care, including maternal and family practices such as those related to frequency of feeding, breastfeeding and weaning.

Some examples of factors involved in the aetiology of PEM are:

- the young child's high needs for both energy and protein per kilogram relative to those of older family members;
- inappropriate weaning practices;
- inappropriate use of infant formula in place of breastfeeding for very young infants in poor families;
- staple diets that are often of low energy density (not infrequently bulky and unappetizing), low in protein and fat content and not fed frequently enough to children;
- inadequate or inappropriate child care because of, for example, time constraints for the mother or lack of knowledge regarding the importance of exclusive breastfeeding;
- inadequate availability of food for the family because of poverty, inequity or lack of sufficient arable land, and problems related to intrafamily food distribution;
- infections (viral, bacterial and parasitic)

which may cause anorexia, reduce food intake, hinder nutrient absorption and utilization or result in nutrient losses;

- famine resulting from droughts, natural disasters, wars, civil disturbances, etc. (Photo 15).

Prematurity or low birth weight may predispose the child to the development of nutritional marasmus. Failure of breastfeeding because of death of the mother, separation from the mother or lack of or insufficient breastmilk may be causes in poor societies where breastfeeding is often the only feasible way for mothers to feed their babies adequately. An underlying cause of PEM is any influence that prevents mothers from breastfeeding their newborn infants when they live in households where proper bottle-feeding may be difficult or hazardous. Therefore promotion of infant formula and insufficient support of breastfeeding by the medical profession and health services may be factors in the aetiology of marasmus. Prolonged exclusive breastfeeding without the introduction of other foods after six months of age may also contribute to growth faltering, PEM and eventually nutritional marasmus.

The view that kwashiorkor is the result of protein deficiency and nutritional marasmus the result of energy deficiency is an oversimplification, as the causes of both conditions are complex. Both endogenous and exogenous causes are likely to influence whether a child develops nutritional marasmus, kwashiorkor or the intermediate form known as marasmic kwashiorkor. In a child who consumes much less food than required for his or her energy needs, energy is mobilized from both body fat and muscle. Gluconeogenesis in the liver is enhanced, and there is loss of subcutaneous fat and wasting of muscles. It has been suggested that under these circumstances, especially when protein intake is very low relative to carbo-

hydrate intake (with the situation perhaps aggravated by nitrogen losses from infections), various metabolic changes take place which contribute to the development of oedema. More sodium and more water are retained, and much of the water collects outside the cardiovascular system in the tissues, which results in pitting oedema. The actual role of infection has not been adequately explained, but certain infections cause major increases in urinary nitrogen, which derives from amino acids in muscle tissue.

There is not yet broad agreement on the actual cause of the oedema that is the hallmark of kwashiorkor. Most researchers agree that potassium deficiency and sodium retention are important in the pathogenesis of oedema. Some evidence supports the classical argument that oedematous malnutrition is a sign of inadequate protein intake. For example, oedema, fatty liver and a kwashiorkor-like condition can be induced in pigs and baboons on a protein-deficient diet. Epidemiological evidence also shows higher rates of kwashiorkor in Uganda, where the staple diet is plantain, which is very low in protein, than in neighbouring areas where the staple food is a cereal.

Recently two new theories have been advanced to explain the cause of kwashiorkor. The first is that kwashiorkor is due to aflatoxin poisoning. The second is that free radicals are important in the pathogenesis of kwashiorkor; it has been hypothesized that most of the clinical features of kwashiorkor could be caused by an excess free radical stress. This new, relatively untested theory also suggests, however, that kwashiorkor, even if produced by free radicals, is likely to occur only in children who have inadequate food intake and are subjected to infection. Thus even if this theory were to be proved correct, it would merely explain a mechanism for the pathogenesis of kwashiorkor. It would not change the fact that improving diet and reducing infection lead to significant reduction in both kwashiorkor and nutritional marasmus. Neither the aflatoxin nor the free radical theory has been proved experimentally, nor is there adequate convincing research to uphold the view of individual dysadaptation as the cause of severe PEM. Surprisingly, no studies have been able to give conclusive proof of either similarities or differences in dietary consumption between children who develop kwashiorkor with oedema and those who show clinical signs of nutritional marasmus without any oedema.

In severe PEM there is usually biochemical evidence, and often clinical evidence, of micronutrient deficiencies, which is not surprising in a child or adult who consumes a grossly inadequate diet. In both nutritional marasmus and kwashiorkor (and also in moderate PEM), clinical examinations or biochemical tests often give clear evidence of, for example, vitamin A deficiency, nutritional anaemia and/or zinc deficiency. However, there is little indication that any one micronutrient deficiency is the main cause of PEM or is by itself responsible for the oedema of kwashiorkor.

Irrespective of which theory of aetiology may be proved correct, improving the quantity of food consumed, taking steps to ensure that diets are nutritionally well balanced and controlling infection all help to prevent PEM.

MANIFESTATIONS AND CLINICAL PICTURE
Mild and moderate PEM
The condition of PEM is often likened to an iceberg, of which 20 percent is visible above the water and about 80 percent submerged. The severe forms of PEM – kwashiorkor, nutritional marasmus and marasmic kwashiorkor – constitute the top, exposed part of the iceberg: they are relatively easy for a doctor or health worker to diagnose simply from their clinical manifestations, described below. On the other hand, children with moderate or mild malnutrition often do not have clear clinical manifestations of malnutrition; rather, they are shorter and/or thinner than would be expected for their age, and they may have deficits in psychological development and perhaps other signs not easy to detect. Mild and moderate PEM are diagnosed mainly on the basis of anthropometry, especially using measurements of weight and height and sometimes other measurements such as arm circumference or skinfold thickness.

As shown by the iceberg diagram (Figure 5), the prevalence of highly visible, serious PEM (kwashiorkor, marasmic kwashiorkor and nutritional marasmus) is usually between about 1 and 5 percent, except in famine areas. In contrast, moderate and mild malnutrition in many countries of sub-Saharan Africa and South Asia add up to 30 to 70 percent. In these areas often only 15 to 50 percent of young children between six months and 60 months of age do not have evidence of PEM. The diagram illustrates that both energy deficiency and protein deficiency play a part, but that energy deficiency is more important. It suggests that protein deficiency plays a greater part in kwashiorkor and energy deficiency in nutritional marasmus.

The percentage of children classified as having severe, moderate and mild PEM depends on how these terms are defined. The two severe forms of malnutrition, kwashiorkor and nutritional marasmus, have very different appearances and clinical features as described below. It is generally agreed that the hallmark of kwashiorkor is pitting oedema, and the overriding feature of nutritional marasmus is severe underweight. Children who have both oedema and severe underweight are diagnosed as having marasmic kwashiorkor.

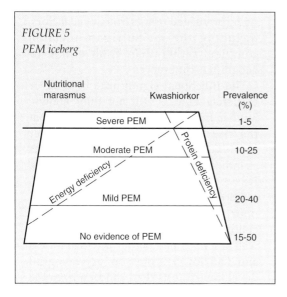

FIGURE 5
PEM iceberg

TABLE 19

Wellcome classification of severe forms of protein-energy malnutrition

Percentage of standard weight for age	Oedema present	Oedema absent
60-80	Kwashiorkor	Undernourishment
<60	Marasmic kwashiorkor	Nutritional marasmus

TABLE 20

The Gomez classification of malnutrition based on weight-for-age standards

Classification	Percentage of standard weight for age
Normal	>90
Grade I (mild malnutrition)	75-89.9
Grade II (moderate malnutrition)	60-74.9
Grade III[a] (severe malnutrition)	<60

[a] J. Bengoa of WHO suggested that all children with oedema be placed in Grade III. This became known as the Bengoa modification.

The so-called Wellcome classification of severe forms of PEM has been widely used for over 20 years (see Table 19). It has the advantage of simplicity because it is based on only two measures, namely the percentage of standard weight for age and the presence or absence of oedema. The category "undernourished" includes children who have moderate or moderately severe PEM but no oedema and whose weight is above 60 percent of the standard. Today a cut-off point using standard deviations (SD) is considered more appropriate than percentage of standard, but not many children would be reclassified.

In the 1950s and 1960s the degree of malnutrition was almost always based on the child's percentage of standard weight for age. In Latin America and elsewhere the Gomez classification was very widely used (Table 20).

In the early 1970s a number of nutrition workers began to suggest that judging the degree of malnutrition only on the basis of weight for age had many disadvantages. A method was suggested that distinguished three categories of mild to moderate PEM based on weight and height

measurements of children. Subsequently these categories came to be known as follows:

- *wasting:* acute current, short-duration malnutrition, where weight for age and weight for height are low but height for age is normal;
- *stunting:* past chronic malnutrition, where weight for age and height for age are low but weight for height is normal;
- *wasting and stunting:* acute and chronic or current long-duration malnutrition, where weight for age, height for age and weight for height are all low.

This classification makes a distinction between current and past influences on nutritional status. It helps the examiner assess the likelihood that supplementary feeding will markedly improve the nutritional status of the child, and it gives the clinician some clue as to the history of the malnutrition in the patient. It also has advantages for nutritional surveys and surveillance. In general, stunting is more prevalent than wasting worldwide.

As is discussed in Chapter 33, which deals with assessment of nutritional status, it is now generally recommended that malnutrition be judged on the basis of SD below the growth standards of the United States National Center for Health Statistics (NCHS) as published by WHO. In country reports published based on weight for age alone, "underweight" is commonly used to denote weight below 2 SD of the NCHS standards in children up to five years of age. In a normal distribution it is expected that 2 to 3 percent of children will fall below the -2 SD cut-off point. Prevalence above that level suggests that there is a nutritional problem in the population assessed. If measurements are also taken of length or height, then the children can be further divided into those who are wasted, stunted, or wasted and stunted.

Policy-makers and health workers need to decide which growth standards to use as a yardstick for judging malnutrition and for surveys, monitoring and surveillance. In recent years the WHO/NCHS growth standards (which do not differ very much from previously used standards, such as the Harvard and Denver growth standards) have gained increasing acceptance. The international growth standards have been found to be applicable for developing countries, as evidence shows that the growth of privileged children in developing countries does not differ importantly from these standards, and that the poorer growth seen among the

underprivileged results from social factors, including the malnutrition-infection complex, rather than from ethnic or geographic differences.

The functional significance of mild or moderate PEM is still not fully known. Studies from several countries show that the risk of mortality increases rather steadily with worsening nutritional status as indicated by anthropometric measures. Recent investigations in Guatemala indicated that teenagers who had manifested poor growth when examined in early childhood were smaller in stature, did less well at school, had poorer physical fitness and had lower scores on psychological development tests than children from the same villages who grew better as young children. These results suggest long-term consequences of PEM in early childhood.

The attempt to control the extent and severity of PEM using many different strategies and actions is at the heart of nutritional programmes and policies in most developing countries. The reduction and eventual prevention of mild or moderate malnutrition will automatically reduce severe malnutrition. Thus, although it may be tempting (particularly for doctors and other health workers) to put major emphasis on the control of nutritional marasmus and kwashiorkor, resources are often better spent on controlling mild and moderate PEM, which will in turn reduce severe PEM.

KWASHIORKOR

Kwashiorkor is one of the serious forms of PEM. It is seen most frequently in children one to three years of age, but it may occur at any age. It is found in children who have a diet that is usually insufficient in energy and protein and often in other nutrients. Often the food provided to the child is mainly carbohydrate; it may be very bulky, and it may not be provided very frequently.

Kwashiorkor is often associated with, or even precipitated by, infectious diseases. Diarrhoea, respiratory infections, measles, whooping cough, intestinal parasites and other infections are common underlying causes of PEM and may precipitate children into either kwashiorkor or nutritional marasmus. These infections often result in loss of appetite, which is important as a cause of serious PEM. Infections, especially those resulting in fever, lead to an increased loss of nitrogen from the body which can only be replaced by protein in the diet.

Clinical signs of kwashiorkor

Kwashiorkor is relatively easy to diagnose based on the child's history, the symptoms reported and the clinical signs observed (Figure 6). Laboratory tests are not essential but do throw more light on each case. All cases of kwashiorkor have oedema to some degree, poor growth, wasting of muscles and fatty infiltration of the liver. Other signs include mental changes, abnormal hair, a typical dermatosis, anaemia, diarrhoea and often evidence of other micronutrient deficiencies (Photos 16 and 17).

Oedema. The accumulation of fluid in the tissues causes swelling; in kwashiorkor this condition is always present to some degree. It usually starts with a slight swelling of the feet and often spreads up the legs. Later, the hands and face may also swell. To diagnose the presence of oedema the medical attendant presses with a finger or thumb above the ankle. If oedema is present the pit formed takes a few seconds to return to the level of the surrounding skin.

Poor growth. Growth failure always occurs. If the child's precise age is known, the child will be found to be shorter than normal and, except in cases of gross

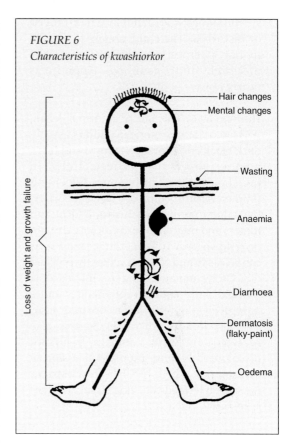

FIGURE 6
Characteristics of kwashiorkor

Loss of weight and growth failure

Hair changes
Mental changes
Wasting
Anaemia
Diarrhoea
Dermatosis (flaky-paint)
Oedema

oedema, lighter in weight than normal (usually 60 to 80 percent of standard or below 2 SD). These signs may be obscured by oedema or ignorance of the child's age.

Wasting. Wasting of muscles is also typical but may not be evident because of oedema. The child's arms and legs are thin because of muscle wasting.

Fatty infiltration of the liver. This condition is always found in post-mortem examination of kwashiorkor cases. It may cause palpable enlargement of the liver (hepatomegaly).

Mental changes. Mental changes are common but not invariably noticed. The child is usually apathetic about his or her surroundings and irritable when moved or disturbed. The child prefers to remain in one position and is nearly always miserable and unsmiling. Appetite is nearly always poor.

Hair changes. The hair of a normal Asian, African or Latin American child is usually dark black and coarse in texture and has a healthy sheen that reflects light. In kwashiorkor, the hair becomes silkier and thinner. African hair loses its tight curl. At the same time it lacks lustre, is dull and lifeless and may change in colour to brown or reddish brown. Sometimes small tufts can be easily and almost painlessly plucked out. On examination under a microscope, plucked hair exhibits root changes and a narrower diameter than normal hair. The tensile strength of the hair is also reduced. In Latin America bands of discoloured hair are reported as a sign of kwashiorkor. These reddish-brown stripes have been termed the "flag sign" or *"signa bandera"*.

Skin changes. Dermatosis develops in some but not all cases of kwashiorkor. It tends to occur first in areas of friction or of pressure such as the groin, behind the knees and at the elbow. Darkly pigmented patches appear, which may peel off or desquamate. The similarity of these patches to old sun-baked, blistered paint has given rise to the term "flaky-paint dermatosis". Underneath the flaking skin are atrophic depigmented areas which may resemble a healing burn.

Anaemia. Most cases have some degree of anaemia because of lack of the protein required to synthesize blood cells. Anaemia may be complicated by iron deficiency, malaria, hookworm, etc.

Diarrhoea. Stools are frequently loose and contain undigested particles of food.

Sometimes they have an offensive smell or are watery or tinged with blood.

Moonface. The cheeks may appear to be swollen with either fatty tissue or fluid, giving the characteristic appearance known as "moonface".

Signs of other deficiencies. In kwashiorkor some subcutaneous fat is usually palpable, and the amount gives an indication of the degree of energy deficiency. Mouth and lip changes characteristic of vitamin B deficiency are common. Xerosis or xerophthalmia resulting from vitamin A deficiency may be seen. Deficiencies of zinc and other micronutrients may occur.

Differential diagnosis

Nephrosis. Oedema is also a feature of nephrosis, which may therefore be confused with kwashiorkor. In nephrosis, however, the urine contains much albumin as well as casts and cells. In kwashiorkor, there is usually only a trace of albumin. If flaky-paint dermatosis or other signs of kwashiorkor are present, the diagnosis is established. Ascites is frequently seen in nephrosis, but only rarely in kwashiorkor. In most developing countries kwashiorkor is a much more common cause of oedema than nephrosis.

Severe hookworm anaemia. Oedema may result from this cause alone. In young children kwashiorkor is often also present. In pure hookworm anaemia there are no skin changes other than pallor. In all cases the stools should be examined.

Chronic dysentery. In this disease oedema is not a feature.

Pellagra. Pellagra is rare in young children. The skin lesions are sometimes similar to those of kwashiorkor, but in pellagra they tend to be on areas exposed to sunlight

TABLE 21
Comparison of the features of kwashiorkor and marasmus

Feature	Kwashiorkor	Marasmus
Growth failure	Present	Present
Wasting	Present	Present, marked
Oedema	Present (sometimes mild)	Absent
Hair changes	Common	Less common
Mental changes	Very common	Uncommon
Dermatosis, flaky-paint	Common	Does not occur
Appetite	Poor	Good
Anaemia	Severe (sometimes)	Present, less severe
Subcutaneous fat	Reduced but present	Absent
Face	May be oedematous	Drawn in, monkey-like
Fatty infiltration of liver	Present	Absent

(not the groin, for example). There may frequently be diarrhoea and weight loss, but no oedema or hair changes.

NUTRITIONAL MARASMUS

In most countries marasmus, the other severe form of PEM, is now much more prevalent than kwashiorkor. In marasmus the main deficiency is one of food in general, and therefore also of energy. It may occur at any age, most commonly up to about three and a half years, but in contrast to kwashiorkor it is more common during the first year of life. Nutritional marasmus is in fact a form of starvation, and the possible underlying causes are numerous. For whatever reason, the child does not get adequate supplies of breast-milk or of any alternative food.

Perhaps the most important precipitating causes of marasmus are infectious and parasitic diseases of childhood. These include measles, whooping cough, diarrhoea, malaria and other parasitic diseases. Chronic infections such as tuberculosis may also lead to marasmus. Other common causes of marasmus are premature birth, mental deficiency and digestive upsets such as malabsorption or vomiting. A very common cause is early cessation of breast-feeding.

Clinical features of nutritional marasmus

The important features of kwashiorkor and nutritional marasmus are compared in Table 21. The following are the main signs of marasmus (Photos 18 and 19).

Poor growth. In all cases the child fails to grow properly. If the age is known, the weight will be found to be extremely low by normal standards (below 60 percent or -3 SD of the standard). In severe cases the loss of flesh is obvious: the ribs are prominent; the belly, in contrast to the rest of the body, may be protuberant; the face has a characteristic simian (monkey-like) appearance; and the limbs are very emaciated. The child appears to be skin and bones. An advanced case of the disease is unmistakable, and once seen is never forgotten.

Wasting. The muscles are always extremely wasted. There is little if any subcutaneous fat left. The skin hangs in wrinkles, especially around the buttocks and thighs. When the skin is taken between forefinger and thumb, the usual layer of adipose tissue is found to be absent.

Alertness. Children with marasmus are quite often not disinterested like those with kwashiorkor. Instead the deep sunken eyes have a rather wide-awake appearance. Similarly, the child may be less miserable and less irritable.

Appetite. The child often has a good appetite. In fact, like any starving being, the child may be ravenous. Children with marasmus often violently suck their hands or clothing or anything else available. Sometimes they make sucking noises.

Anorexia. Some children are anorexic.

Diarrhoea. Stools may be loose, but this is not a constant feature of the disease. Diarrhoea of an infective nature, as mentioned above, may commonly have been a precipitating factor.

Anaemia. Anaemia is usually present.

Skin sores. There may be pressure sores, but these are usually over bony prominences, not in areas of friction. In contrast to kwashiorkor, there is no oedema and no flaky-paint dermatosis in marasmus.

Hair changes. Changes similar to those in kwashiorkor can occur. There is more frequently a change of texture than of colour.

Dehydration. Although not a feature of the disease itself, dehydration is a frequent accompaniment of the disease; it results from severe diarrhoea (and sometimes vomiting).

MARASMIC KWASHIORKOR

Children with features of both nutritional marasmus and kwashiorkor are diagnosed as having marasmic kwashiorkor. In the Wellcome classification (see above) this diagnosis is given for a child with severe malnutrition who is found to have both oedema and a weight for age below 60 percent of that expected for his or her age. Children with marasmic kwashiorkor have all the features of nutritional marasmus including severe wasting, lack of subcutaneous fat and poor growth, and in addition to oedema, which is always present, they may also have any of the features of kwashiorkor described above. There may be skin changes including flaky-paint dermatosis, hair changes, mental changes and hepatomegaly. Many of these children have diarrhoea.

LABORATORY TESTS

Laboratory tests have a limited usefulness for the diagnosis or evaluation of PEM. Some biochemical estimations are used, and give different results for children with kwashiorkor and nutritional marasmus than for normal children or those with moderate PEM.

In kwashiorkor there is a reduction in total serum proteins, and especially in the albumin fraction. In nutritional marasmus the reduction is usually much less marked. Often, because of infections, the globulin fraction in the serum is normal or even raised. Serum albumin drops to low or very low levels usually only in clinically evident kwashiorkor. Serum albumin levels are not useful in predicting imminent kwashiorkor development in moderate PEM cases. It is often true that the more severe the kwashiorkor, the lower the serum albumin, but serum albumin levels are not useful in evaluating less severe PEM.

There is general agreement that serum albumin concentrations below 3 g/dl are

TABLE 22

Levels of serum albumin concentrations in malnourished children

Concentration (g/dl)	Interpretation
≥3.5	Normal
3-3.4	Subnormal
2.5-2.9	Low
≤2.5	Pathological

Source: Alleyne *et al.*, 1977.

low and that those below 2.5 g/dl are seriously deficient (see Table 22). It has also been suggested that serum albumin levels below 2.8 g/dl should be considered deficient and indicate a high risk.

Serum albumin determinations are relatively easy and cheap to perform, and unlike the other biochemical tests mentioned below, they can be done in modest laboratories in many developing countries.

Levels of two other serum proteins, pre-albumin and serum transferrin, are also of use and not too difficult to determine. Levels of both are reduced in kwashiorkor and may be useful in judging its severity. However, serum transferrin levels are also influenced by iron status, which reduces their usefulness as an indicator of kwashiorkor.

Levels of retinol binding protein (RBP), which is the carrier protein for retinol, also tend to be reduced in kwashiorkor and to a lesser degree in nutritional marasmus. However, other diseases, such as liver disease, vitamin A and zinc deficiencies and hyperthyroidism, may also influence RBP levels.

Other biochemical tests that have been used or recommended for diagnosing or evaluating PEM have limited usefulness. These include tests for:

• fasting serum insulin levels, which are

elevated in kwashiorkor and low in marasmus;

• ratio of serum essential amino acids to non-essential amino acids, which is low in kwashiorkor but not much influenced by nutritional marasmus;

• hydroxyproline and creatinine levels in urine, which if low may indicate current growth deficits and nutritional marasmus.

These tests are not specific, and most cannot be performed in ordinary hospital laboratories.

TREATMENT OF SEVERE PEM
Hospitalization

All children with severe kwashiorkor, nutritional marasmus or marasmic kwashiorkor should, if possible, be admitted to hospital with the mother. The child should be given a thorough clinical examination, including careful examination for any infection and a special search for respiratory infection such as pneumonia or tuberculosis. Stool, urine and blood tests (for haemoglobin and malaria parasites) should be performed. The child should be weighed and measured.

Often hospital treatment is not possible. In that case the best possible medical treatment available at a health centre, dispensary or other medical facility is necessary. If the child is still being breast-fed, breastfeeding should continue.

Diet. Treatment is often based on dried skimmed milk (DSM) powder.[1] DSM may most simply be reconstituted in hospital by adding one teaspoonful of DSM powder to 25 ml of boiled water and mixing thoroughly. The child should receive 150 ml of this mixture per kilogram of

---

[1] There is a risk if non-vitaminized DSM is used. Attention to providing all micronutrients is important.

body weight per day, given in six feeds at approximately four-hour intervals. For example, a 5-kg child should receive 5 × 150 ml per day = 750 ml per day, divided into six feeds = 125 ml per feed. Each feed is made by adding five teaspoonfuls of DSM powder to 125 ml of water.

The milk mixture should be fed to the child with a feeding cup or a spoon. If cup- or spoon-feeding is difficult – which is possible if the child does not have sufficient appetite and is unable to cooperate or if the child is seriously ill – the same mixture is best given through an intragastric tube. The tube should be made of polyethylene; it should be about 50 cm long and should have an internal diameter of 1 mm. It is passed through one nostril into the stomach. The protruding end should be secured to the cheek either with sticky tape or zinc oxide plaster. The tube can safely be left in position for five days. The milk mixture is best given as a continuous drip, as for a transfusion. Alternatively, the mixture can be administered intermittently using a large syringe and a needle that fits the tube. The milk mixture is then given in feeds at four-hour intervals. Before and after each feed, 5 ml of warm, previously boiled water should be injected through the lumen of the tube to prevent blockage.

There are better mixtures than plain DSM. They can all be administered in exactly the same way (by spoon, feeding cup or intragastric tube). Most of these mixtures contain a vegetable oil (e.g. sesame, cottonseed), casein (pure milk protein), DSM and sugar. The vegetable oil increases the energy content and energy density of the mixture and appears to be tolerated better than the fat of full cream milk. Casein increases the cost of the mixture, but as it often serves to reduce the length of the hospital stay, the money is well spent. A good and easily remembered formula for the sugar/casein/oil/

milk (SCOM) mixture is: one part sugar, one part casein, one part oil and one part DSM, with water added to make 20 parts. A stock of the dry SCOM mixture can be stored for up to one month in a sealed tin. To make a feeding, the desired quantity of the mixture is placed in a measuring jug, and water is added to the correct level. Stirring or, better still, whisking will ensure an even mixture. As with the plain DSM mixture, 150 ml of liquid SCOM mixture should be given per kilogram of body weight per day; a 5-kg child should receive 750 ml per day in six 125-ml feeds, each made by adding five teaspoonfuls of SCOM mixture to 125 ml of boiled water. A 30-ml portion of made-up liquid feed provides about 28 kcal, 1 g protein and 12 mg potassium.

Rehydration. Children with kwashiorkor or nutritional marasmus who have severe diarrhoea or diarrhoea with vomiting may be dehydrated. Intravenous feeding is not necessary unless the vomiting is severe or the child refuses to take fluids orally. Rehydration should be achieved using standard oral rehydration solution (ORS), as is described for the treatment of diarrhoea (see Chapter 37). For severely malnourished children, unusually dilute ORS often provides some therapeutic advantage. Thus if standard ORS packets are used which are normally added to 1 litre of boiled water, in a serious case a packet might be added to 1.5 litres of water.

Treatment of hypothermia. Even in tropical areas temperatures at night often drop markedly in hospital wards and elsewhere. The seriously malnourished child has difficulty maintaining his or her temperature and may easily develop a lower than normal body temperature, termed hypothermia. Untreated hypothermia is a common cause of death in malnourished children. At home the child may have been kept warm sleeping in bed with the mother, or the windows of the house may have been kept closed. In the hospital ward the child may sleep alone, and the staff may keep the windows open. If the child's temperature is below 36°C, efforts must be made to warm the child. He or she must be kept in warm clothes and must be kept covered with warm bedding, and there must be an effort to ensure that the room is adequately warm. Sometimes hot-water bottles in the bed are used. The child's temperature should be checked frequently.

Medication. Although it is useful to establish standard procedures for treating kwashiorkor and nutritional marasmus in any hospital or other health unit, each case should nevertheless be treated on its own merits. No two children have identical needs.

Infections are so common in severely malnourished children that antibiotics are often routinely recommended. Benzyl-penicillin by intramuscular injection, 1 million units per day in divided doses for five days, is often used. Ampicillin, 250 mg in tablet form four times a day by mouth, or amoxycillin, 125 mg three times a day by mouth, can also be given. Gentamycin and chloramphenicol are alternative options but are less often used.

In areas where malaria is present an antimalarial is desirable, e.g. half a tablet (125 mg) of chloroquine daily for three days, then half a tablet weekly. In severe cases and when vomiting is present, chloroquine should be given by injection.

If anaemia is very severe it should be treated by blood transfusion, which should be followed by ferrous sulphate mixture or tablets given three times daily.

If a stool examination reveals the presence of hookworm, roundworm or other intestinal parasites, then an appropriate anthelmintic drug such as albenda-zole should be given after the general condition of the child has improved.

Severely malnourished children not infrequently have tuberculosis and should be examined for it. If the disease is found to be present, specific treatment is needed.

Recovery

On the above regime, a child with serious kwashiorkor would usually begin to lose oedema during the first three to seven days, with consequent loss in weight. During this period, the diarrhoea should ease or cease, the child should become more cheerful and alert, and skin lesions should begin to clear.

When the diarrhoea has stopped, the oedema has disappeared and the appetite has returned, it is desirable to stop tube-feeding if this method has been used. The same SCOM or plain DSM mixture can be continued with a cup and spoon or feeding bowl. A bottle and teat should not be used. If anaemia is still present, the child should now start a course of iron by mouth, and half a tablet (125 mg) of chloroquine should be given weekly.

Children with severe nutritional maras-mus may consume very high amounts of energy, and weight gain may be quite rapid. However, the length of time needed in hospital or for full recovery may be longer than for children with kwashiorkor.

In both conditions, as recovery conti-nues, usually during the second week in hospital, the patient gains weight. While feeding of milk is continued, a mixed diet should gradually be introduced, aimed at providing the energy, protein, minerals and vitamins needed by the child.

If the disease is not to recur, it is important that the mother or guardian participate in the feeding at this stage. She must be told what the child is being fed and why. Her cooperation with and follow-up of this regime is much more likely if the hospital diet of the child is based mainly on products that are used at home and that are likely to be available to the family. This is not feasible in every case in a large hospital, but the diet should at least be based on locally available foods. Thus in a maize-eating area, for example, the child would now receive maize gruel with DSM added. For an older child, crushed groundnuts can be added twice a day, or, if preferred by custom, roasted groundnuts can be eaten. A few teaspoonfuls of ripe papaya, mango, orange or other fruit can be given. At one or two meals per day, a small portion of the green vegetable and the beans, fish or meat that the mother eats can be fed to the child, after having been well chopped. Protein-rich foods (e.g. beans, peas, groundnuts, meat, sour milk or eggs) can be given. If eggs are available and custom allows their consumption, an egg can be boiled or scrambled for the child; the mother can watch as it is prepared. Alternatively, a raw egg can be broken into some simmering gruel. Protein-rich foods of animal origin are often relatively expensive. They are not essential; a good mixture of cereals, legumes and vegetables serves just as well. If suitable vitamin-containing foods are not available, then a vitamin mixture should be given, because the DSM and SCOM mixtures are not rich in vitamins.

The above maize-based diet is just an example. If the diet of the area is based on rice or wheat, these can be used instead of maize. If the staple food is plantain or cassava, then protein-rich supplements are important.

After discharge, or if a moderate case of kwashiorkor has been treated at home and not in the hospital, the child should be followed if possible in the out-patient department or a clinic. It is much better if such cases can visit separately from other patients (i.e. on a particular afternoon or at a child welfare or growth monitoring clinic) to avoid the tumult of most out-patient sessions. A relaxed atmosphere is desirable, and the medical attendant should have time to explain matters to the mother and to see that she understands what is expected of her. It is useless just to hand over a bag of milk powder or other supplement, or simply to weigh the child but not provide simple guidance.

Satisfactory weight gain is a good measure of progress. At each visit the child should be weighed. Weight is plotted on a chart to provide a picture for the health worker and the mother.

Out-patient treatment should be based on the provision of a suitable dietary supplement, but in most cases it is best that this supplement be given as part of the diet. The mother should be shown a teaspoon and told how many teaspoonfuls to give per day based on the child's weight. Many supplements, especially DSM, are best provided by adding them to the child's usual food (such as cereal gruel) rather than by making a separate preparation. The mother should be asked how many times a day she feeds the child. If he or she is fed only at family mealtimes and the family eats only twice a day, then the mother should be told to feed the child two extra times.

If facilities exist and it is feasible, the SCOM mixture can be used for out-patient treatment. It is best provided ready mixed in sealed polyethylene bags.

PROGNOSIS

Most deaths in children hospitalized for kwashiorkor or nutritional marasmus occur in the first three days after admission. Case fatality rates depend on many factors including the seriousness of the child's illness at the time of admission and the adequacy of the treatment given. In some societies sick children are taken to hospital very late in the disease, when they are almost moribund. In this situation fatality rates are high.

The cause and the severity of the disease determine the prognosis. A child with severe marasmus and lungs grossly damaged by tuberculous infection obviously has poor prospects. The prospects of a child with mild marasmus and no other infection are better. Response to treatment is likely to be slower with marasmus than with kwashiorkor.

It is often difficult to know what to do when the child is cured, especially if the child is under one year of age. There may be no mother or she may be ill, or she may have insufficient or no breastmilk. Instruction and nutrition education are vital for the person who will be responsible for the child. If the child has been brought by the father, then some female relative should spend a few days in the hospital before the child is discharged. She should be instructed in feeding with a spoon or cup and told not to feed the child from a bottle unless he or she is under three months of age. The best procedure is usually to provide a thin gruel made from the local staple food plus two teaspoonfuls of DSM (or some other protein-rich supplement) and two teaspoonfuls of oil per kilogram of body weight per day. Instruction regarding other items in the diet must be given if the child is over six months old. The mother or guardian should be advised to attend the hospital or clinic at weekly intervals if the family lives near enough (within about 10 km) or at monthly intervals if the distance is greater. Supplies of a suitable supplement to last for slightly longer than the interval between visits should be given at each visit. The child can be put on other foods, as mentioned in the discussion of infant feeding in Chapter 6.

It is essential that the diet provide adequate energy and protein. Usually 120 kcal and 3 g of protein per kilogram of body weight per day are sufficient for long-term treatment. Thus a 10-kg child should receive about 1 200 kcal and 30 g of protein

daily. It should be noted that a marasmic child during the early part of recovery may be capable of consuming and utilizing 150 to 200 kcal and 4 to 5 g of protein per kilogram of body weight per day.

PROTEIN-ENERGY MALNUTRITION IN ADULTS
Adult kwashiorkor

There is little doubt that a disorder due mainly to energy deficiency does occur in adults; it is more common in communities suffering from chronic protein deficiency. The patient is markedly underweight for his or her height (unless grossly oedematous), the muscles are wasted, and subcutaneous fat is reduced. Mental changes are common: the patient is usually disinterested and appears to be in a dream world. It is difficult to attract the patient's attention and equally hard to keep it. Appetite is reduced, and the patient is very weak.

Some degree of oedema is nearly always present, and this may mask the weight loss, wasting and lack of subcutaneous fat. Oedema is most common in the legs, and in male patients also in the scrotum, but any part of the body may be affected. The face is often puffy. This condition has been termed "famine oedema" because it occurs where there is starvation resulting from famine or other causes. It was commonly reported in famines in Indonesia and Papua New Guinea.

Frequent, loose, offensive stools may be passed. The abdomen is often slightly distended, and on palpation the organs can be very easily felt through the thin abdominal wall. During palpation there is nearly always a gurgling noise from the abdomen, and peristaltic movements can often be detected with the fingertips. It is not uncommon for adult kwashiorkor patients to regard their physical state as a consequence of abdominal upset. For this reason, strong purgatives, either proprietary or herbal, and peppery enemas are sometimes used by these patients before they reach hospital, which may greatly aggravate the condition.

The hair frequently shows changes. The skin is often dry and scaly, and may have a crazy-pavement appearance, especially over the tibia. Swelling of both parotid glands is frequent. On palpation the glands are found to be firm and rubbery.

Anaemia is nearly always present and may be severe. The blood pressure is low. There is usually only a trace of albumin in the urine.

Oedema may also be caused by severe anaemia. In adult PEM there is less dyspnoea than in anaemia and usually no cardiomegaly. Other features such as hair changes and parotid swelling are common in adult PEM but not in anaemia. However, the two conditions are closely related.

Nutritional marasmus in adults

In contrast to adult kwashiorkor or famine oedema, which is not very prevalent, the adult equivalent of nutritional marasmus is very common. There are five major causes.

Insufficient food. Any older child or adult whose diet is grossly deficient in energy will develop signs almost exactly like those of nutritional marasmus, and if the condition progresses it may often be fatal. In the case of famines, the condition may be termed starvation (see Chapter 24). Famines and severe food shortages resulting from war, civil disturbance or natural disasters such as droughts, floods and earthquakes may result in nutritional marasmus in children and a similar condition in adults, who suffer from weight loss, wasting, diarrhoea, infectious diseases, etc.

Infections. The second major cause of severe wasting or severe PEM in adults is infections, especially chronic, untreated or untreatable infections. The most common of these now is acquired immunodefi-ciency syndrome (AIDS) resulting from infection with the human immunodefi-ciency virus (HIV). As the disease progresses there is marked weight loss and severe wasting. As mentioned in Chapter 3, in Uganda the name "slim disease" is given to AIDS because of the thinness of its victims. Advanced tuberculosis and many other long-term chronic infections also lead to wasting and weight loss.

Malabsorption. A number of malabsorption conditions cause PEM in adults and children. These diseases, of which some are hereditary, result in the inability of the body to digest or absorb certain foods or nutrients. Examples are cystic fibrosis, coeliac disease and adult sprue.

Malignancies. Another cause of wasting in people of any age is malignancy or cancer of any organ once it progresses to a stage not treatable by surgical excision. Cachexia is a feature of many advanced cancers.

Eating disorders. A group of eating disorders cause weight loss leading to the equivalent of PEM. The most widely described is anorexia nervosa, which occurs much more commonly in females than males, in adolescents or younger adults rather than older persons and in affluent rather than poor societies. Other psychological conditions may also result in poor food intake and lead to PEM.

Treatment

Treatment of adult PEM includes therapy related to the underlying cause of the condition and therapy related to feeding and rehabilitation, when the cause makes that feasible. Thus infections such as tuberculosis or chronic amoebiasis require specific therapy which when effective will eliminate the cause of the weight loss and wasting. In contrast, curative treatment is not applicable in advanced AIDS or cancer.

Dietary treatment for adult PEM should be based on principles similar to those described for the treatment of severe PEM in children, including those recovering from kwashiorkor or marasmus. Emergency feeding and the rehabilitation of famine victims (described in Chapter 24) have relevance to adult PEM.

PREVENTION AND CONTROL OF PEM

The prevention of PEM in Asia, Africa and the Americas presents a huge challenge. It is much more difficult than controlling, for example, iodine deficiency disorders (IDD) and vitamin A deficiency, because the underlying and basic causes, as described above, are often numerous and complex, and because there is no single, universal, cheap, sustainable strategy that can be applied everywhere to reduce the prevalence or severity of PEM.

Part V of this book includes various strategies to reduce the prevalence of PEM. Appropriate nutrition policies and programmes are suggested, and separate chapters deal with, for example, improving food security, protection and promotion of good health, and appropriate care practices to ensure good nutrition. These chapters provide guidance on how to deal with the three underlying causes of malnutrition, namely inadequate food, health and care, which in Chapter 1 were included in the conceptual framework for malnutrition. Other chapters in Part V discuss solutions to particular aspects of the problem, including improving the quality and safety of foods, promoting appropriate diets and healthy lifestyles, procuring food in different ways and incorporating nutrition objectives into development policies and programmes. Throughout Part V there is an emphasis on improving the quality of life of people, especially by reducing poverty, improving diets and promoting good health. Improving the energy intakes of those at risk of PEM is vital.

In the late 1950s and 1960s it was thought that most PEM was caused mainly by inadequate intake of protein. A great deal of emphasis was placed on protein-rich foods as a major solution to the huge problem of malnutrition in the world. This inappropriate strategy diverted attention from the first need, which is adequate food intake by children. There is now much less emphasis on high-protein weaning foods and on nutrition education efforts to ensure greater consumption of meat, fish and eggs, which are economically out of the reach of many families who have children with PEM.

Protein is an essential nutrient, but PEM is more often associated with deficient food intake than with deficient protein intake. In general, when commonly consumed cereal-based diets meet energy needs, they usually also meet protein needs, especially if the diet also provides modest amounts of legumes and vegetables. Primary attention needs to be given to increasing total food intake and reducing infection.

Sensible efforts are needed to protect and promote breastfeeding and sound weaning; to increase the consumption by young children of cereals, legumes and other locally produced weaning foods; to prevent and control infection and parasitic disease; to increase meal frequency for children; and, where appropriate, to encourage higher consumption of oil, fat and other items that reduce bulk and increase the energy density of foods fed to children at risk. These measures are likely to have more impact if accompanied by growth monitoring, immunization, oral rehydration therapy for diarrhoea, early treatment of common diseases, regular deworming and attention to the underlying causes of PEM such as poverty and inequity. Some of these measures can be implemented as part of primary health care. Readers planning strategies to control PEM should consult Part V of this book.

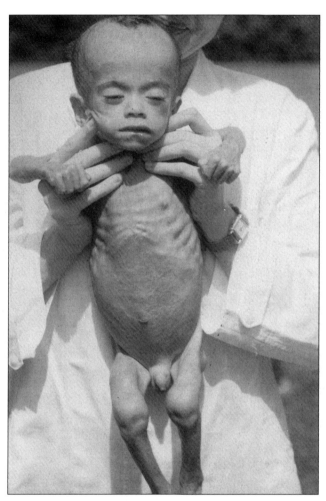

PHOTO 15
Nutritional marasmus with extreme wasting in a child
from Rotterdam, the Netherlands, during the Second
World War

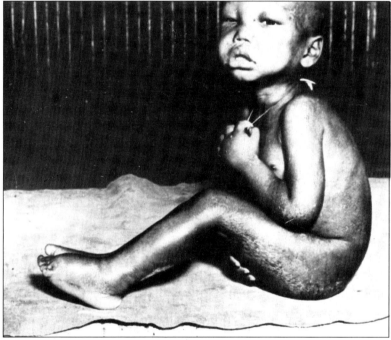

PHOTO 16
*A child with kwashiorkor shows dermatosis of the thigh, arm and back
and oedema of the legs and face which masks muscle wasting and growth
failure*

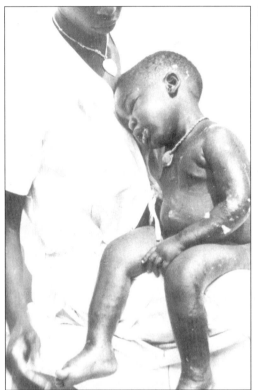

PHOTO 17
*Oedema, skin changes and an ulcer
near the elbow seen in kwashiorkor*

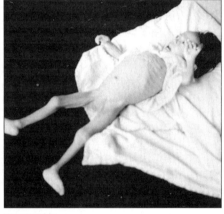

PHOTO 18
*A Colombian child with nutritional
marasmus*

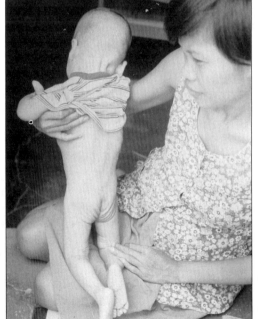

PHOTO 19
*Evident loss of subcutaneous fat in a
child with nutritional marasmus
from the Philippines*

Chapter 13
Iron deficiency and other nutritional anaemias

Nutritional anaemias are extremely prevalent worldwide. Unlike protein-energy malnutrition (PEM), vitamin A deficiency and iodine deficiency disorders (IDD), these anaemias occur frequently in both developing and industrialized countries. The most common cause of anaemia is a deficiency of iron, although not necessarily a dietary deficiency of total iron intake. Deficiencies of folates (or folic acid), vitamin B_{12} and protein may also cause anaemia. Ascorbic acid, vitamin E, copper and pyridoxine are also needed for production of red blood cells (erythrocytes). Vitamin A deficiency is also associated with anaemia.

Anaemias can be classified in numerous ways, some based on the cause of the disease and others based on the appearance of the red blood cells. These classifications are fully discussed in medical textbooks.

Some anaemias do not have causes related to nutrition but are caused, for example, by congenital abnormalities or inherited characteristics; such anaemias, which include sickle cell disease, aplastic anaemias, thalassaemias and severe haemorrhage, are not covered here.

Based on the characteristics of the blood cells or other features, anaemias may be classified as microcytic (having small red blood cells), macrocytic (having large red blood cells), haemolytic (having many ruptured red blood cells) or hypochromic (having pale-coloured cells with less haemoglobin). Macrocytic anaemias are often caused by folate or vitamin B_{12} deficiencies.

In anaemia the blood has less haemoglobin than normal. Haemoglobin is the pigment in red cells that gives blood its red colour. It is made of protein with iron linked to it. Haemoglobin carries oxygen in the blood to all parts of the body. In anaemia either the amount of haemoglobin in each red cell is low (hypochromic anaemia) or there is a reduction in the total number of red cells in the body. The life of each red blood cell is about four months, and the red bone marrow is constantly manufacturing new cells for replacement. This process requires adequate amounts of nutrients, especially iron, other minerals, protein and vitamins, all of which originate in the food consumed.

Iron deficiency is the most prevalent important nutritional problem of humans. It threatens over 60 percent of women and children in most non-industrialized countries, and more than half of these have overt anaemia. In most industrialized countries in North America, Europe and Asia, 12 to 18 percent of women are anaemic.

Although deficiency diseases are usually considered mainly as consequences of a lack of the nutrient in the diet, iron deficiency anaemia occurs frequently in people whose diets contain quantities of iron close to the recommended allowances. However, some forms of iron are absorbed better than others; certain items in the diet enhance or detract from iron absorption; and iron can be lost because of many conditions, an important one in many tropical countries being hookworm infection, which is very common.

Nutritional anaemias have until recently been relatively neglected and not infrequently remain undiagnosed. There are many reasons for the lack of attention, but the most important are probably that the symptoms and signs are much less obvious than in severe PEM, IDD or xerophthalmia, and that although anaemias do contribute to mortality rates they do not often do so in a dramatic way, and death is usually ascribed to another more conspicuous cause such as childbirth. However, research now indicates that iron deficiency has very important implications, including poorer learning ability and behavioural abnormalities in children, lower ability to work hard and poor appetite and growth.

CAUSES AND EPIDEMIOLOGY

To maintain good iron nutritional status each individual needs to have an adequate quantity of iron in the diet. The iron has to be in a form that permits a sufficient amount of it to be absorbed from the intestines. The absorption of iron may be enhanced or inhibited by other dietary substances.

Human beings have the ability both to store and to conserve iron, and it must also be transported properly within the body. The average male adult has 4 to 5 g of iron in his body, most of it in haemoglobin, a little in myoglobin and in enzymes and around 1 g in storage iron, mainly ferritin in the cells, especially in the liver and bone marrow. Losses of iron from the body must not deplete the supply to less than that needed for manufacture of new red blood cells.

To produce new cells the body needs adequate quantities and quality of protein, minerals and vitamins in the diet. Protein is needed both for the framework of the red blood cells and for the manufacture of the haemoglobin to go with it. Iron is essential for the manufacture of haemoglobin, and if a sufficient amount is not available, the cells produced will be smaller and each cell will contain less haemoglobin than normal. Copper and cobalt are other minerals necessary in small amounts. Folates and vitamin B_{12} are also necessary for the normal manufacture of red blood cells. If either is deficient, large abnormal red blood cells without adequate haemoglobin are produced. Ascorbic acid (vitamin C) also has a role in blood formation. Providing vitamin A during pregnancy has been shown to improve haemoglobin levels.

Of the dietary deficiency causes of nutritional anaemias, iron deficiency is clearly by far the most important. Good dietary sources of iron include foods of animal origin such as liver, red meat and blood products, all containing haem iron, and vegetable sources such as some pulses, dark green leafy vegetables and millet, all containing non-haem iron. However, the total quantity of iron in the diet is not the only factor that influences the likelihood of developing anaemia. The type of iron in the diet, the individual's requirements for iron, iron losses and other factors often are the determining factors.

Iron absorption is influenced by many factors. In general, humans absorb only about 10 percent of the iron in the food they consume. The adult male loses only about 0.5 to 1 mg of iron daily; his daily requirement for iron is therefore about 10 mg per day. On an average monthly basis, the adult pre-menopausal woman loses about twice as much iron as a man. Similarly, iron is lost during childbirth and lactation. Additional dietary iron is needed by pregnant women and growing children.

The availability of iron in foods varies greatly. In general, haem iron from foods of animal origin (meat, poultry and fish) is well absorbed, but the non-haem iron in vegetable products, including cereals such as wheat, maize and rice, is poorly absorbed. These differences may be modified when a mixture of foods is consumed. It is well known that phytates and phosphates, which are present in cereal grains, inhibit iron absorption. On the other hand, protein and ascorbic acid (vitamin C) enhance iron absorption. Recent research has shown that ascorbic acid mixed with table salt and added to cereals increases the absorption of intrinsic iron in the cereals two- to fourfold. The consumption of vitamin C-rich foods such as fresh fruits and vegetables with a meal may therefore promote iron absorption. Egg yolk impairs the absorption of iron, even though eggs are one of the better sources of dietary iron. Tea consumed with a meal may reduce the iron absorbed from the meal.

The normal child at birth has a high haemoglobin level (usually at least 18 g per 100 ml), but during the first few weeks many cells are haemolysed. The iron liberated is not lost but is stored in the body, especially in the liver and spleen. As milk is a poor source of iron, this reserve store is used during the early months of life to help increase the volume of blood, which is necessary as the baby grows. Premature infants have fewer red blood cells at birth than full-term infants, so they are much more prone to anaemia. In addition, iron deficiency in the mother may affect the infant's vital iron store and render the infant more vulnerable to anaemia. A baby's store of iron plus the small quantity of iron supplied in breast-milk suffice for perhaps six months, but then other iron-containing foods are needed in the diet. Although it is desirable that breastfeeding should continue well beyond six months, it is also necessary that other foods containing iron be introduced into the diet at this time.

Although most solid diets, both for children and adults, provide the recommended allowances for iron, the iron may be poorly absorbed. Many people have increased needs because of blood loss from hookworm or bilharzia infections, menstruation, childbirth or wounds. Women have increased needs during pregnancy, when iron is needed for the foetus, and during lactation, for the iron in breastmilk. It is stressed that iron from vegetable products, including cereal grains, is less well absorbed than that from most animal products.

Anaemia is common in premature infants; in young children over six months of age on a purely milk diet; in persons infected with certain parasites; and in those who get only marginal quantities of iron, mainly from vegetable foods. It is more common in women, especially pregnant and lactating women, than in men.

In most of the world, both North and South, the greatest attention to iron deficiency anaemia is directed at women during pregnancy, when they have increased needs for iron and often become anaemic. Pregnant women form the one group of the healthy population who are advised to take a medicinal dietary supplement, usually iron and folic acid. Pregnant and lactating women are a group at especially high risk of developing anaemia.

It is only in recent years that the prevalence and importance of iron deficiency apart from anaemia has been widely discussed. Clearly, however, if the causes of iron deficiency are not removed, corrected or alleviated then the deficiency will lead to anaemia, and gradually the anaemia will become more serious. Increasing evidence suggests that iron deficiency as manifested by low body iron stores, even in the absence of overt anaemia, is associated with poorer learning and decreased cognitive development.

International agencies now claim that iron deficiency anaemia is the most common nutritional disorder in the world, affecting over 1 000 million people. In females of child-bearing age in poor countries prevalence rates range from 64 percent in South Asia to 23 percent in South America, with an overall mean of 42 percent (Table 23). Prevalence rates are usually considerably higher in pregnant women, with an overall mean of 51 percent. Thus half the pregnant women in these regions, whose inhabitants represent 75 percent of the world's population, have anaemia. Unlike reported figures for PEM and vitamin A deficiency, which are declining, estimates suggest that anaemia prevalence rates are increasing.

In most of the developing regions, and particularly among persons with anaemia or at risk of iron deficiency, much of the iron consumed is non-haem iron from staple foods (rice, wheat, maize, root crops or tubers). In many countries the proportion of dietary iron coming from legumes and vegetables has declined, and rather small quantities of meat, fish and other good sources of haem iron are consumed. In some of the regions with the highest prevalence of anaemia the poor are not improving their dietary intake of iron, and in some areas the per caput supply of dietary iron may even be decreasing year by year.

In many parts of the world where iron deficiency anaemia is prevalent it is due as much to iron losses as to poor iron intakes. Whenever blood is lost from the body, iron is also lost. Thus iron is lost in menstruation and childbirth and also when pathological conditions are present such as bleeding peptic ulcers, wounds and a variety of abnormalities involving blood loss from the intestinal or urinary tract, the skin or various mucous membrane surfaces. Undoubtedly one of the most prevalent and important causes of blood loss is hookworms (Photo 20), which can be present in very large numbers. The worms suck blood and also damage the intestinal

TABLE 23
Prevalence of iron deficiency anaemia among females of child-bearing age

Region	Prevalence rate (%)
South Asia	64
Southeast Asia	48
Sub-Saharan Africa	42
Near East and North Africa	33
Central America and the Caribbean	28
China	26
South America	23
Overall mean	**42**

Source: UN ACC/SCN, 1992a.

wall, causing blood leakage. Some 800 million people in the world are infested with hookworms. Other intestinal parasites such as *Trichuris trichiura* may also contribute to anaemia. Schistosomes or bilharzias, which are of several kinds, also cause blood loss either into the genito-urinary tract (in the case of *Schistosoma haematobium*) or into the gut. Malaria, another very important parasitic infection, causes destruction of red blood cells that are parasitized, which can lead to what is termed haemolytic anaemia rather than to iron deficiency anaemia. In programmes to reduce anaemia actions may be needed to control parasitic infections and to reduce blood loss resulting from disease as well as to improve dietary intakes of iron.

Anaemia resulting from folate deficiency is less prevalent than that from iron deficiency or iron loss. It occurs when folate intakes are low and when red cells are haemolysed or destroyed in conditions like malaria. The anaemia of both folate and vitamin B_{12} is macrocytic, with larger than normal red blood cells. Folic acid or folates are present in many foods including foods of animal origin (e.g. liver and fish) and of vegetable origin (e.g. leafy vegetables). Vitamin B_{12} is present only in foods of animal origin. In most countries vitamin B_{12} deficiency is uncommon.

CLINICAL MANIFESTATIONS

Haemoglobin in the red blood cells is necessary to carry oxygen, and many of the symptoms and signs of anaemia result from the reduced capacity of the blood to transport oxygen. The symptoms and signs are:

- tiredness, fatigue and lassitude;
- breathlessness following even moderate exertion;
- dizziness and/or headaches;
- palpitations, with the person complaining of being aware of his or her heartbeat;
- pallor of the mucous membranes and beneath the nails;
- oedema (in chronic, severe cases).

These symptoms and signs are not confined to iron deficiency anaemia but are similar in most forms of anaemia. Most occur also in some other illnesses and thus are not specific to anaemia. Because none of the symptoms seem severe, dramatic or life threatening, at least in the early stages of anaemia, the disorder tends to be neglected.

An experienced health worker can sometimes make a preliminary diagnosis by examining the tongue, the conjunctiva of the lower eyelid and the nailbed, which may all appear paler than normal in anaemia. The examiner can compare the redness or pinkness below the nail of the patient with the colour beneath his or her own nails. Enlargement of the heart may result and can be detected in advanced severe anaemia. Oedema usually occurs first in the feet and at the ankles. There may also be an increased pulse rate or tachycardia. Occasionally the nails become relatively concave rather than convex and become brittle. This condition is termed koilonychia. Anaemia is also reported to lead both to abnormalities of the mouth such as glossitis and to pica (abnormal consumption of earth, clay or other substances).

What is surprising is that many persons with very low haemoglobin levels, especially women in developing countries, appear to function normally. With chronic anaemia they have adapted to low haemoglobin levels. They may indeed do reduced work, have fatigue and walk more slowly, but they still give the appearance of performing their normal duties even though severely anaemic. Severe anaemia can progress to heart failure and death.

Anaemia, as well as producing the symptoms and signs discussed above, also leads to a reduced ability to do heavy work for long periods; to slower learning and more difficulty in concentration by children in school or elsewhere; and to poorer psychological development.

A very important aspect of anaemia in women is that it markedly increases the risk of death of the mother during or after childbirth. The woman may bleed severely, and she has low haemoglobin reserves. There is also an increased risk for her infant.

LABORATORY TESTS

The diagnosis of anaemia requires a laboratory test. In this respect it differs from the serious manifestations of PEM, vitamin A deficiency and IDD; kwashiorkor, nutritional marasmus, advanced xerophthalmia, goitre and cretinism can all be diagnosed with some degree of certainty by skilled clinical observation. Consequently, whereas few district hospitals and practically no health centres have laboratories set up to test, for example, levels of serum vitamin A or urinary iodine, most are able to do haemoglobin or haematocrit determinations. These tests require quite cheap apparatus and can be performed by a trained technician, nurse or other health worker.

Determinations of haemoglobin or haematocrit levels are the most widely used in the diagnosis of anaemia. It is now realized that although these tests provide information on the absence, presence or severity of anaemia, they do not provide information on the iron stores of the individual. In terms of nutritional assessment to guide nutrition planning and interventions, or for research, it may be important to know more about the iron status of an individual than can be gained from haemoglobin and haematocrit determinations.

Many methods are used to measure haemoglobin levels. These range from simple colorimetric tests to more advanced tests which require a proper laboratory. Some new portable colorimeters can be used in the field; they are simple to use and provide reasonably accurate measurements. In the laboratory of even a moderate-sized hospital the so-called cyanmethaemoglobin method is frequently used; it is accurate and can be used to test blood collected by finger prick in the field. The different methods and their advantages are discussed in various books, of which some are included in the Bibliography.

Haematocrit level or packed cell volume (PCV), i.e. the percentage of the blood that is packed cells rather than straw-coloured serum, can also be determined by a simple test. Blood (also obtained from a finger prick) is placed in a capillary tube and centrifuged, usually at 3 000 rpm. The centrifuge can be electric (run if necessary from a vehicle battery) or hand operated.

A thin blood film examined under the microscope can be used to judge if the red blood cells are smaller (microcytic) or larger (macrocytic) than normal (normo-cytic). In iron deficiency they are microcytic and in folate or vitamin B_{12} deficiency they are macrocytic. Pale cells are termed hypochromic.

Cut-off points taken from the World Health Organization (WHO) suggestions for the diagnosis of anaemia based on haemoglobin and haematocrit determinations are given in Table 24.

Certain other laboratory tests are useful in judging iron nutritional status rather than for diagnosing anaemia or its severity. In recent years it has been increasingly recognized that iron status is important because mild or moderate iron deficiency, prior to the development of anaemia, may adversely influence human behaviour, psychological development and temperature control. A person whose diet is low in iron or who is losing iron goes through a period when body iron stores (which are mainly in the liver) are gradually depleted before he or she develops anaemia as judged by low haemoglobin or haematocrit levels (see Figure 7). Anaemia is the end stage after iron stores have been depleted. To monitor iron stores it is useful to determine serum ferritin levels, because they are the first to decline. This is not a simple or cheap test to do, and few small

TABLE 24

Suggested criteria for diagnosis of anaemia using haemoglobin (Hb) and haematocrit (PCV) determinations

Subject	Hb below (g/dl)	PCV below (%)
Adult male	13	42
Adult female (non-pregnant)	12	36
Pregnant female	11	30
Child 6 months to 6 years	11	32
Child 6 to 14 years	12	32

Source: WHO, 1975a.

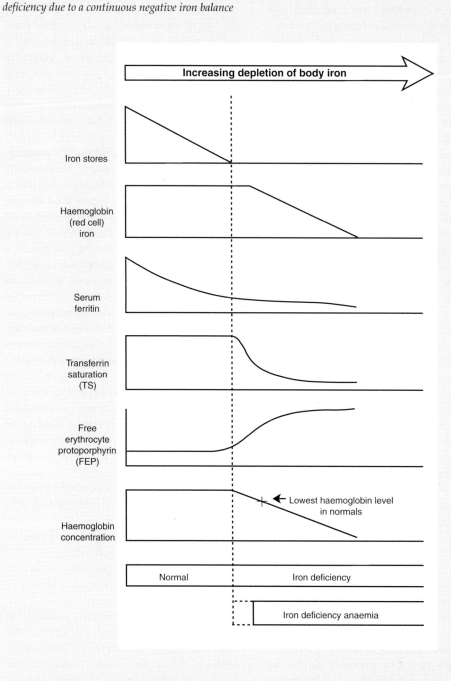

FIGURE 7

Changes in body iron compartments and laboratory parameters of iron status during development of iron deficiency due to a continuous negative iron balance

Increasing depletion of body iron

Iron stores

Haemoglobin
(red cell)
iron

Serum
ferritin

Transferrin
saturation
(TS)

Free
erythrocyte
protoporphyrin
(FEP)

Haemoglobin
concentration

← Lowest haemoglobin level
in normals

Normal

Iron deficiency

Iron deficiency anaemia

Source: International Nutritional Anemia Consultative Group, 1977

or medium-sized hospitals in developing countries have the ability to do it, but teaching hospitals and nutrition research laboratories sometimes can. Unfortunately serum ferritin levels are influenced by infections, which are common in developing countries. Other determinations that may be done to evaluate iron status and which are described in textbooks include free erythrocyte protoporphyrin (FEP) and transferrin saturation (TS) (Figure 7).

TREATMENT

The treatment of anaemia depends on the cause. Iron deficiency anaemia is relatively easy and very cheap to treat. There are many different iron preparations on the market; ferrous sulphate is among the cheapest and most effective. The recommended dose of ferrous sulphate is usually 300 mg (providing 60 mg of elemental iron) twice daily between meals for adults. Iron tends to make the stools black. Because side-effects can occur, particularly involving the intestinal tract, sometimes people do not take their iron tablets regularly. Slow-release iron capsules have become available and seem to be associated with fewer side-effects. Most capsules contain ferrous sulphate in small pellets, so the iron is slowly released. Only one capsule or dose needs to be taken each day, but the capsules cost much more than ferrous sulphate tablets. Therefore it is unlikely that slow-release preparations will replace standard ferrous sulphate tablets for use in clinics in developing countries.

New research conducted in China suggests that ferrous sulphate is as effective when given once every week as when given once a day. If further trials confirm this observation, the finding will alter both the treatment of anaemia and the efforts to prevent it using medicinal iron supplements in prenatal clinics. In Indonesia, where vitamin A deficiency is a problem, it has been shown recently that giving vitamin A as well as iron improves the haemoglobin levels of pregnant women more than iron tablets alone.

Severely anaemic patients who are very ill, vomiting, unable to tolerate oral iron, uncooperative or unlikely to be seen by the doctor again can be given injectable iron preparations and/or treated with packed cell transfusion if facilities are available. In all cases the underlying cause of the anaemia should be sought and treated if possible.

Iron dextran is the injectable preparation most commonly used. Intravenous injection is preferable. The standing rule is to give a very small test dose initially and to wait for five minutes for any sign of an anaphylactic reaction. If there is no reaction, then 500 mg can be given from a syringe over a period of five to ten minutes. These injections may be given at intervals over a few days.

Alternatively, a total dose infusion can be provided at one time. This procedure must be employed only by doctors experienced in the technique and in calculating dosage levels.

It is common during pregnancy to provide folate as well as iron, or combined with iron, as part of the treatment of or prophylaxis against anaemia. For prevention, where anaemia is prevalent, doses of 120 mg of iron and 5 mg of folate daily are recommended. For treatment of established anaemia, doses of 180 mg of iron and 10 mg of folate are suggested.

In vitamin B_{12} deficiency an oral dose of 1 µg vitamin B_{12} daily is needed.

Successful treatment usually leads to a response in haemoglobin levels within four weeks.

Persons with iron deficiency anaemia on very poor diets should be advised to consume more fresh fruits and vegetables at mealtimes. These foods contain vitamin C, which enhances the absorption of non-haem iron in cereals, root crops and legumes. They also contain folic acid and an array of other vitamins and minerals. If it is feasible and in line with the anaemic patient's budget and culinary habits, he or she could also be advised to consume, even in small quantities, more foods rich in haem iron such as meat, especially liver or kidney. Creating awareness of the nutritional needs of different family members and helping household decision-makers to understand how these needs can best be met from available resources are important steps in preventing iron deficiency.

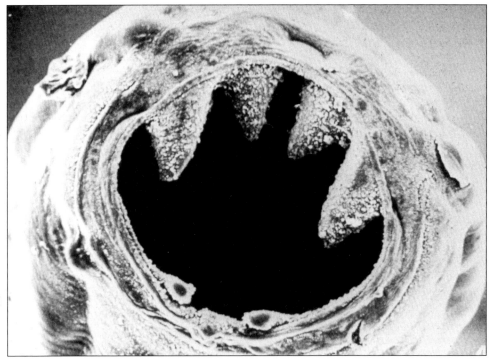

PHOTO 20
The face of a hookworm; hookworms cause blood and iron loss from the intestines and are an
important cause of anaemia

Chapter 14
Iodine deficiency disorders

Iodine deficiency is responsible not only for very widespread endemic goitre and cretinism, but also for retarded physical growth and intellectual development and a variety of other conditions. These conditions together are now termed iodine deficiency disorders (IDD). They are particularly important because:

- perhaps one-quarter of the world's people consume inadequate amounts of iodine;
- the disorders have a major impact on the individual and on society;
- of the four major deficiency diseases, IDD is the easiest to control.

In fact, as H.R. Labouisse wrote in 1978 when he was Executive Director of the United Nations Children's Fund (UNICEF), "Iodine deficiency is so easy to prevent that it is a crime to let a single child be born mentally handicapped for this reason" (quoted in Hetzel, 1989). Nonetheless this crime persists.

Endemic goitre and severe cretinism are the exposed part of the IDD iceberg. These are abnormalities that are visible to the populations where they are prevalent, and they can be diagnosed relatively easily by health professionals without the use of laboratory or other tests. The submerged and larger part of the iceberg includes smaller, less visible enlargements of the thyroid gland and an array of other abnormalities. In many areas of Latin America, Asia and Africa iodine deficiency is a cause of mental retardation and of children's failure to develop psychologically to their full potential. It is also associated with higher rates of foetus loss (including spontaneous abortions and stillbirths), deaf-mutism, certain birth defects and neurological abnormalities.

For several decades the main measure used to control IDD has been the iodization of salt, and when properly conducted and monitored it has proved extremely effective in many countries. It is also relatively cheap. Several international meetings, including the International Conference on Nutrition held in Rome in 1992, called for the virtual elimination of IDD by the year 2000. This goal is achievable, provided the effort receives international support and real national commitment in each of the many countries where the disorders remain prevalent.

CAUSES

The most important cause of endemic goitre and cretinism is dietary deficiency of iodine. The amount of iodine present in the soil varies from place to place and this influences the quantity of iodine present in the foods grown in different places and in the water. Iodine is leached out of the soil and flows into streams and rivers which often end in the ocean. Many areas where endemic goitre is or has been highly prevalent are plateau or mountain areas or inland plains far from the sea. These areas include the Alps, the Himalayas and the Rocky Mountains; smaller mountain ranges or highland areas in countries such as China, the United Republic of Tanzania, New Zealand, Papua New Guinea and countries of Central Africa; and inland areas and plains in the United States, Central Asia and Australia (Figure 8).

A less important cause of IDD is the consumption of certain foods which are

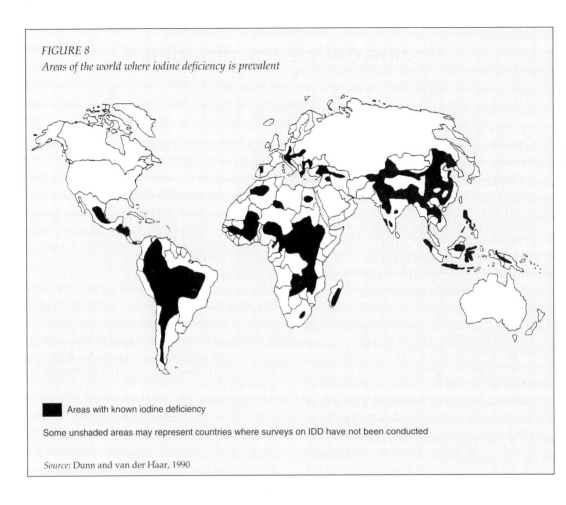

FIGURE 8
Areas of the world where iodine deficiency is prevalent

■ Areas with known iodine deficiency

Some unshaded areas may represent countries where surveys on IDD have not been conducted

Source: Dunn and van der Haar, 1990

said to be goitrogenic or to contain goitrogens. Goitrogens are "antinutrients" which adversely influence proper absorption and utilization of iodine or exhibit antithyroid activity. Foods from the genus *Brassica* such as cabbage, kale and rape and mustard seeds contain goitrogens, as do certain root crops such as cassava and turnips. Unlike goitrogenic vegetables, cassava is a staple food in some areas, and in certain parts of Africa, for example Zaire, cassava consumption has been implicated as an important cause of goitre.

EPIDEMIOLOGY

Any enlargement of the thyroid gland is called a goitre. The thyroid is an endocrine gland centrally situated in the lower front part of the neck. It consists of two lobes joined by an isthmus. In an adult each lobe of the normal thyroid gland is about the size of a large kidney bean. In areas of the world or communities where only sporadic goitre occurs or where health workers see only an occasional patient with an enlarged thyroid gland, the cause is not likely to be related to the individual's diet. Sporadic goitre may for example be due to a thyroid tumour or thyroid cancer. However, if goitre is common or endemic in a community or district, then the cause is usually nutritional. Endemic goitre is almost certainly caused by iodine deficiency, and where goitre is endemic other iodine deficiency disorders can also be expected to be prevalent.

Where goitre is endemic, often large numbers of people have an enlargement of the thyroid gland, and some have enormous unsightly swellings of the neck. The condition is usually somewhat more prevalent in females, especially at puberty and during pregnancy, than in males. The enlarged gland may be smooth (colloid goitre) or lumpy (adenomatous or nodular goitre).

The iodine content of foods varies widely, but the amount of iodine present in common staple foods such as cereals or root crops depends more on the iodine content of the soil where the crop is grown than on the food itself. Because the amount of iodine in foods such as rice, maize, wheat or legumes depends on where they are grown, food composition tables cannot provide good figures for their iodine content. Foods from the ocean, including shellfish, fish and plant products such as seaweed, are generally rich in iodine.

In many populations, particularly in the industrialized countries of the North and among affluent groups almost everywhere, diets do not depend mainly on locally grown foods. As a result many of the foods purchased and consumed may contribute substantially to iodine intakes. For example, persons living in the Rocky Mountains of North America, where goitre used to be endemic, now do not rely much on locally produced foods; they may consume bread made from wheat grown in the North American central plains, rice from Thailand, vegetables from Mexico or California, seafood from the Atlantic coast and so on. Similarly, affluent segments of society in La Paz, Bolivia consume many foods not grown in the altiplano, and these imported foods will have adequate quantities of iodine. In contrast, the poor in the Bolivian highlands eat mainly locally grown foods and do develop goitre.

Many countries of Asia, Africa and Latin America have major iodine deficiency problems, although some countries have made great progress in reducing the prevalence of IDD. China and India, with their vast populations, still have a high prevalence of IDD. Not all African countries have been surveyed, but it is known that IDD is prevalent in Ethiopia, Nigeria, Tanzania, Zaire, Zimbabwe and many smaller nations. In the Americas, endemic goitre has been largely controlled in the United States and Canada, but many Andean countries including Bolivia, Colombia, Ecuador and Peru still have relatively high endemic goitre and cretinism rates. IDD is also encountered in the Central American countries and in parts of Brazil.

During a survey conducted by the author in the 1960s in the Ukinga Highlands of Tanzania, 75 percent of the people examined had goitre. This was the highest prevalence yet reported in Africa. Prevalence rates of over 60 percent have been reported from communities in many African, Asian and Latin American countries.

Generally goitre prevalence rates of 5 to 19.9 percent are considered mild, 20 to 29.9 percent moderate and 30 percent and over severe. But even with rates of 10 to 15 percent the need for action is important. Where prevalence rates are moderate, urgent action is needed. Where rates are severe, early action is critical (see Table 25).

CLINICAL MANIFESTATIONS
Endemic goitre

Enlargement of the thyroid gland is the most frequently described and most obvious clinical manifestation of iodine deficiency (Photos 21 and 22). It is believed that when dietary intakes of iodine fall below about 50 µg per day in adults, the thyroid gland begins to compensate by enlarging slowly over time. Where there is

TABLE 25

Severity and public health significance of IDD

Severity	Clinical features[a]			Typical goitre prevalence (%)	Median urinary iodine (μg/litre)	Need for correction
	Goitre	Hypothyroidism	Cretinism			
Mild (Stage I)	+	0	0	5.0-19.9	>50-99	Important
Moderate (Stage II)	++	+	0	20-29.9	20-49	Urgent
Severe (Stage III)	+++	+++	++	>30	<20	Critical

Source: Adapted from WHO, 1994.
[a] 0 = absent; + = mild/least severe; ++ = moderate/more severe; +++ = most severe.

a chronic dietary deficiency of iodine the thyroid often begins to enlarge during childhood, and it becomes more markedly enlarged around the time of puberty, particularly in girls. In many areas where goitre is endemic the majority of people have some evidence of thyroid enlargement.

The thyroid gland secretes hormones vital to metabolism and growth. The gland is made mainly of follicles called acini, minute sacs filled with colloid. Each sac manufactures thyroid hormones, stores them and secretes them into the bloodstream as needed. The main thyroid hormone is thyroxine. The amount of thyroxine secreted is controlled by another endocrine gland, the anterior pituitary, and its hormone, called thyroid stimulating hormone (TSH) or thyrotrophic hormone. The function of the thyroid gland is somewhat similar to that of the thermostat of the heating system in a house. It controls the rate of metabolism and influences the Basal metabolic rate (BMR), to some extent the heart rate and also growth in children.

The normal adult thyroid gland contains about 8 mg of iodine. In simple goitres the total iodine content might be only 1 or 2 mg even though the gland is larger than normal. Thyroxine contains 64 percent iodine.

A lack of dietary iodine makes it increasingly difficult for the thyroid to manufacture enough thyroxine. The gland enlarges to try to compensate and make more thyroxine. This enlargement is described by pathologists as a hyperplasia of the gland. It is triggered by increased production of TSH by the pituitary gland. Microscopic examination of a gland undergoing hyperplasia shows ingrowths or invaginations of the lining epithelium into the normal architecture of the colloid-containing acini. There is an intense multiplication of cells, with an excess of colloid. This compensatory reaction is an attempt to trap more iodine, and it is partly successful. Many people with colloid goitres show no evidence of poor thyroid function.

Investigation of goitre prevalence is one of the most important means of assessing whether there is an IDD problem of public health importance. Examination of well-chosen samples of schoolchildren has often been recommended as the first step; this survey is relatively easy because schoolchildren are collected together in one place and are usually disciplined, so large numbers can be examined over a short time. To get a full picture of the prevalence in the area, however, it is important at some stage to examine a representative sample of community members of all ages and both sexes.

The thyroid gland of each person should be examined both visually and by palpation to judge its size. Visual examination informs the examiner whether a goitre is visible with the head in normal position or with the head tilted back. Palpation is usually done with the examiner sitting or standing facing the person being examined; the examiner's eyes should be level with the person's neck. By placing and rolling the thumbs on either side of the trachea below the Adam's apple or voice box, the examiner can feel the gland and judge its size. A normal thyroid gland is considerably smaller than the last joint (terminal phalanx) of the thumb. (In fact a normal thyroid lobe is perhaps one-fifth that size.) If each lobe is larger than this joint, then there is a goitre. Palpation from behind is recommended by some because the fingertips are then used to determine gland size, and they are more sensitive than the tips of the thumbs.

It is useful to classify the goitre size using an accepted classification system. Such a system was recommended by the World Health Organization (WHO) over 30 years ago and, as modified by WHO, UNICEF and the International Council for Control of Iodine Deficiency Disorders (ICCIDD), is still used (Table 26). Use of the system assures reasonable comparisons by different observers and in different regions. The main use of grading goitres is for survey purposes and to allow comparisons of goitre prevalence rates between areas. It is not possible to be completely objective, and there will seldom be complete agreement between two examiners, but there will be a reasonable measure of agreement.

Persons with goitre are more likely than others to have manifestations of poor thyroid function, especially hypothyroidism. A large goitre, and especially one that

TABLE 26
WHO/UNICEF/ICCIDD simplified classification of goitre

Grade	Thyroid gland size
0	No palpable or visible goitre
1	A mass in the neck that is consistent with an enlarged thyroid that is palpable but not visible when the neck is in normal position. It moves upwards in the neck as the subject swallows. Nodular alteration(s) can occur even when the thyroid is not visibly enlarged.
2	A swelling in the neck that is visible when the neck is in normal position and is consistent with an enlarged thyroid when the neck is palpated.

Source: WHO, 1994.

enlarges behind the upper part of the sternum, may cause pressure on the trachea and oesophagus, which may interfere with breathing, cause an irritative cough or voice changes and occasionally affect swallowing.

Moderate and large goitres also create an undesirable appearance and possibly difficulty with wearing certain clothes. It has been reported that in some areas where endemic goitre is highly prevalent, goitres may be accepted as the normal condition or as a sign of beauty and people without a goitre may be considered abnormal. However, in the Ukinga Highlands of Tanzania, where prevalence was over 70 percent, the author found that the people were not pleased to have large neck swellings. Many people had symmetrical small scars in the skin covering the goitre, which was clear evidence that they had sought local medical treatment; in East Africa treatment frequently consists of cuts and scarification of the offending area, sometimes with herbal medicines rubbed into the cuts (Photo 23). Clearly these people hoped their goitres would disappear.

Hypothyroidism

If for any reason too little thyroid hormone is produced, the BMR goes down and a condition called hypothyroidism develops, which may lead to the clinical condition called myxoedema. In the adult this condition is characterized by coarsened features, dry skin and sometimes puffiness of the face. The person is often somewhat overweight, has a slow pulse and feels sluggish. Testing would reveal a low BMR and low levels of thyroid hormones in the blood.

In contrast, an overactive thyroid gland producing more thyroid hormone than necessary produces a condition known as hyperthyroidism or Graves' disease. The adult with this condition tends to be thin and asthenic, to be nervous and to have a rapid pulse rate, particularly during sleep. Tests reveal high thyroid hormone levels and high BMR.

As stated above, persons with endemic goitre often have good compensation and do not have evidence of either hypothyroidism or hyperthyroidism. They are said to be euthyroid, which means that they have normal thyroid function despite thyroid enlargement. However, in endemic areas rates of hypothyroidism are elevated. In many cases the hypothyroidism is mild and not as obvious as classical myxoedema, but thyroid hormone levels are low, and low BMR, lower productivity and slower mental functioning may be chronic.

It is hypothyroidism in children, however, that is of most concern for developing countries, because of the strong evidence that it causes both mental retardation and slowing of physical growth. Mental retardation ranges from very severe, which is easy to recognize, to mild, which may be difficult to diagnose. In areas with a high prevalence of IDD large numbers of children may fail to reach their intellectual potential because of impaired school performance and lower IQ than in matched groups from areas without iodine deficiency. These children may later, as adults, fail to make as great a contribution to society and to national development as they would have made if they and their mothers had always consumed adequate amounts of iodine.

Endemic cretinism

Endemic cretinism, including deaf-mutism and mental retardation, begins in infancy. Iodine deficiency in a woman during pregnancy can lead to the birth of a cretinous child. The infant may appear normal at birth but is slow to grow and to develop, small in size, mentally dull, slow to learn and retarded in reaching normal development milestones. Many of these children are deaf mutes. As the child gets older he or she may have the typical appearance of a cretin (Photos 24 and 25), which includes a thick skin, coarse features, a depressed nose, a large protruding tongue and frequently strabismus (the medical term for eyes that look in different directions, cross-eye or squint). At two years of age the child may still be unable to walk unassisted, and at three years he or she may not be able to talk or understand simple commands.

Cretinism may occur in two forms, namely the neurological form and the hypothyroid form. However, many cretins have some manifestations of both. Features of the neurological form include profound mental deficiency; the characteristic appearance; an inability to walk or a shuffling gait; difficulty in controlling exact movements of the hands and feet (spasticity); and sometimes, but not always, an enlarged thyroid gland. Signs of hypothyroidism may or may not be obvious.

In contrast, the hypothyroid cretin by definition has evidence of low levels of thyroid hormone. The child usually has a slow pulse, a puffy face and thick skin; is very retarded in physical growth, in bone age and in mental development; and has low BMR. In much of Asia and in South America (and formerly in Europe) neurological cretinism predominates, whereas in eastern Zaire the myxoedematous form is more widespread. It is not certain if this occurrence is associated with cassava consumption.

In both forms of cretinism the neurological damage, the mental retardation and the dwarfing are not reversible by treatment. Worsening of the condition may be halted, but permanent damage has been done during pregnancy. Therefore the importance of prevention must be emphasized; it is imperative to ensure that women of child-bearing age are not iodine deficient.

Mental retardation

A consequence of iodine deficiency in communities that is perhaps more important than endemic goitre or overt cretinism is the failure of a large number of persons to grow optimally, either physically or mentally, even though they do not have the classical feature of cretinism. In some, neurological functioning may also be abnormal (Photo 26). Increasing evidence suggests that iodine deficiency is a major cause of children's failure to reach their intellectual potential, even for those who are not cretins or severely mentally retarded. School performance may be impaired.

Iodine deficiency in an area may have adverse effects on domestic animals as well as humans. Iodine-deficient cattle, goats and poultry may exhibit poor growth and reproduction.

LABORATORY TESTS

The most widely used laboratory test of iodine nutritional status is determination of urinary iodine. Measurement of urinary iodine excretion should ideally be done on 24-hour urine samples. In the field it is difficult to collect all urine passed over a 24-hour period, so casual urine samples are collected and the amount of iodine in the urine is related to the amount of creatinine and expressed as micrograms of iodine per gram of creatinine (μg/g). If mean iodine excretion is below 50 μg/g creatinine then it is usually concluded that iodine deficiency is a problem in the population. Levels below 20 μg/g creatinine are considered very low. When 24-hour urine collection is done, or where creatinine determinations are not conducted, urinary iodine levels below 5 μg/dl suggest iodine deficiency. Relatively few laboratories in developing countries have the equipment or trained personnel to do urinary iodine determinations. This is not a test that ordinary district or even regional hospitals can perform.

Other laboratory tests that are used are not measures of iodine status, strictly speaking, but of thyroid function. Serum thyroxine (T_4) is measured and if low is evidence of poor thyroid function, which may be related to goitre. An alternative determination which is increasingly recommended is measurement of blood levels of TSH. Radioimmunoassay (RIA) techniques are now preferred for both T_4 and TSH determinations. In most industrialized countries blood is taken from the umbilical cord or heel of all infants born in hospital and sent on filter paper to a special laboratory for determination of thyroxine or TSH. This test is done because about one in 4 000 infants born is hypothyroid because the thyroid gland did not develop properly. If the condition is not diagnosed and treated soon after birth there will be serious consequences, including poor brain development. Congenital hypothyroidism, however, is not related to IDD. Generally T_4 levels below 4 μg percent are considered low, requiring treatment. As with urinary iodine, few hospitals in most developing countries are equipped to do T$_4$ and TSH determinations.

Another test of thyroid function is measurement of radioactive iodine uptake levels, usually using I^{131}, to assess the avidity or "hunger" of the subject's thyroid gland for iodine. In persons with hypothyroidism caused by iodine deficiency, most of the dose of iodine is taken up by the thyroid gland, and less than 10 percent remains.

In the past, protein bound iodine (PBI) in blood plasma was a widely used test.

Some practitioners recommend the use of ultrasonography to produce an image of the thyroid gland, which allows more accurate judgement of the size of the gland than is possible by visual examination and palpation. Ultrasound is being used increasingly in medicine to examine different organs of the body. It is an attractive method because it is non-invasive and does not involve subjection to X-rays. However, in developing countries ultrasonography will seldom be practical for surveys or for assessing IDD problems. The equipment is expensive, and a well-trained technologist is required to operate it and to interpret the results.

It is important for those seriously concerned with IDD assessment and control in Asia, Africa and Latin America to make wise judgements about how best to determine the extent of the problem and to evaluate the effectiveness of control measures. Often it will not be feasible to opt for the use of the more difficult and expensive laboratory methods for assessment of the problem or for evaluation, and even if it is feasible, it may not be a good use of limited financial and personnel resources. These methods, if available in a national or teaching hospital in the capital city or in a national nutrition laboratory, should usually be used mainly for diagnostic purposes for certain patients with metabolic diseases, for well-designed research projects and for subsamples of populations being intensively studied for IDD. They are usually completely inappropriate for mass use in goitre surveys conducted either to assess the extent of IDD or to judge effectiveness of control measures.

TREATMENT

The treatment of goitre caused by iodine deficiency is easy and satisfying in the case of a simple goitre or a colloid goitre that is not very large. Usually either potassium iodide (6 mg daily) or Lugol's iodine (one drop daily for ten days, then one drop weekly) will lead to a fairly rapid reduction in the size of the goitre. One drop of Lugol's iodine provides about 6 mg of iodine. Alternatively, Lugol's iodine can be diluted in any small hospital laboratory so that one teaspoonful of the dilute solution yields 1 mg of iodine. Lugol's solution is very cheap and is widely available. Of primary-school children treated in Tanzania, over 60 percent with Grade 1 goitre had no goitre after 12 weeks of receiving Lugol's iodine, and most larger goitres had improved markedly. An alternative treatment which is also effective but which needs careful medical supervision is the use of thyroid extract or medicinal thyroxine.

Large nodular goitres and some other goitres that do not respond to treatment with either iodine or thyroxine can only be properly treated by surgical excision. Surgery is especially needed if the goitre is causing symptoms because it is retrosternal or pressing on the trachea. Thyroidectomy requires a good well-trained surgeon and good medical management afterwards. Patients who have had total thyroidectomy must receive thyroxine or thyroid hormones for the rest of their lives.

PREVENTION OF IDD

Clearly, rather than treating each individual who has goitre caused by iodine deficiency, it is much preferable to take measures to control iodine deficiency in the community, the district or the nation. The most common, and often the best, measure is iodization of salt, which will reduce the prevalence and also the severity of goitre over a relatively short period among those who consume the salt. Control measures are discussed in detail in Chapter 39.

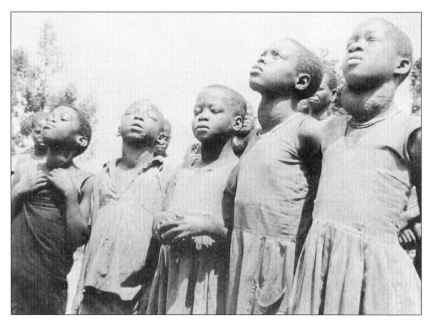

PHOTO 21
Goitre in children in the Ukinga Highlands of Tanzania

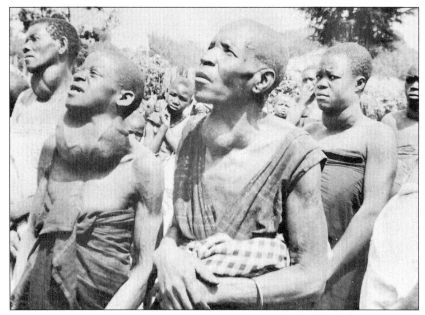

PHOTO 22
Goitre in adults in the Ukinga Highlands of Tanzania

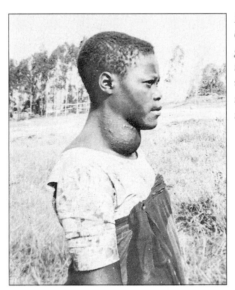

PHOTO 23
Goitre in an adolescent girl, showing patterned marks over the swelling where cuts have been made and traditional medicine applied

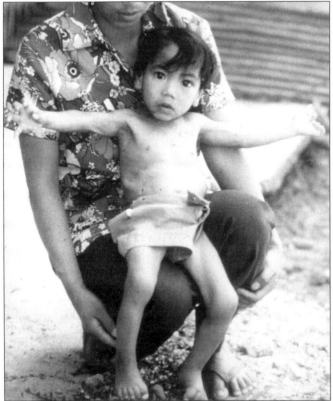

PHOTO 24
Cretin from Asia

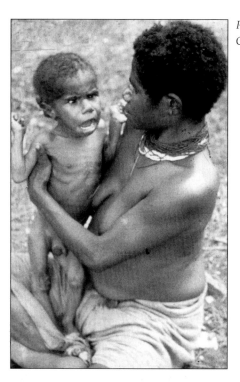

PHOTO 25
Cretin from Africa

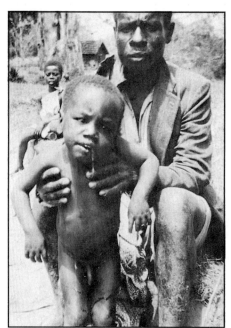

PHOTO 26
*Mental deficiency in a
child of a goitrous
mother*

Chapter 15
Vitamin A deficiency

Vitamin A was discovered in 1913 when experiments showed that if the only fat present in diets of young animals was lard, their growth was retarded, and when butter was substituted the animals grew and thrived. A substance in butter but not in lard was found also in egg yolk and cod-liver oil. It was named vitamin A. It was later established that many products of vegetable origin had nutritional properties similar to those presented by vitamin A in foods of animal origin; they were found to contain a yellow pigment, carotene, which is converted to vitamin A in the body. Preformed vitamin A or retinol is a fat-soluble vitamin found only in animal products. Carotenes or carotenoids can act as a provitamin. There are many carotenoids in plants, but the most important for human nutrition is beta-carotene, which can be converted to vitamin A by enzymatic action in the intestinal wall. Breastmilk is an important source of vitamin A for infants.

Dietary deficiency of vitamin A most commonly and importantly affects the eyes, and it can lead to blindness. Xerophthalmia, meaning drying of the eyes (from the Greek word *xeros*, meaning dry), is the term now used to cover the eye manifestations resulting from vitamin A deficiency. Vitamin A deficiency also has a role in a variety of clinical conditions not related to the eyes, and it may contribute to higher child mortality rates, especially in children who develop measles. It has been demonstrated that laboratory animals on diets deficient in vitamin A have increased rates and severity of infections. Vitamin A deficiency also adversely affects epithelial surfaces apart from the eye and is associated with an increased incidence of certain cancers, including cancer of the colon. The serious eye manifestations of vitamin A deficiency leading to corneal destruction and blindness are mainly seen in young children (Photo 27). This condition is sometimes called keratomalacia.

Until recently vitamin A deficiency was a relatively neglected condition, probably for the following four reasons:

- Public health and nutrition efforts were concentrated on the control of protein-energy malnutrition (PEM), with which vitamin A deficiency is associated, and which is the most important form of malnutrition in non-industrialized countries.
- Where xerophthalmia is prevalent there were few eye specialists or health workers who could correctly diagnose the condition.
- The condition occurs in the very young child behind closed eyelids, or it does not appear to the parents to warrant medical attention until too late, when the cornea is irreversibly damaged.
- Because the fatality rates from advanced xerophthalmia are high, relatively few blind children survive in the community, which reduces the social significance and visibility of the problem.

However, recently the World Summit for Children (1991) and the International Conference on Nutrition (1992) called for the virtual elimination of vitamin A deficiency and its consequences, including blindness, by the year 2000. Much more emphasis is now being placed on the control of vitamin A deficiency.

CAUSES

An inadequate intake of carotene or preformed vitamin A, poor absorption of the vitamin or an increased metabolic demand can all lead to vitamin A deficiency. Of these three, dietary deficiency is by far the most common cause of xerophthalmia.

Good sources of retinol, or preformed vitamin A, are liver, fish-liver oils, egg yolks and dairy products. In most non-industrialized countries, however, the majority of poor people get most, often 80 percent or more, of their vitamin A from carotene in foods of vegetable origin. The yellow colour of carotene may be masked by chlorophyll in many dark green leafy vegetables. Carotenes are present in good quantities in a wide variety of green and yellow vegetables and fruits, in yellow maize and in yellow root crops, e.g. sweet potatoes. A rich source is red palm oil, which is eaten extensively in West Africa and widely grown but infrequently consumed in many other areas, e.g. Malaysia. In many tropical diets important sources are dark green leafy vegetables [e.g. amaranth, cassava and drumstick (*Moringa oleifera*) leaves], mangoes, papayas, tomatoes and sometimes local yellow pumpkins, squash and yellow maize. The wet tropics often abound in both cultivated and wild food sources of carotene, but the poor often consume too little of these foods, and young children often dislike green vegetables. In some seasons the main sources of vitamin A may be less available or more expensive.

The biological activity of vitamin A is now usually expressed as retinol equivalents (RE) rather than in international units (IU). One RE is equal to 1 μg of retinol or 6 μg of beta-carotene. The World Health Organization (WHO) has recommended an intake of 300 RE daily for infants and 750 RE for adults.

Vitamin A, either preformed (retinol) or converted from carotene, is stored in the liver. Retinol is transported from the liver to other sites in the body by retinol binding protein (RBP), a specific carrier protein. Protein deficiency may influence vitamin A status by reducing the synthesis of RBP.

Low intake of vitamin A and carotene over an extended period is the most common cause of xerophthalmia. The condition may be influenced by other factors, however, e.g. intestinal parasitic infections, gastro-enteritis or malabsorption. Measles often precipitates xerophthalmia because it leads to lowered food intake (in which anorexia and stomatitis may be factors) and to increased metabolic demands for vitamin A. The virus may also affect the eye, aggravating lesions caused by vitamin A deficiency. PEM is also important as a cause or accompaniment of xerophthalmia. Data from Indonesia and elsewhere suggest that serious corneal involvement in xerophthalmia seldom occurs except in children who have moderate or severe PEM.

EPIDEMIOLOGY

Vitamin A deficiency is the most common cause of blindness in children in many endemic areas. Xerophthalmia occurs almost entirely in children living in poverty. It is extremely rare to find cases in more affluent families, even in areas where xerophthalmia is prevalent. It is a disease related to low socio-economic status, low levels of female literacy, land shortages, inequity, poor availability of curative and preventive primary health care, high rates of infectious and parasitic diseases (often related to poor sanitation and water supplies) and grossly inadequate family food security. As with PEM, three essentials for prevention of vitamin A deficiency are adequate food security, care and health.

It is always frustrating and extremely sad to see a child with advanced xerophthalmia that includes a perforated cornea when a few days earlier the sight of the child could easily have been saved. A few days and a few cents could have prevented a whole lifetime of blindness. The parents are often poor and uneducated. They love their children, but they may be resigned about the illness because they have inadequate access to good health care, and they may be fatalistic or suspicious of Western medicine. Therefore a small eye problem may not lead the parents to seek early health care even if it is easily available.

In recent decades xerophthalmia has been especially prevalent in children of poor rice-eating families in South and Southeast Asia (e.g. Bangladesh, India, Indonesia and the Philippines). There is a high incidence in some African countries (e.g. Burkina Faso, Ethiopia, Malawi, Mozambique and Zambia), whereas other countries, especially in West Africa, seem to have a lower prevalence in part because of the consumption of red palm oil, which is high in carotene. In the Western Hemisphere, Haiti and northeastern Brazil are areas where xerophthalmia is highly prevalent. It occurs also in many poorer areas of Central and South America. Vitamin A deficiency used to be a problem in the Near East, but few recent data on its prevalence there are available. In poor developing countries where vitamin A deficiency is endemic, it is also prevalent among lactating mothers. In Europe and North America, and in affluent people everywhere, vitamin A deficiency may occur in alcoholics, in those with malabsorption or anorexia nervosa and in persons who for any reason consume diets low in carotene or vitamin A.

Prevalence rates of five different signs have been recommended as criteria for judging whether xerophthalmia is a significant public health problem in a given population (Table 27). It is suggested that

TABLE 27

Prevalence criteria for determining public health significance of vitamin A deficiency

Sign	Prevalence above (%)
Night blindness	1
Bitot's spots	0.5
Corneal xerosis/corneal ulceration/keratomalacia	0.01
Corneal scar	0.05
Plasma vitamin A <10 µg/dl	5

Source: WHO, 1982.

if the prevalence of any one sign (i.e. the percentage of children examined having the sign) in children aged six months to six years in a vulnerable population is above the cut-off, then xerophthalmia should be considered a public health problem in that population.

It is believed that worldwide between 500 000 and 1 million children each year develop active xerophthalmia with some corneal involvement. Of these, perhaps half will become blind or have serious visual impairment, and a large proportion will die. In addition, many millions of children are vitamin A deficient or at risk but do not have xerophthalmic eye manifestations. Deficiency is manifested by low liver stores of retinol and low serum vitamin A levels.

CLINICAL MANIFESTATIONS

Clinical signs of xerophthalmia are illustrated in Figure 9. WHO and others have accepted a classification of the disease according to these signs (Table 28). The classification is now widely used in surveys.

Night blindness (XN) is often the first evidence of vitamin A deficiency; the individual has a reduced ability to see in

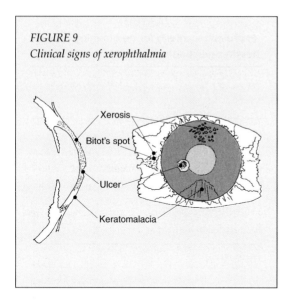

FIGURE 9
Clinical signs of xerophthalmia

dim light. In many countries where xerophthalmia is endemic, there are local terms for night blindness. Parents may notice that their young child is clumsy in the dark or fails to recognize people in a poorly lit room. Night blindness occurs because vitamin A deficiency reduces the rhodopsin in the rods of the retina.

TABLE 28
Classification of xerophthalmia

Ocular signs	Classification
Night blindness	XN
Conjunctival xerosis	X1A
Bitot's spots	X1B
Corneal xerosis	X2
Corneal ulceration/keratomalacia <1/3 corneal surface	X3A
Corneal ulceration/keratomalacia ≥1/3 corneal surface	X3B
Corneal scar	XS
Xerophthalmia fundus	XF

The next sign is drying of the conjunctiva, which is known as conjunctival xerosis (X1A). Patches of xerosis give the appearance of sandbanks at receding tide. The conjunctiva loses its shiny lustre and often becomes thickened, wrinkled and sometimes pigmented.

Sometimes accompanying the conjunctival xerosis are Bitot's spots (X1B), which are usually triangular-shaped, raised whitish plaques that occur in both eyes (Photos 28 and 29). When examined closely they look like a fine foam with many tiny bubbles. This foamy, sticky material can be wiped away. Bitot's spots in the absence of xerosis may have a cause other than vitamin A deficiency.

The next stage is corneal xerosis (X2), drying of the corneal surface, which first appears hazy and then granular on simple eye examination. The drying is followed by a softening of the cornea, often with ulceration and areas of necrosis.

Corneal ulcers are usually circular and punched out in appearance. They may initially be small (X3A), but they may extend centrally to involve much of the cornea (X3B). Ulceration may lead to perforation of the cornea, prolapse of the iris, loss of ocular contents and perhaps destruction of the eye, a condition termed keratomalacia (Photo 30). Although the lesions usually occur in both eyes, the corneal ulceration may be more advanced in one eye. With these severe manifestations the child is also usually seriously ill, sometimes with a high fever.

If treatment is instituted when a corneal ulcer is still small, it will heal, forming a corneal scar (XS). The size of the scar and the limits it imposes on future vision will depend on how large or advanced the corneal ulceration was and its location.

Xerophthalmia of the fundus (XF) is sometimes seen early in the disease under examination with an ophthalmoscope. The retina has white dots around the periphery of the fundus. They disappear following treatment.

The ocular signs of xerophthalmia allow diagnosis on clinical grounds, especially when the condition is moderately advanced. Corneal xerosis and ulceration are easily detected and cannot be mistaken easily for trachoma, which usually begins on the conjunctival surface of the upper lid. A history of night blindness in areas where vitamin A deficiency occurs provides strong evidence of the deficiency. The diagnosis is often missed because the sick child presents with serious PEM (kwashiorkor or nutritional marasmus), measles, tuberculosis, dehydration or some other condition that occupies the attention of the medical attendant. A failure to look into the eyes of a sick child is a common, sad and inexcusable reason for missing xerophthalmia and preventing blindness. The eyes of sick children must always be examined. The only requirement is good natural light or a simple torch or flashlight.

Non-ocular effects of vitamin A deficiency have been described better in experimental animals than in humans. In young animals growth retardation is marked. It is likely that vitamin A deficiency in children has similar consequences, but the association has not been clearly shown. Although vitamin A deficiency depresses immune response, recent detailed studies in Ghana, India, Indonesia, Nepal, the Sudan and the United Republic of Tanzania did not show lower prevalence of most common infections in children receiving regular doses of vitamin A. The prevalence and severity of diarrhoea and respiratory infections were not significantly reduced by vitamin A supplementation. In contrast, there is much evidence that providing vitamin A to children with measles is highly beneficial. Research in several countries showed that providing vitamin A supplements reduced young child mortality by 20 to 40 percent, but a few other studies showed no impact on mortality rates. In areas where supplements reduced mortality significantly, rates of PEM were usually high, measles immunization rates were low and primary health care was poor.

LABORATORY TESTS

Since vitamin A is stored in the liver, a diet deficient in vitamin A results eventually in low hepatic stores. Thus the best way to judge vitamin A nutritional status is to obtain an estimate of the level of vitamin A in the liver. This level can be measured easily only at autopsy.

Determination of serum vitamin A levels is useful for community surveys. Serum retinol levels often fall from normal levels of 30 to 50 µg per 100 ml of plasma to low or deficient levels below 20 µg per 100 ml of plasma. Children with xerophthalmia will usually have levels below 10 µg per 100 ml. Ocular manifestations of xerophthalmia seldom occur before serum vitamin A levels are deficient.

Techniques known as the relative dose response and the modified dose response are now favoured but are more complex. They give a better picture of liver vitamin A stores than does the simple measure of serum vitamin A levels. RBP levels may also be low. Conjunctival impression cytology, in which conjunctival cells are stained and examined microscopically, holds promise for early detection of vitamin A deficiency.

TREATMENT

Effective treatment depends on early diagnosis, immediate dosing with vitamin A and proper treatment of other illnesses such as PEM, tuberculosis, infections and dehydration. Severe cases with corneal involvement should be treated as emergencies. Sometimes hours, and certainly days, may make the difference between reasonable vision and total blindness.

Treatment for children one year of age or over should consist of 110 mg of retinyl palmitate or 66 mg of retinyl acetate (200 000 IU of vitamin A) orally or preferably 33 mg (100 000 IU) of water-miscible vitamin A (retinyl palmitate) by intramuscular injection. Vitamin A in oil should not be used for injection. The oral dose should be repeated on the second day and again on discharge from hospital or seven to 30 days after the first dose. These doses should be halved for infants.

When there is corneal involvement it is desirable to apply an antibiotic ointment such as topical bacitracin to both eyes six times per day. Appropriate systemic antibiotics should also be administered.

Night blindness and conjunctival xerosis are completely reversible and respond quickly to treatment using oral doses of vitamin A on an out-patient basis. Corneal ulceration is arrested by treatment and will heal within a week or two but will leave scars. The case fatality rate is often high because of accompanying PEM and infections.

PREVENTION

In the long term, sustainable control will be achieved by increasing the production and consumption of foods rich in vitamin A and carotene by at-risk populations. Other methods include medicinal supplements, often consisting of high doses of vitamin A every four to six months; fortification of foods; and nutrition education. Control methods are discussed in detail in Chapter 39.

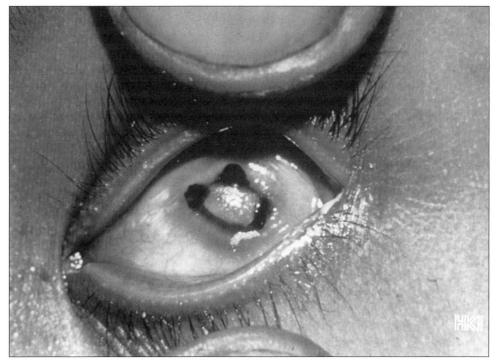

PHOTO 27
Advanced xerophthalmia has destroyed the cornea and blinded the eye

PHOTO 28
Bitot's spots: note abnormal area on temporal side of the eye

PHOTO 29
Under magnification Bitot's spots appear as small white foamy bubbles

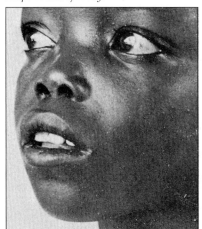

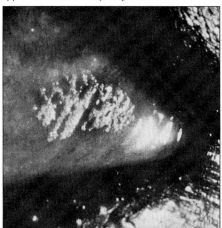

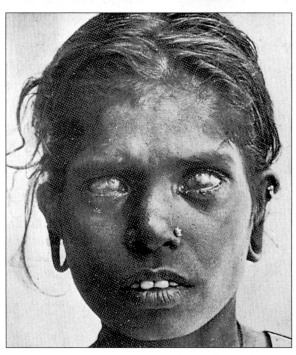

PHOTO 30
Keratomalacia

Chapter 16
Beriberi and thiamine deficiency

Beriberi is a serious disease which was extremely prevalent, particularly in poor rice-eating people in Asia, around the end of the nineteenth century and the beginning of the twentieth. Beriberi, which takes different clinical forms, is caused mainly by thiamine deficiency. Classical cases of beriberi are now reported only sporadically. Because the disease was controlled in the highly endemic areas of Asia some years ago, medical practitioners and public health officials now give less attention to thiamine deficiency and are less familiar than in the past with its manifestations. However, thiamine deficiency leading to a variety of clinical signs, sometimes in conjunction with deficiencies of other vitamins, is not uncommon, but is under-reported. Thiamine deficiency is prevalent in chronic alcoholics in industrialized and developing countries, with manifestations different from beriberi.

CAUSES AND EPIDEMIOLOGY

Experimental investigations in Japan, Indonesia and Malaysia led to medical discoveries that proved that beriberi was a deficiency disease, leading to the discovery of its actual cause (see Chapter 11). Beriberi can be said to be a disease in part caused by new technologies: it became a scourge as the milling industry expanded throughout Asia, providing poor people with highly milled polished rice deprived of its thiamine content, at a financial cost no higher than that of home-pounded rice, but at the cost of many thousands of lives. In Asian countries such as China, Indonesia, Japan, Malaysia, Myanmar, the Philippines and Thailand, beriberi used to

be a major cause of morbidity and mortality in those whose diet consisted mainly of rice. In contrast, people in many parts of the Indian subcontinent were relatively protected from beriberi because they consumed mainly parboiled rice, which conserves enough thiamine. There have been authenticated cases of beriberi in wheat eaters in the Canadian province of Newfoundland and elsewhere, and also in those consuming other staple foods, but high prevalence rates have been confined to rice-eating people.

It has been suggested that an outbreak of disease in Cuba in 1993 may have been caused in part by thiamine deficiency. The manifestations included neurological signs and optic neuritis including loss of sight (see Chapter 22).

Chapter 26 provides details about the nutritional consequences of milling cereals including rice, wheat and maize.

CLINICAL MANIFESTATIONS

There are various ways of dividing beriberi into clinical types. Here it is grouped into three forms: wet beriberi, dry beriberi and infantile beriberi. These conditions have many different features, yet they appear to be caused by the same dietary deficiencies and they occur in the same endemic areas. Wet beriberi is the cardiac form and dry beriberi is the neurological form.

Early clinical features common to both wet and dry beriberi

Wet and dry beriberi usually begin in a similar mild way. The person feels unwell. The legs become tired and heavy and appear to have less power, with some swelling towards evening. There may be a little numbness and some feeling of pins and needles in the legs, as well as occasional palpitations. Activity may continue to be normal, although movement at home or at work may often be reduced, but the person seldom reports to a doctor. Examination would reveal a little loss of motor power of the legs, perhaps some alteration in gait and areas of mild anaesthesia, often over the shin. The condition would improve either with a better diet or with thiamine. If left untreated the condition might continue for months or years, but it could at any stage progress to either wet or dry beriberi. No satisfactory explanation has been given as to why one case develops one way and a second case the other.

Wet beriberi

The patient does not usually appear either particularly thin or wasted. The main feature is pitting oedema, which is nearly always present in the legs but may also be seen in the scrotum, face and trunk of the body. The patient usually complains of heart palpitations and chest pain. Other symptoms include dyspnoea (breathlessness); a rapid, sometimes irregular pulse; and distended neck veins with visible pulsations. The heart is found to be enlarged. The urine, which tends to be diminished in volume, should always be tested for albumin, either in the hospital ward or in a small dispensary. In beriberi no albumin is present, and this feature is an important help in diagnosing a case with oedema.

A patient with wet beriberi, even if he or she looks reasonably well, is in danger of very rapid physical deterioration with the development of sudden coldness of the skin, cyanosis, increased oedema, severe dyspnoea, acute circulatory failure and death.

Dry beriberi

The patient is thin, with weak, wasted muscles. Anaesthesia and pins and needles

in the feet and arms may increase, and the patient gradually develops difficulty in walking, until it is not possible to walk at all. Before this stage is reached, the patient may develop a peculiar ataxic gait. Foot drop and wrist drop commonly occur.

On examination, the main features are wasting, anaesthetic patches (especially over the tibia), tenderness of the calves to pressure and difficulty in rising from the squatting position.

The disease is usually chronic, but at any stage improvement may occur if a better diet is consumed or if treatment is begun. Otherwise, the patient becomes bedridden and frequently dies of chronic infections such as dysentery, tuberculosis or bedsores.

Infantile beriberi

Beriberi is the only serious deficiency disease that commonly occurs in otherwise normal infants under six months of age who receive adequate quantities of breastmilk. It results from inadequate thiamine in the milk of mothers who are deficient in this vitamin, though the mother often has no overt signs of beriberi.

Infantile beriberi usually occurs at two to six months of age. In the acute form, the infant develops dyspnoea and cyanosis and soon dies of cardiac failure. In the more chronic variety, the classical sign is aphonia: the child goes through the motions of crying but, like a well-rehearsed mime, emits no sound or at most the thinnest of whines. The infant becomes wasted and thin, develops vomiting and diarrhoea and, as the disease advances, becomes marasmic because of deficiency of energy and nutrients. Oedema is occasionally seen, and convulsions have been described in the terminal stages.

DIAGNOSIS AND LABORATORY TESTS

The diagnosis of wet, dry and infantile beriberi is difficult when only the early manifestations are present. Evidence of a diet deficient in thiamine in an endemic area and of an improvement on a good diet both help to establish the diagnosis.

Wet beriberi must be distinguished from oedema resulting from kidney disease or congestive cardiac failure. In both of these conditions there is albuminuria. A wrong diagnosis of dry beriberi may sometimes be made in a case of neuritic leprosy that has no obvious skin lesions. In neuritic leprosy the affected nerves, especially the ulnar and peroneal nerves, are palpably thickened and cordlike, whereas in beriberi there is no enlargement. It is often extremely difficult to differentiate infective and toxic neuropathies from dry beriberi, but a full investigation into the patient's history is essential.

In acute infantile beriberi the course of the disease is so rapid that diagnosis is very difficult. In the more chronic form, loss of voice is one of the characteristic signs of the disease. In either form the mother should be examined for signs of thiamine deficiency.

In nutrition status surveys thiamine levels in urine are sometimes used to determine the thiamine status of the community. If 24-hour urine specimens are used or thiamine levels are related to urinary creatinine levels, urine testing can provide evidence of thiamine status. However, for the individual subject urinary thiamine reflects amounts of dietary thiamine consumed in the last 48 hours, and levels may be low without the person's thiamine status being low.

Another method has been to test for elevated blood pyruvate levels following a dose of glucose. The most sensitive test to date is measurement of erythrocyte transketolase activity levels. This test is made more sensitive with the addition of thiamine pyrophosphate (TPP). These tests are usually only available in well-equipped laboratories.

In wet beriberi and infantile beriberi the response to medicinal thiamine is usually dramatic. Non-response is a good indication that the condition is not beriberi.

TREATMENT
Wet beriberi

In wet beriberi the following treatment is recommended:

- absolute bed rest;
- thiamine by intramuscular injection (or intravenously), 50 to 100 mg daily until improvement is shown;
- after injections are discontinued, 10 mg daily by mouth;
- a full nutritious diet rich in foods known to contain thiamine (perhaps supplemented with the vitamin B complex) but low in carbohydrate.

Severe wet beriberi is a most gratifying disease to treat, for the response is in most cases rapid and dramatic. Diuresis and lessening of dyspnoea is observed, and after a few days oedema disappears.

Dry beriberi

Treatment of dry beriberi consists of the following:

- rest in bed;
- 10 mg thiamine daily by mouth;
- a full nutritious diet rich in thiamine and supplemented with the vitamin B complex;
- physiotherapy or splinting of joints, depending on the individual case.

Response to treatment tends to be rather slow, but deterioration of the condition is arrested.

Infantile beriberi

Treatment of infantile beriberi is as follows:

- intramuscular or intravenous injection of 25 mg thiamine when the disease is first seen (can be repeated);
- 10 mg thiamine twice daily by mouth to the mother if the child is being breast-fed, and/or 5 mg to the child;

• provision of thiamine-rich foods or supplements (such as yeast-based products) to the child if the mother is unavailable or the child is not being breastfed.

PREVENTION

People should be encouraged to consume a varied diet containing adequate quantities of vitamin B. If highly milled white rice is the staple diet, part of the rice should be replaced by a lightly milled cereal such as millet, and the diet should be supplemented with foods rich in thiamine such as nuts, groundnuts, beans, peas and other pulses, whole-grain cereals or cereal brans and yeast-based products.

The sale of thiamine-deficient rice and other cereals should be prevented by:

• encouraging the consumption of lightly milled rice and other cereals;
• legislation or other inducement to ensure that all rice put up for sale is lightly milled, parboiled or enriched;
• legislation to ensure vitamin enrichment of cereals made deficient by milling.

Instruction should be given in the most satisfactory ways of preparing and cooking foods to minimize thiamine loss.

Thiamine should be administered in natural food, yeast products, rice polishings or as tablets to certain vulnerable groups in the community.

Nutrition education should be implemented to stress the cause of the disease and to indicate the foods that should be consumed and the ways of minimizing vitamin loss during food preparation.

It is important to strive for early diagnosis of cases of thiamine deficiency and appropriate measures of treatment and prevention.

THIAMINE DEFICIENCY IN ALCOHOLICS

Although classical beriberi is uncommon in industrialized countries, thiamine deficiency is by no means a rarity. It is prevalent in the alcoholic population in countries both North and South. Alcoholism is an increasingly prevalent condition, and several clinical features previously believed to be due to chronic alcoholic intoxication are now known to be the result of nutritional deficiencies. The most common of these conditions is probably alcoholic polyneuropathy, which has similarities to neuritic beriberi and is believed to result mainly from thiamine deficiency.

Alcoholics who get much of their energy from alcoholic drinks often consume insufficient food and do not get adequate amounts of thiamine and other micronutrients. They may develop a peripheral neuritis, which can influence both the motor and the sensory systems, often affecting the legs more than the arms. The various manifestations include muscle wasting, abnormal reflexes, pain and paraesthesia. These symptoms often respond to treatment with thiamine or B-complex vitamins taken orally.

Another condition resulting from thiamine deficiency in alcoholics is Wernicke-Korsakoff syndrome. Wernicke's disease is characterized by eye signs such as nystagmus (rapid involuntary oscillation of the eyeball), diplopia (double vision arising from inequal action of the eye muscles), paralysis of the external rectus (one of the muscles of the eyeball) and sometimes ophthalmoplegia (paralysis of the muscles of the eye). It is also characterized by ataxia (loss of coordination of body movements) and mental changes. Korsakoff's psychosis involves a loss of memory of the immediate past and often elaborate confabulation which tends to conceal the amnesia. It is now generally agreed that any distinction between Wernicke's disease and Korsakoff's psychosis in the alcoholic patient may be artificial; Korsakoff's psychosis may be regarded as the psychotic component of Wernicke's disease. This view is supported by the fact that many patients who appear with ocular palsy, ataxia and confusion, and who survive, later show loss of memory and other signs of Korsakoff's psychosis. Similarly, psychiatric patients with Korsakoff's psychosis often show the stigmata of Wernicke's disease even years after the illness. Pathological evidence also indicates the unity of the two conditions.

That Wernicke-Korsakoff syndrome is caused by thiamine deficiency and not by chronic alcohol intoxication is shown by the fact that the condition responds to thiamine alone, even if the patient continues to consume alcohol. Of overriding importance in this syndrome is the rapid occurrence of irreversible brain damage; early recognition and treatment are therefore vital. A patient at all suspected of having the syndrome should immediately receive 5 to 10 mg of thiamine by injection, even before a definitive diagnosis is made.

Prevention

The prevention of Wernicke-Korsakoff syndrome calls for considerable public health ingenuity. Several possible measures have been suggested:

- the "immunization" of alcoholics with large doses of thiamine at regular intervals (the development of a suitable depot carrier to reduce the frequency of these injections would be very helpful);
- the fortification of alcoholic beverages with thiamine;
- a provision by public health authorities that thiamine-impregnated snacks be made available on bar counters.

The cost of any of these measures would almost certainly be less than the present enormous expenditure on institutional care of those who have suffered from Wernicke-Korsakoff syndrome.

OTHER THIAMINE DEFICIENCY STATES

An optic or retrobulbar neuritis, also known as nutritional amblyopia, that occurred in prison camps during the Second World War was probably caused at least in part by thiamine deficiency not associated with alcoholism. This occurrence may be similar to the serious outbreak of neuropathy disease in Cuba in 1993.

Chapter 17
Pellagra

CAUSES AND EPIDEMIOLOGY

Pellagra, caused mainly by a deficiency of dietary niacin, is generally associated with a maize diet in the Americas, just as beriberi is associated with a rice diet in East Asia.

As mentioned in the discussion of niacin in Chapter 11, a number of factors have at different times been suggested as the cause of pellagra. Each theory seemed, when first expounded, to oppose another. Three of the principal theories appear to have an element of truth. Pellagra was first thought to be caused by a toxin in maize, then by a protein deficiency and finally by a lack of niacin in the diet.

It has now been found that maize contains more niacin than some other cereal foods, but it is believed that the niacin in maize is in a bound form. In Mexico, Guatemala and elsewhere where maize has traditionally been treated with alkalis such as lime water to make tortillas and other foods, consumers have been protected from pellagra. It is possible that lime treatment followed by cooking makes the niacin more available, or perhaps it improves amino acid balance. The human body can convert the amino acid trypto-phan into niacin; thus a high-protein diet, if the protein contains good quantities of tryptophan, will prevent pellagra. None-theless, niacin is still the most important factor in pellagra, and any programme to prevent the disease should aim at pro-viding adequate niacin in the diet. Simi-larly, all cases of pellagra should receive niacin therapeutically.

Pellagra used to be a very prevalent disease in the southern United States, particularly among poor sharecroppers in the early part of the twentieth century. The disease, unknown in Europe in earlier times, became prevalent in the eighteenth and nineteenth centuries as maize for the first time began to be widely eaten in Italy, Portugal, Spain and parts of eastern Europe. In the twentieth century pellagra has been common in Egypt and parts of southern and eastern Africa, and sporadic cases have been reported in India. In each of these areas the disease was associated with maize becoming the staple diet of poor people who could afford very little else to supplement the diet.

The highest prevalence in recent times has probably been in South Africa, where conditions for some agricultural and industrial workers until 1994 were not unlike those in the southern United States between 1900 and 1920. A report from South Africa suggested that 50 percent of patients seen at a clinic in the Transvaal had some evidence of pellagra, and that the majority of adults admitted to the mental hospital in Pretoria had the disease.

Pellagra regrettably has also been widely reported in refugee camps and in famine situations where maize has been the relief food and relief agencies have given too little attention to providing a balanced diet or adequate micronutrient intakes. An outbreak of pellagra occurred during a drought in central Tanzania in the 1960s when the affected people were consuming mainly donated maize from the United States. The pellagra was quickly controlled using niacin supplements.

CLINICAL MANIFESTATIONS

Persons suffering from pellagra usually appear poorly nourished. They are often rather weak and underweight. The disease is characterized by "the three Ds": dermatitis, diarrhoea and dementia (Figure 10). Mild sensory and motor changes such as diminished sensitivity to gentle touch, some muscular weakness and tremor all occur. A wide variety of other signs have been described. Paralysis, however, is rare. Untreated cases of pellagra may die of the disease.

Dermatitis

The disease is most often diagnosed from the appearance of the skin, which has characteristic lesions (Photo 31). The lesions occur on areas of the skin exposed to sunlight, such as the face, the back of the hands, the neck, the forearms and exposed portions of the leg. This pellagrous dermatitis begins with a deepening of the pigmentation. The hyperpigmented areas lose the oily sheen of healthy skin and become dry, scaly and eventually cracked. There is usually a definite line of demarcation between these lesions and the healthy skin, and this line can be felt, for the affected area is rough to the touch. The skin condition may remain static, heal or progress. If it progresses, desquamation commonly occurs; there may be cracking and fissuring, or occasionally the skin may blister. The blisters contain a colourless exudate. Areas that have shed a layer of skin are sometimes shiny, thin and rather depigmented. All these skin lesions are usually more or less symmetrical.

In white subjects the skin lesions initially look like the erythema of sunburn. In both black and white patients, the lesions of pellagra produce burning sensations and pain when exposed to the direct rays of the sun, just as sunburn does in a person with pale skin. The lesions may also correspond with a hole or holes in a

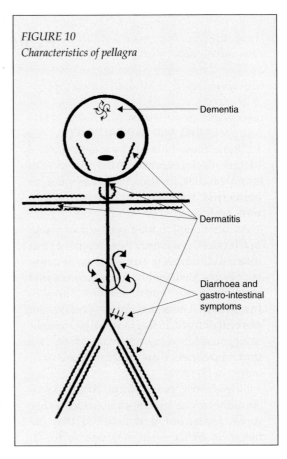

FIGURE 10
Characteristics of pellagra

Dementia

Dermatitis

Diarrhoea and gastro-intestinal symptoms

frequently worn garment which allowed the sunlight to reach the skin. For example, the classic Casal's necklace around the neck and upper chest (Photo 32) results from the sun playing on this part of the body in a subject wearing an open-necked shirt.

The tongue and other parts of the mouth are often sore, red, smooth and raw-looking. Angular stomatitis and cheilosis, usually associated with riboflavin deficiency, are frequently observed.

Diarrhoea

Bouts of abdominal pain, diarrhoea and other digestive upsets are frequently associated with pellagra. It is believed that changes similar to those that occur in and around the mouth are present in various other parts of the alimentary tract, and these may be the cause of abdominal discomfort and intestinal burning. Few if any of these symptoms and signs are specific to pellagra, but if they accompany skin changes or mental symptoms or respond to niacin, a diagnosis of pellagra is supported.

Dementia

Involvement of the nervous system is manifested by extremely variable symptoms and signs. The most common are irritability, loss of memory, anxiety and insomnia. These symptoms may lead to dementia, and it is not uncommon in practice for persons with dementia resulting from pellagra to be admitted to mental institutions. All cases of insanity, especially where maize is the staple food and where pellagra occurs, should therefore be examined for other signs of pellagra.

DIAGNOSIS AND LABORATORY TESTS

The skin lesions are usually characteristic in appearance. Lesions that are symmetrical and on surfaces of the body exposed to sunlight substantiate the diagnosis. The symptoms and signs involving the alimentary canal and nervous system are not often specific. The dietary history, the presence of skin changes, the appearance of the mouth and above all a good response to niacin are indicative. In children the stunted growth or wasting of protein-energy malnutrition may also be present.

Assessment of urinary excretion of N-methylnicotinamide is used both in nutritional surveys and in evaluation of individual patients for niacin deficiency. In six-hour urine collections, nicotinamide levels between 0.2 and 0.5 mg are considered low, and a level below 0.2 mg indicates niacin deficiency. In random urine specimens, deficiency is suggested by less than 0.5 mg nicotinamide per gram of creatinine. Urinary levels are more useful for providing information on recent consumption of niacin and tryptophan, however, than for the diagnosis of pellagra. Nevertheless, normal amounts of N-methylnicotinamide in urine may help rule out pellagra as the diagnosis.

TREATMENT

The following treatment is recommended for pellagra.

- Admission to hospital and rest in bed are desirable for serious cases. Milder cases may be treated as out-patients.
- The patient should be given 50 mg of niacin (nicotinic acid, nicotinamide) three times a day by mouth.
- The diet should contain at least 10 g per day of good protein (if possible, meat, fish, milk or eggs; if not, groundnuts, beans or other legumes) and should be high in energy (3 000 to 3 500 kcal per day).
- Because the patient may also have a deficiency of other B vitamin components, a vitamin B complex preparation or a yeast product should be prescribed.
- Sedation for a few days is recommended. Those with mental disturbances benefit greatly from any of a number of tranquillizers, for example, valium. The sedative should be given orally, but if the patient is uncooperative more potent tranquillizers may be needed by injection.

Pellagra is often a very gratifying disease to treat. Violent, almost uncontrollable mental patients can become normal, rational, peaceful human beings within a few days of taking a few tablets of nicotinamide. In persons with severe skin lesions, a sore mouth and severe diarrhoea with frequent watery stools, dramatic improvements occur within 48 hours. The skin redness and pain on exposure to sunlight improves; pain in the mouth abates and eating becomes a pleasure for the patient; and most gratifying for the patient, the intractable diarrhoea disappears.

PREVENTION

The following steps can help in the prevention of pellagra.

- Diversity in the diet is important. Reliance on maize as the sole staple foodstuff should be discouraged, and the consumption of other cereals in place of part of the maize should be encouraged. This is less necessary in those parts of the Americas where maize is treated with lime.
- Production and consumption of foods known to prevent pellagra, i.e. those rich in niacin, such as groundnuts, and those rich in tryptophan, such as eggs, milk, lean meat and fish, should be increased.
- Legislation or other inducement should be put in place to ensure the enrichment of milled maize meal with niacin.
- Niacin tablets should be administered as a prophylaxis in prisons and institutions in areas where pellagra is endemic, and to refugees and in famine relief.
- Nutrition education should be provided to teach people what foods can prevent the disease.

An important lesson to be learned from past experience in the southern United States and current experience in South Africa is that pellagra will be controlled if the conditions for poor agricultural and industrial workers are improved. In the United States the end of slavery, the reduction of sharecropping on southern farms and improvements in wages, working conditions and food supplies had more impact in reducing pellagra than did fortification or medicinal nicotinamide supplements. Recent political changes in South Africa are likely to change and improve the working conditions and diets of poor Bantu in that country and to reduce the prevalence of pellagra there.

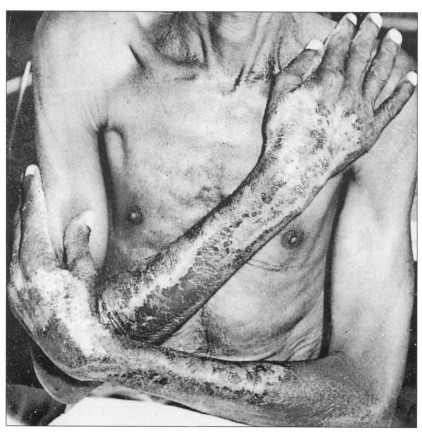

PHOTO 31
Dermatitis affecting exposed surfaces in pellagra

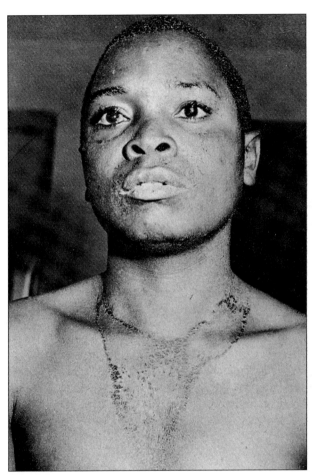

PHOTO 32
Casal's necklace in pellagra

Chapter 18
Rickets and osteomalacia

CAUSES AND EPIDEMIOLOGY

The main feature of both rickets and osteomalacia is a lack of calcium in the bones; rickets occurs in children whose bones are still growing, and osteomalacia in adults who have formed bones. The conditions are, however, caused mainly by a deficiency of vitamin D and not by a dietary lack of calcium. As described in Chapters 10 and 11, vitamin D is obtained both from animal foodstuffs in the diet and from exposure of the skin to sunlight. Vitamin D functions like a hormone in regulating calcium metabolism.

Because the body can obtain adequate amounts of vitamin D from even moderate exposure to sunlight, rickets and osteomalacia are uncommon in most African, Asian and Latin American countries, where sunlight is abundant. Where the diseases do occur, they are usually caused in part by a particular cultural practice or local circumstance. For example, in some Muslim societies women practising purdah wear clothes that cover most of the skin, and they and their babies may rarely leave the household. Rickets is reported in some large, densely populated cities (e.g. Calcutta, India; Johannesburg, South Africa; Addis Ababa, Ethiopia), presumably mainly in children who do not get out in the sunlight. Rickets and osteomalacia are now being diagnosed in immigrant families of Asian origin in the United Kingdom. However, nowhere in the tropics or subtropics is rickets a highly prevalent disease, as it was in Europe in the nineteenth century (see Chapter 11).

Severe rickets usually occurs in children under four years of age who consume only small quantities of foods of animal origin and who for any reason do not have much exposure to sunlight. The bony deformities, however, may be most obvious in older children. Osteomalacia is most common in women who have had several children, who have become depleted of calcium as a result of successive pregnancies and lactation, and who have insufficient vitamin D.

CLINICAL MANIFESTATIONS
Rickets

Children with rickets, unlike those with most other deficiency diseases, often are plump and appear well fed because their energy intake is usually adequate. The appearance frequently misleads the mother into thinking all is well. The child, however, tends to be miserable, and closer examination will reveal the flabby toneless state of the muscles that causes a pot-belly. Another feature of the disease is a general impairment of normal development. The child is late in reaching all the milestones of early life, such as learning to sit, walking and teething. Other generalized symptoms include gastro-intestinal upsets and excessive sweating of the head.

The main signs of the disease, however, and those on which the diagnosis of rickets is made are bone deformations (Photo 33). The first and main feature is a swelling at the growing ends (epiphyses) of the long bones. This swelling may first be found at the wrist, where the radius is affected. Another classic site is the junction of the ribs with the costal cartilage, where swelling produces a beadlike appearance known as "rickety rosary".

Swellings of the epiphyses of the tibia, fibula and femur may also be seen. In infants with rickets the anterior fontanelle closes late, and in older children a bossing of the frontal bone is found.

Once a child with rickets begins to stand, walk and become active, she or he develops new deformities because of the soft, weak character of the bones. The most common deformity is bow-legs (Photo 34); less frequently knock-knees are seen. More serious, however, are deformities of the spine. Changes in the pelvis, though often not visible, may lead to difficulty in childbirth in women who have had rickets in childhood.

Rickets can be diagnosed from the clinical and X-ray appearance of the bones and by laboratory tests.

Osteomalacia

Osteomalacia is characterized by pain, sometimes severe, in bones, particularly in the pelvis, lower back and legs. Tenderness may sometimes be felt in the shins and in other bones. The patient usually walks with feet rather widely separated and may appear to waddle. Deformities of the pelvis may be obvious. Tetany may occur; it may be manifested by involuntary twitching of the muscles of the face or by carpopedal spasm (in which the hand goes into rigid spasm with the thumb pressed into the palm). Spontaneous fractures may be a feature. Before the deformities are clinically detectable, diagnosis may be made by X-ray examination, which will show rarefaction or decalcification of bones all over the body. Osteomalacia should not be confused with osteoporosis, a disease of ageing, in which decalcification is also a feature.

LABORATORY FINDINGS

Levels of vitamin D metabolites and sterols in blood, which can now be measured in sophisticated laboratories, are always very low in cases of both rickets and osteomalacia. Low serum phosphorus and high serum alkaline phosphatase levels are also seen. Usually the amount of calcium in urine will be low.

TREATMENT
Rickets

The basis of treatment is to provide vitamin D and calcium. Vitamin D may be given as cod-liver oil. Three teaspoonfuls three times a day will supply about 3 000 IU, which is adequate. Synthetic calciferol can also be used. Calcium is best given as milk, at least half a litre a day. Cows' milk contains 120 mg calcium per 100 ml.

Tablets containing vitamin D and calcium are available. One of these may be given twice a day to a child under five years of age, and one tablet three times a day to an older child.

While the child is being treated, the mother should be educated regarding the value of sunshine. Rickets, unless severe, is not usually a fatal disease *per se*, although the child may be more prone to infectious diseases.

Mild bone deformities tend to right themselves with treatment, but in more severe cases some degree of deformity may persist. One of the more serious consequences is obstructed childbirth due to pelvic abnormalities, which may necessitate Caesarean section in hospital.

Osteomalacia

The treatment of osteomalacia is similar to that for rickets. A dose of 50 000 IU vitamin D should be given daily as cod-liver oil or in some other preparation. Calcium should be provided either as milk or, if milk is not available, in some medicinal form such as calcium lactate.

In women with pelvic deformity regular antenatal care is essential, and in some cases Caesarean section before term may be necessary.

PREVENTION

The prevention of rickets and osteomalacia will depend on the reasons for their occurrence in the particular communities where they are now seen. Usually there is a cultural or environmental cause which may be locally specific and which may need particular attention.

Rickets

Measures should be taken to ensure that all children get adequate amounts of sunlight. In temperate climates such measures include slum clearance; smoke abatement; the provision of parks, play-grounds, open yards and gardens; and regular outings for the young.

Children should have adequate calcium and vitamin D in their diets. Milk and milk products are especially valuable.

Where it is not possible to expose children to adequate sunlight, vitamin D supplements such as cod-liver oil should be given.

Children should attend clinics regularly so that early diagnosis of rickets can be made and curative measures taken.

Nutrition education should be provided regarding the needs for calcium and vitamin D and the methods by which adequate amounts of them can be obtained.

Osteomalacia

The body should be exposed to adequate sunlight. (This need may conflict with religious or social customs, e.g. those requiring women to be heavily covered or veiled, or those forbidding women to go out in public.)

It is important to ensure that a diet containing adequate quantities of calcium and vitamin D is consumed, especially by pregnant and lactating women.

Clinics or home visiting should be established to allow examination of pregnant and lactating women and, where necessary, to issue cod-liver oil or other vitamin D supplements. Advice should be given regarding the consumption of calcium-rich foods. Sometimes medicinal calcium (e.g. calcium lactate) will have to be prescribed.

Nutrition education should be provided, and it should include the topic of child spacing.

PHOTO 33
Ethiopian child with rickets

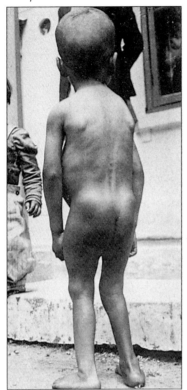

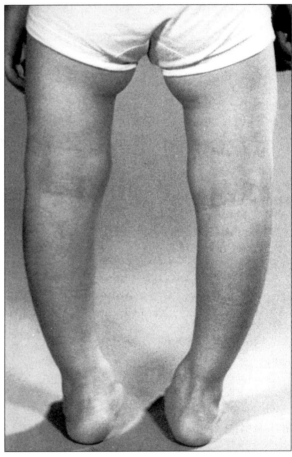

PHOTO 34
Bowing of the legs in a European child with rickets

Chapter 19
Vitamin C deficiency and scurvy

CAUSES AND EPIDEMIOLOGY

Dietary surveys in many countries in Asia, Africa and Latin America indicate that large segments of their populations consume much lower amounts of vitamin C than is considered essential or desirable. Nevertheless scurvy, the classical and serious disease that results from severe deficiency of vitamin C, now appears to be relatively uncommon. No country reports scurvy as a major health problem, but outbreaks are seen in refugee camps, during famines and occasionally in prisons.

Scurvy was first recognized in the fifteenth and sixteenth centuries as a serious disease of sailors on long sea voyages who had no access to fresh foods including fruits and vegetables (see Chapter 11). Before the era of vitamin research it became practice in the British navy to provide limes and other citrus fruit to prevent scurvy.

Vitamin C or ascorbic acid is an essential nutrient and is necessary for the formation and healthy upkeep of intercellular material (see Chapter 11); it is like a cement that binds cells and tissues. In scurvy the walls of the very small blood vessels, the capillaries, lack solidity and become fragile, and bleeding or haemorrhage from various sites results. Moderate vitamin C deficiency may result in poor healing of wounds.

As discussed in Chapter 13, vitamin C enhances the absorption of iron and thus has a role in reducing iron deficiency anaemia.

Some oral contraceptives lead to lowered plasma vitamin C levels.

CLINICAL MANIFESTATIONS

The following symptoms and signs may occur:
- tiredness and weakness;
- swollen gums which bleed easily at the base of the teeth (Photo 35);
- haemorrhages in the skin (Photo 36);
- other haemorrhages, e.g. nosebleeds, blood in the urine or faeces, splinter haemorrhages below the fingernails or subperiosteal haemorrhages;
- delayed healing of wounds;
- anaemia.

A patient who has scurvy and exhibits some of the above symptoms, though not appearing very seriously ill, may suddenly die of cardiac failure.

Although scurvy is a relatively rare disease, swelling and bleeding of the gums occur fairly frequently in certain regions and may be due to vitamin C deficiency. Subclinical vitamin C deficiency may also result in the slow healing of wounds or ulcers. Patients who are to undergo surgery should be given vitamin C if they may be deficient.

Vitamin C deficiency may also contribute to anaemia in pregnancy.

Infantile scurvy (Barlow's disease)

Scurvy sometimes occurs in infants, usually aged two to 12 months, who are bottle-fed with inferior brands of processed milk. During the processing of the milk, the vitamin C is frequently destroyed by heat. Good brands of processed milk are fortified with vitamin C to prevent scurvy.

The first sign of infantile scurvy is usually painful limbs. The infant cries when the limbs are moved or even touched. The child usually lies with the legs bent at the knees and hips, widely separated from each other and externally rotated, in what has been termed the "frog-leg position". Bruising of the body may be seen, although it is difficult to detect in darkly pigmented African skin. Swellings may be felt, especially in the legs. Haemorrhages may occur from any of the sites mentioned above, but bleeding does not take place from the gums unless the child has teeth.

DIAGNOSIS AND LABORATORY TESTS

The capillary fragility test is not specific for scurvy but may be useful. It is simple to perform in any health facility. The cuff of a blood pressure machine or sphygmomanometer is placed around the upper arm. It is inflated to a pressure approximately midway between the subject's systolic and diastolic pressure (perhaps 100 mm Hg) and left in place for four to six minutes. In a positive test, numerous small red spots appear in the skin below the cuff; these are petechial haemorrhages arising from capillary fragility. The test is a little more difficult in very dark-skinned people, but usually the anterior surface of the lower arm is pale enough for recognition of petechial haemorrhages.

Ascorbic acid levels can be determined in blood plasma or in white blood cells. These levels provide evidence of body reserves of vitamin C. If the level of ascorbic acid in either the blood plasma or the white blood cells is within the normal range, the condition almost certainly is not scurvy.

In infantile scurvy X-ray examination will reveal periosteal haemorrhages, which together with clinical signs provide the diagnosis.

TREATMENT

Because of the risk of sudden death, it is inadvisable to treat scurvy with only a vitamin C-rich diet. It is advisable rather to give 250 mg ascorbic acid by mouth four times a day as well as to put the patient on a diet with plenty of fresh fruit and vegetables. It is only necessary to inject ascorbic acid if the patient is vomiting.

Increased intake of vitamin C with meals can have a manifest effect on the absorption of iron. In many iron-deficient populations, increasing vitamin C intake will help reduce the incidence and severity of iron deficiency anaemia.

PREVENTION

Vitamin C deficiency can most easily be prevented in all societies by consumption of adequate amounts of fresh foods, particularly generous intakes of fruits and vegetables, including green leaves. Guavas and various other tropical fruits, for example, are high in vitamin C. (These foods are described in Chapter 28, and the vitamin C content of foods is given in Annex 3.)

Recommended preventive measures are as follows:

- increased production and consumption of vitamin C-rich foods, such as fruit and vegetables;
- provision of vegetables, fruit and fruit juice to all members of the community, including children, beginning in the sixth month of life;
- provision of vitamin C concentrates if for any reason the previous two measures are not possible;
- improved horticulture, including the provision of village and household gardens, orchards and vegetable allotments in towns and school gardens;
- encouragement of the wide use of edible wild fruits and vegetables known to be rich in vitamin C (e.g. amaranth, baobab fruit);
- action to avoid and discourage the replacement of fresh vegetables, fruit and other foods by canned and pre-

served foodstuffs, and encouragement of the greater use of fresh fruit and juices in place of bottled products;

- nutrition education, which should cover the reasons and need for eating fresh foods, and instruction in means of minimizing vitamin C loss in cooking and food preparation.

PHOTO 35
In scurvy the gums are swollen between the teeth and bleed easily

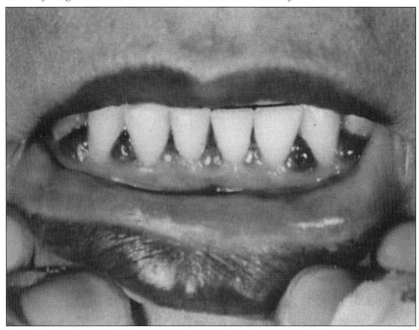

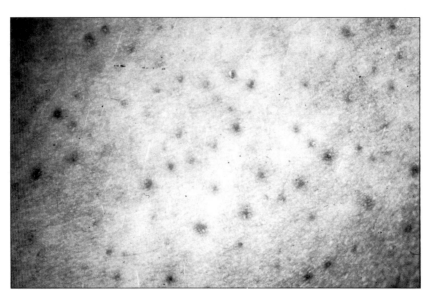

PHOTO 36
Petechial haemorrhages in the skin resulting from vitamin C deficiency

Chapter 20
Zinc deficiency

Zinc is an essential nutrient (see Chapter 10) and is apparently deficient in the diets of many people in both industrialized and non-industrialized countries. In nutrition journals in the 1990s more is published on zinc and zinc deficiency than on protein-energy malnutrition (PEM). However, zinc deficiency is not claimed as a major public health problem in any country in the world, and no clear disease syndrome is described for zinc deficiency. In Egypt and the Islamic Republic of Iran a condition in males characterized by dwarfism and hypogonadism (poor development of sexual organs) is associated with zinc deficiency. In the United States and elsewhere, low zinc status in children has been associated with retarded growth, poor appetite and impaired sense of taste.

An extremely rare congenital disease known as acrodermatitis enteropathica results in the child's inability to absorb zinc properly. The condition used to be fatal but is now known to respond to zinc therapy. It is characterized by a serious dermatitis, poor growth and diarrhoea.

Laboratory animals on zinc-deficient diets (usually more severely deficient in zinc than any normal human diet) have exhibited anorexia, decreased efficiency of feed utilization, poor growth, depressed gonadal function, impaired immunity, poor healing of wounds and dermatitis. When a zinc-deficient diet was fed to pregnant rats and monkeys, poor behavioural development was observed in their offspring. It is likely that any or all of these signs and symptoms would occur in humans on a very deficient diet, but apparently most human diets provide enough zinc to prevent these more serious manifestations.

It is not surprising that zinc deficiency is often associated with PEM. A diet that is deficient in total amounts of energy and protein is also likely to be deficient in zinc and many other micronutrients. Many children with PEM have low levels of zinc in blood and hair, but these low levels do not prove that their PEM is due to zinc deficiency. A better diet, including more food, would prevent both PEM and zinc deficiency.

Research currently being conducted in several countries may show that in certain populations zinc supplementation can improve poor growth, perhaps by improving appetite which leads to improved dietary intake and better growth. It may also be shown that zinc can improve the functioning of the immune system and in this way reduce morbidity due to infections, thus reducing PEM.

Zinc is present in most foods of vegetable and animal origin. Good sources include flesh from chicken, fish or mammals (pork, beef, mutton), legumes and whole-grain cereals. The United States recommended dietary allowance (RDA) for zinc for an adult is 15 mg daily. It is unlikely that signs of zinc deficiency would arise if intakes were 5 to 8 mg daily, but absorption of zinc, like that of iron (see Chapter 13), is quite variable. In cases of kwashiorkor and nutritional marasmus treated in hospital, oral zinc supplements may be recommended. Some paediatricians claim that the zinc supplementation speeds recovery, and it can do no harm.

Chapter 21
Dental caries and fluorosis

Dental caries is not a deficiency disease. However, it is human beings' most prevalent disease and it is one of the most expensive diseases to treat and to prevent. Dental disease is the only disease that a medical doctor is not trained to treat; its treatment is left to a special category of health professionals.

Fluorosis is a condition that arises from excess intake of a mineral nutrient, not a deficiency. It is also discussed in this chapter because it is a nutritionally related condition of teeth (and bones). The properties of fluoride and its role in malnutrition were discussed in Chapter 10. Fluoride in water, in toothpaste or painted on the teeth makes the tooth enamel more resistant to dental caries.

DENTAL CARIES
Dental caries is the medical term for tooth decay, including cavities in teeth. It begins as a loss or destruction of the outer mineral layers of the tooth. Decay tends to be progressive, with loss of minerals and then loss of tooth protein and formation of tooth cavities (Photo 37). The decay may lead to pain, tooth destruction and sometimes infection of surrounding tissues (abscess). Dental caries is an example of an interaction of nutrition and infection.

Three factors contribute to dental caries (Figure 11):
- host factors, namely a susceptible tooth surface;
- the presence of bacterial flora, usually the pathogenic organism *Streptococcus mutans*, which is cariogenic;
- the presence of a suitable substrate, that is carbohydrate adherent to or

between the teeth which allows the bacteria to survive and flourish.

Carbohydrates are broken down and produce organic acids such as lactic acid which lead to demineralization of the teeth. Formerly sucrose was considered particularly culpable. Recent studies have highlighted the fact that caries prevalence correlates well with sucrose consumption in communities where oral hygiene is poor and where fluoride is absent, but not elsewhere. It is now recognized that any fermentable carbohydrate is equally able to lead to dental caries.

Control of dental caries can in theory involve attempts to control or moderate

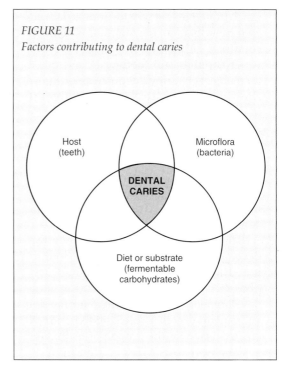

FIGURE 11
Factors contributing to dental caries

any of the three factors that contribute to the disease. Adequate intakes of fluoride make the tooth surface less vulnerable to caries; mouthwashes can reduce the bacterial presence; and appropriate eating habits can reduce the contact of teeth with sticky carbohydrate, while tooth brushing can remove carbohydrate adherent to the teeth.

In surveys dental caries is assessed by counting the number of decayed (D), missing (M) and filled (F) teeth in each person examined. The total number of D, M and F teeth gives a DMF index. In a survey conducted in the United Republic of Tanzania in 1964, schoolchildren aged six to 14 years had a DMF index of 0.2; that is, an average of one child in five had one affected tooth. In contrast, in a ten-state survey in the United States in 1968, the DMF index for children aged six to 14 years was 7; that is, the average child had seven decayed, missing or filled teeth.

Twenty-five years ago it would have been true to say that dental caries was much more prevalent in the industrialized countries than in the non-industrialized countries. However, with fluoridation of water supplies and toothpaste and other methods of ensuring adequate amounts of fluoride, and with improved dental hygiene and education, dental caries has declined in Western countries. In contrast, with modernization, changing diets and more frequent consumption of fermentable carbohydrates, dental caries has increased in the developing countries, particularly in urban areas of Africa, Asia and Latin America.

Many nutrients are necessary for the development of teeth and their surrounding structures. Vitamin D, calcium and phosphorus, which are important in bone development, are also essential for the development of teeth. Protein and vitamin A are necessary for the growth of teeth, and as has been described, vitamin C is

essential for healthy gums. In terms of preventing or reducing dental caries, however, fluoride is the most important nutrient.

In the 1930s it was observed that persons who had access to drinking-water that contained one to two parts per million (ppm) of fluoride had considerably less tooth decay than those whose water supply had much lower amounts of fluoride. It was subsequently found that in areas where the water had very little fluoride, it was possible to reduce the incidence of dental caries by 60 to 70 percent by adjusting the fluoride level of the water to about 1 ppm.

Figure 12 shows a comparison of DMF teeth in two cities in the state of New York, United States: Kingston, where there was

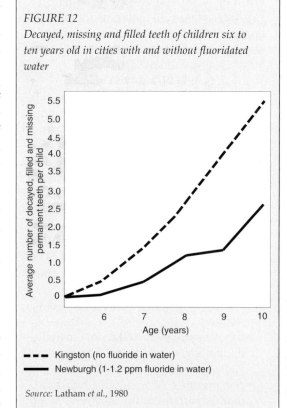

FIGURE 12

Decayed, missing and filled teeth of children six to ten years old in cities with and without fluoridated water

- - - Kingston (no fluoride in water)
——— Newburgh (1-1.2 ppm fluoride in water)

Source: Latham *et al.,* 1980

no fluoride in the municipal water, and Newburgh, which had optimum amounts of fluoride. It can be seen that at age ten years children not receiving fluoride in drinking-water had 5.5 DMF teeth compared with 2.5 in those receiving fluoride. Other studies have shown even larger reductions as a result of fluoridation (Figure 13).

It is now generally agreed that the appropriate amount of fluoride needed in urban water supplies is about 1 ppm, but each city should decide on the level appropriate to its population.

There is no doubt that the fluoridation of water supplies is a public health measure of very great importance. Every physician, dentist and health worker has a responsibility to urge and support fluoridation of the water supply where needed. Fluoridation has been found to be absolutely safe at 1 ppm for people of all ages and in every state of health. Fluoridation is not a form of medication, only an adjustment of the level of a nutrient, like the fortification of bread with vitamins. It is not an infringement of individual rights.

There are substitutes for fluoridation such as pills, drops and fluoridated toothpaste, but none combine the efficiency, practicality, effectiveness and economy of fluoridation for the general public. It should be appreciated that the increased rates of dental caries where water is not fluoridated have the most serious implications for the poor, who cannot afford, or do not have access to, good dental care.

Another means to reduce dental caries is nutrition education to teach parents and children about cariogenic diets and associated risks; education can encourage better dental hygiene, including brushing of teeth and removal of food from between teeth with toothpicks, dental floss or, as is common in much of Africa, a traditional cleaning stick.

In older people the main cause of tooth

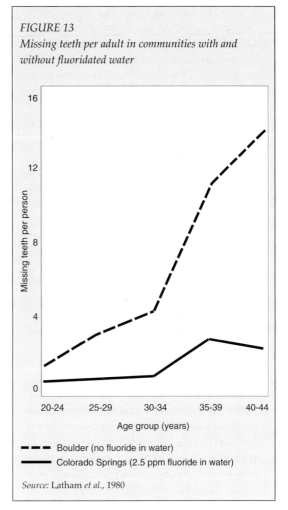

FIGURE 13
Missing teeth per adult in communities with and without fluoridated water

Missing teeth per person vs Age group (years)

- ▬ ▬ Boulder (no fluoride in water)
- ▬▬ Colorado Springs (2.5 ppm fluoride in water)

Source: Latham *et al.*, 1980

loss is periodontal or gum disease. This condition usually begins with the formation of plaque (sometimes called tartar or calculus) by bacteria that survive on carbohydrate adhering to the teeth. Plaque between the teeth and close to the gums may lead to secondary infection, to receding and bleeding gums and eventually to loss of supporting bone and loss of teeth. Cleaning teeth, scraping away plaque and chewing fibrous foods help reduce periodontal disease. In a study of poor women in the United States, some 40 percent between 40 and 50 years of age had lost all of their teeth. In contrast, few Africans living in rural areas have had periodontal disease rampant enough to cause such a loss of teeth. Traditional diets are often relatively protective against both dental caries and plaque formation. Western diets are a risk factor.

FLUOROSIS

In some parts of the world, including certain areas of India, Kenya and Tanzania, natural water supplies contain much higher than desirable levels of fluoride. Intake of water that contains more than about 4 ppm will result in widespread dental fluorosis in the population. In this condition the teeth become mottled and discoloured (Photo 38). At first the teeth have chalky white patches, but soon brownish discoloured areas develop. Fluorosis is not a serious condition, but local people may not like it.

Of more seriousness is skeletal fluorosis, which may result from prolonged intake of water containing high fluoride levels of 4 to 15 ppm. A survey in northern Tanzania revealed a high incidence of fluorotic bone abnormalities in older subjects who normally drank water containing high levels of fluoride. X-ray examinations showed that the bones were very dense or sclerotic and that abnormal calcification was common in ligaments between the vertebra, where tendons link muscles to bones, and in interosseous areas, for example in the forearm (Photo 39). Skeletal fluorosis may cause back pain and rigidity and neurological abnormalities.

DENTAL CARE

In most poor developing countries there are too few dentists to meet the needs of the population. Usually the ratio of dentists per 100 000 people is much higher in the large cities and extremely low in rural areas. Many countries have acknowledged that most of the dental care needed,

including diagnosis and treatment such as fillings, extractions and plaque removal, does not need to be provided by a dentist. New Zealand pioneered the use of dental auxiliaries, and now many developing countries train dental assistants or other dental health workers. These workers have much shorter training than dentists and cost much less to employ, but they are fully able to take adequate care of most dental conditions. The few dentists are treated in the same way as other medical specialists; particularly complicated or difficult cases are referred to them. In many countries strong dental associations have opposed the use of dental auxiliaries and have prevented them from doing much of the dental work. This bar is a disservice, especially when even in rich countries like the United States the poor often cannot get adequate dental care.

PHOTO 37
Dental caries

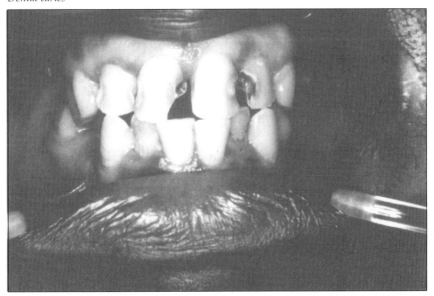

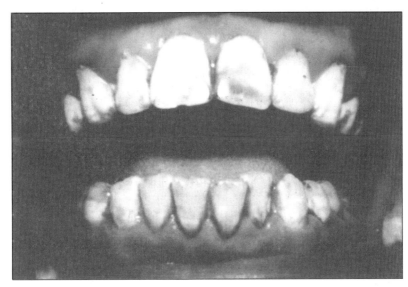

PHOTO 38
Mottling of the teeth in dental fluorosis

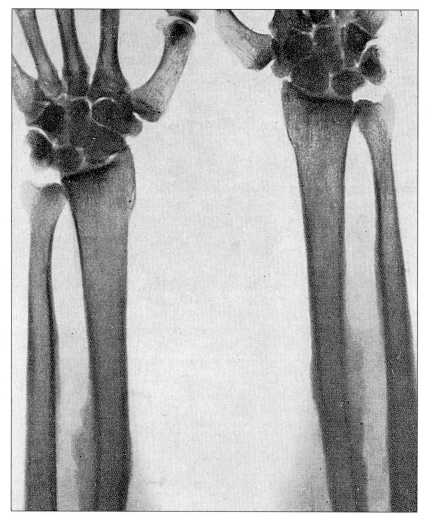

PHOTO 39
X-ray of the forearms of a person with skeletal fluorosis, showing increased bone density and calcification between the radius and ulna

Chapter 22

Other micronutrient deficiencies and minor nutritional disorders

NUTRITIONAL NEUROPATHIES

The nervous system is the communications system within the body, and it is a highly complicated mechanism. If it does not function properly there can be important consequences. The nervous system needs oxygen and nutrients and obtains its energy from carbohydrates. A range of complex enzymes controls its functioning. These enzymes are proteins, and their activities require the participation of a number of vitamins. It is not surprising therefore that dietary deficiencies can cause symptoms and signs indicating impairment or damage to the nervous system.

The relationship between diet and the nervous system is still not fully understood, and the subject is beyond the scope of this book. Nevertheless it is important for all medical persons to keep in mind that any disease of the nervous system may have a nutritional origin. If it is impossible to obtain a proper diagnosis of a nutritional disease, the sufferer should be advised and helped to eat a balanced diet.

The B group of vitamins has a special place in relation to the nervous system. These vitamins are commonly found in the outer layers of cereal grains. Milling tends to reduce the quantity of B vitamins in cereal flours. Deficiencies of B vitamins are therefore common, and cases of various neuropathies are likely to increase. For example, an outbreak of a neuropathy in a Tanzanian institution was caused by a change in diet from lightly milled to highly milled maize meal as the main source of energy.

Neuropathies may lead to weakness and pins and needles in the feet, severe burning pains, ataxia, nerve deafness, disturbances of vision, absent or exaggerated reflexes and other symptoms. There is much overlap in the causation of many of these conditions, and classification is difficult.

The neurological signs of dry beriberi and of thiamine deficiency in alcoholics (alcoholic polyneuropathy and the so-called Wernicke-korsakoff syndrome) were described in Chapter 16, and the burning feet syndrome in pantothenic acid deficiency was mentioned in Chapter 11. These are all either polyneuropathies affecting the peripheral nerves or are caused by lesions of the central nervous system (in Wernicke's encephalopathy). It is likely that patients with mixed forms are often not correctly diagnosed. It can be difficult to distinguish accurately between neurological complications resulting from nutrient deficiencies and those resulting from toxins (for example, lathyrism, described in Chapter 34) or drugs.

As discussed below, vitamin B_6 deficiency secondary to treatment of tuberculosis with isoniazid leads to a polyneuritis. The cause of a recent outbreak of optic neuritis and an epidemic neuropathy in Cuba has not been definitively determined. The outbreak has subsided but was almost certainly the result of a nutrient deficiency, most probably a dietary deficiency of thiamine. Konzo, an epidemic neurological disease, occurs as a result of excessive cyanide intake in those eating toxic cassava (see Chapters 26 and 34).

RIBOFLAVIN DEFICIENCY (ARIBOFLAVINOSIS)

A dietary deficiency of riboflavin resulting in clinical signs is very prevalent worldwide, in both industrialized and non-industrialized countries. In the United States a ten-state nutrition survey showed poor riboflavin status in over 12 percent of all subjects and in 27 percent of black people examined. In most studies in poor countries riboflavin deficiency is found to be much more prevalent, often affecting 40 percent of the people. As described below, the main clinical features are lesions of the mouth. A deficiency does not cause either life-threatening disease or serious morbidity.

The most frequently seen abnormalities in riboflavin deficiency are angular stomatitis and cheilosis of the lips (Photo 40). Angular stomatitis consists of fissures or cracks in the skin radiating from the angles of the mouth. Sometimes the lesions extend to the mucous membrane inside the mouth. The cracks have a raw appearance but may become yellowish as a result of secondary infection. In cheilosis there are painful cracks on the upper and lower lips. The lips may be swollen and denuded at the line of closure. The lesions may be red and sore or dry and healing.

Glossitis (inflammation of the tongue) occasionally develops involving a patchy denudation, papillary atrophy and so-called magenta tongue. These conditions are not caused exclusively by riboflavin deficiency.

Scrotal dermatitis in males and vulval dermatitis in females have been particularly well described in experimentally induced riboflavin deficiency. The affected skin is usually intensely itchy and tends to desquamate.

Abnormalities in the eyes including redness and vascularization (visible blood vessels), photophobia and lacrimation have been associated with riboflavin deficiency.

A skin condition named dyssebacia may occur near the nose.

Affected persons often have several signs of deficiency at the same time (Figure 14).

In surveys laboratory assessment of riboflavin status has usually been based (as with other water-soluble vitamins) on urinary excretion of the vitamin. A level below 30 µg of riboflavin per gram of creatinine is considered low. Riboflavin status in the individual is better determined by measuring the increased activation of red blood cell (erythrocyte) glutathione reductase. Few hospital laboratories in developing countries are able to do these tests.

Treatment consists of large oral doses of riboflavin for a few days, followed by lower doses which may need to be taken for a long time unless a diet rich in

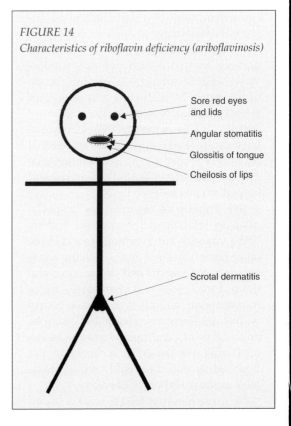

FIGURE 14

Characteristics of riboflavin deficiency (ariboflavinosis)

Sore red eyes and lids

Angular stomatitis

Glossitis of tongue

Cheilosis of lips

Scrotal dermatitis

riboflavin is consumed. A dose of 10 mg riboflavin twice a day for one week, followed by 4 mg daily for several weeks, is recommended. Dietary intakes of around 1 to 1.5 mg daily will be protective. Milk is a particularly rich source of riboflavin.

PYRIDOXINE OR VITAMIN B$_6$ DEFICIENCY

A primary dietary deficiency of vitamin B$_6$ resulting in symptoms of disease is very rare, because even poor diets contain adequate quantities of this vitamin.

Pyridoxine deficiency occurs in developing countries mainly secondary to treatment of tuberculosis with the medicine isoniazid. This drug, which is highly effective and can be taken by mouth, was introduced as a treatment for tuberculosis in the early 1950s and became widely used, in part replacing injection of streptomycin which was until then the most common treatment. Despite the development of other medicines, isoniazid is still widely used. Tuberculosis, largely controlled in industrialized countries in the 1970s, is now in resurgence, with drug-resistant cases and cases related to acquired immunodeficiency syndrome (AIDS) worrying public health officials. In many African and Asian countries tuberculosis has remained prevalent and is an important cause of morbidity and mortality.

Isoniazid taken in large doses over long periods is very likely to precipitate vitamin B$_6$ deficiency. It is said to increase vitamin B$_6$ needs.

The deficiency is usually manifested by neurological abnormalities, including a peripheral neuritis which may involve severe pain in the extremities, including the legs. Experience in East Africa showed that because of the pain rural patients were often unable to walk to health centres for examination or to obtain their medicine.

It is strongly recommended that tuberculosis patients being treated with isoniazid be given 10 to 20 mg pyridoxine by mouth

daily. Unfortunately, pyridoxine is much more expensive than isoniazid, so providing the vitamin greatly increases the cost of treatment.

It has been suggested that in certain parts of the world, particularly in Thailand, low intakes of vitamin B$_6$ may be responsible for bladder stones. It is known that vitamin B$_6$ increases oxalate excretion in urine and that vitamin B$_6$ deficiency leads to an increased risk of oxalate stone formation in the kidney or bladder.

Hormonal contraceptive pills have been associated with both folate and vitamin B$_6$ deficiencies. However, the newer birth control pills have not been shown to result in vitamin B$_6$ deficiency. Oral vitamin B$_6$ tablets have been claimed to reduce the nausea of some women in the first months of pregnancy.

An extremely rare congenital disease called pyridoxine-responsive genetic disease leads to hyperirritability, convulsions and anaemia in the first few days of life. Unless treated very early with vitamin B$_6$ the child develops serious permanent mental retardation.

MINOR NUTRITIONAL DISORDERS AND CLINICAL SIGNS

The most important and serious diseases resulting from nutritional deficiencies have already been covered. They have been described in terms of syndromes or disease entities and have not been classified according to their aetiology. Other clinical conditions may also arise from dietary deficiencies, and some of them may lead to the diseases described earlier. Some have physical signs that can be observed but cause little disfigurement or disability. Some conditions have a specific, known aetiology. Other conditions, although they may occur commonly in malnourished persons, may not have had their exact cause elucidated. All are of some importance and should be looked for because they can lead a medical worker into an investigation of the diet of a patient and can thus serve to prevent the onset of more serious disease. They should especially be sought in routine examinations of groups of persons, such as those carried out in schools, prisons and institutions, or during medical surveys of a community. These minor disorders can serve as indicators of the dietary status of the community as a whole.

Dry scaly skin or xerosis

Normal skin is smooth and slightly oily and has a healthy sheen. In xerosis the skin loses these characteristics and becomes dry, scaly and rather rough to the touch. Pieces of the skin tend to flake off much as in dandruff of the scalp. This condition is thought to be caused mainly by vitamin A deficiency. However, lack of protein and fat may also have a part.

Crazy-pavement or cracked skin (mosaic dermatosis)

This condition is commonly found on the lower leg. The skin resembles a paved walk or the sun-baked and cracked bed of a dried-up mud swamp. There are islands of fairly normal skin, each surrounded by a shallow crack. The edges may be scaly or desquamating. Protein and vitamin A deficiencies may have a part in causing the disorder; dirt and alternate exposure to dryness and moisture under hot conditions may also be causative factors.

Follicular hyperkeratosis

Type I follicular hyperkeratosis consists of lesions that feel spiky to the touch, consisting of multiple horny dry papules. They are most commonly seen on the backs of the arms. On close inspection they are seen to arise from the hair follicles. This condition is associated with a deficiency of vitamin A and possibly also of riboflavin.

Type II follicular hyperkeratosis is similar in appearance and occurs commonly on the trunk or thighs. The surrounding skin is less dry, and the mouths of the hair follicles are seen to contain brown-pigmented denatured blood. This condition is possibly caused by vitamin C deficiency.

Dyssebacia (naso-labial seborrhoea)

This condition, in which plugs of yellowish keratin stand out from the follicles, is usually seen on each side of the nose but sometimes extends to other parts of the face. It is believed to be caused by riboflavin deficiency.

Scrotal (or genital) dermatitis

The skin of the scrotum (or the genital region in females) is affected, becoming dry and irritated. There may be desquamation, intense itching and secondary infection. Riboflavin deficiency (and possibly deficiency of other B vitamins) seems to be the cause.

Oedema of the tongue

The tongue is swollen, with notches on the sides corresponding to the teeth. The papillae are usually prominent. This condition is associated with deficiency of riboflavin and niacin.

Atrophic tongue

The tongue is much smoother than normal, usually reddened (magenta-coloured) and denuded of normal papillae. It may be painful. This condition may be caused by a lack of niacin and other B vitamins.

Patchy glossitis

In patchy glossitis the tongue shows patchy desquamation; the patches are often red and inflamed oval areas. This condition is usually the result of riboflavin deficiency and may sometimes be accompanied by oedema of the tongue.

Parotid swelling

Swelling of the parotid gland can be felt as a firm area just in front of and slightly below the meatus (hole) of the ear. The swelling is usually bilateral. It may disappear completely after a balanced diet is consumed for six to 12 months. The condition is possibly associated with protein deficiency.

Tropical ulcers

Tropical ulcers affect the lower leg and may be single or multiple. They are chronic, sometimes large and often grossly infected. The cause has not been fully elucidated but is possibly nutritional. Tropical ulcers are rare in well-nourished persons.

THE NUTRITION EXAMINATION

At the nutrition examination, the name, sex and age of the individual should be recorded. If the subject is female, it should be noted if she is pregnant or lactating. Table 29 summarizes the signs to look for in the examination. The following measurements should also be taken:

- height,
- weight,
- skinfold thickness (for which special callipers are necessary),
- haemoglobin,
- haematocrit,
- serum ferritin,
- arm circumference,
- chest circumference,
- head circumference.

It is also important to note other observations that may have a bearing on the case, e.g. parasitic infection or scarred cornea.

A list of deficiency disorders is given in Table 30.

TABLE 29

Signs to look for in a nutrition examination

Part of body examined	Possible changes or disorders
Hair	Colour change Texture change
Eyes	Bitot's spots Xerosis and xerophthalmia Keratomalacia Pallor of the conjunctiva of the lower lid Vascularization of the cornea
Mouth	Angular stomatitis Cheilosis Glossitis Atrophic tongue Oedema of tongue Mottled teeth Carious teeth Swollen or bleeding gums Pallor of tongue
Skin	Oedema Follicular hyperkeratosis Crazy-pavement skin Dry scaly skin Hyperpigmentation Ulcers Haemorrhages Pallor beneath nails
Central nervous system	Apathy Irritability Anaesthesia or sensory changes Calf tenderness Abnormal gait Loss of reflexes Poor mental development Dementia
Skeleton	Deformity (e.g. knock-knees) Rickety rosary Bony swelling Skeletal fluorosis
Other	Thyroid enlargement

TABLE 30

Deficiencies and associated signs

Deficiency	Associated disorder	Deficiency	Associated disorder
Vitamin A	Follicular hyperkeratosis, Type I Night blindness Bitot's spots Conjunctival xerosis Corneal xerosis Keratomalacia Possibly also dry scaly skin and crazy-pavement skin	Vitamin D	Deformity Rickety rosary Bony swelling Bow-legs Knock-knees
		Protein-energy	Muscle wasting Apathy Irritability

Riboflavin
(ariboflavinosis)
	Angular stomatitis
	Cheilosis of lips
	Scrotal or genital dermatitis
	Possibly also follicular
	   hyperkeratosis, oedema of the
	   tongue, magenta tongue and
	   patchy glossitis
	Vascularization of the cornea
			Oedema
			Dermatosis
			Hair changes
			Weight reduction
			Height reduction
			Small arm circumference
			Reduced skinfold thickness

		Iodine	Enlargement of thyroid Cretinism Deaf-mutism Mental retardation
Thiamine	Oedema Anaesthesia Calf tenderness Abnormal gait Various central nervous system signs	Fluorine	Dental caries Mottled teeth[a] Bone changes[a]
Niacin	Hyperpigmentation Pellagrous dermatitis Atrophic tongue Diarrhoea Mental signs	Iron	Anaemia Pale conjunctiva of lower lid Pallor of tongue Pallor of nailbed Poor growth Poor appetite
Vitamin C	Swollen or bleeding gums Petechial or other skin haemorrhages Other haemorrhages Follicular hyperkeratosis, Type II Tender subperiosteal swellings		

[a] From excess, not deficiency, of fluorine.

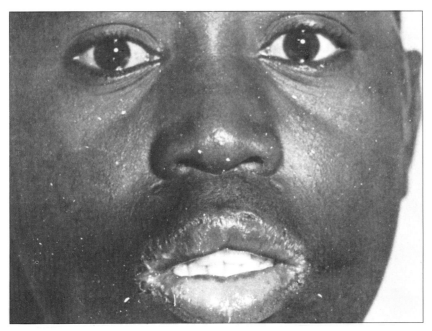

PHOTO 40
Angular stomatitis and cheilosis of the lips resulting from riboflavin deficiency

Chapter 23
Chronic diseases with nutritional implications

In the relatively wealthy industrialized countries most nutrition research, teaching and action relates to certain chronic diseases in which diet has a role. These include obesity, arteriosclerosis and coronary heart disease, hypertension or high blood pressure (which may lead to stroke), certain cancers, osteoporosis, dental caries and tooth loss, some liver and kidney diseases, diabetes mellitus, alcoholism and other diseases. Most of these diseases have known dietary or nutritional factors in their aetiology or in their treatment, or in both. It is now evident that the incidence of many of these chronic diseases or conditions is increasing in developing countries, especially in more affluent sections of their populations. Some countries are witnessing a transition from the major nutritional problems related to poverty and underconsumption, which are covered in detail in other chapters of this book, to nutrition-associated diseases related to overconsumption and affluence. In other countries there is less a transition than a situation in which one part of the population has problems related to poverty and undernutrition and another has problems related to affluence, more sedentary lifestyles and overconsumption of energy or of certain foods.

The implications of the transition or of the coexistence of different nutritional conditions in two parts of the population present significant public health problems for these nations. It is important that the countries consider appropriate agricultural, public health and other policies that could mitigate or even avert the bad effects of these changes.

It is striking that in the United Kingdom between about 1942 and 1947, when very strict rationing was imposed as a result of the Second World War, the British people were probably better nourished than ever before or after. Severe restrictions were put on each family, particularly regarding the amount of meat, butter, eggs, edible fat and other foods of animal origin in their diets. Fruits and vegetables were not rationed. Rationing applied to both the rich and the poor, and it is believed to have been rather fairly implemented. The rich certainly reduced their intake of foods of animal origin, and the poor received their fair share. Both groups of the population benefited nutritionally. Even mortality rates from diabetes were markedly lowered.

Rationing of foods is not suggested as a strategy in normal times. However, the British experience suggests that more equitable consumption of certain foods may be nutritionally beneficial to both segments of the population, reducing both undernutrition and overnutrition.

It has been recognized that excessive intake of energy, certain fats, cholesterol, alcohol and sodium (mainly salt) and decreased consumption of fruits, vegetables and fibres coupled with sedentary lifestyles contribute importantly to increased incidence of chronic diseases in the affluent sectors of most communities around the world. These diseases are often described as nutritional diseases of affluence, which is an easy but misleading description. Factors other than income influence the changing incidence of these diseases, and in many more affluent countries it is the poor who suffer most from these diseases.

This chapter provides a brief discussion of the causes, manifestations and prevention of some of the more important nutrition-associated chronic diseases:

- arteriosclerotic heart disease,
- hypertension or high blood pressure,
- diabetes mellitus,
- cancer,
- osteoporosis,
- other conditions.

In some of these diseases the cause is clearly dietary; in others diet may be important in contributing to the cause or in treatment; and in some the relationship to diet is suspected but not proven.

These very important diseases and their nutritional implications are described in detail in major textbooks of nutrition and medicine used in industrial nations of the North. Because the aim of this book is mainly to assist developing countries of the South with their major nutritional problems, only minor attention is given here to these chronic diseases. Readers wanting more detailed information on these conditions are advised to refer to other publications, especially the major nutrition textbooks, some of which are included in the Bibliography.

ARTERIOSCLEROTIC HEART DISEASE

Coronary heart disease caused by arteriosclerosis is one of the leading causes of deaths in most industrialized countries in North America, Europe and elsewhere. Over half a million people die of arteriosclerotic heart disease in the United States each year. Working in three different rural hospitals in the United Republic of Tanzania in the 1960s, the author did not see a single case of coronary thrombosis in an African patient. Arteriosclerotic disease

is associated with many risk factors which appear to be common in middle-aged and older men and post-menopausal women living in industrialized countries of the North; they are apparently much less common in traditional rural societies in countries of the South. The situation is changing, however, and heart disease and stroke are becoming important causes of mortality in many Asian and Latin American countries.

Causes

The actual cause of arteriosclerosis and the coronary thrombosis that may result is not exactly known. Various factors lead to deposits of lipid material in the arteries. The deposits may at first be lipid streaks, but they may then be followed by atheromatous plaques and often a narrowing of the coronary arteries.

Even if the exact cause of arteriosclerosis is not known, risk factors that increase the likelihood of serious arteriosclerosis are recognized:

- Hypertension or high blood pressure adds to the risk of serious arteriosclerosis and coronary thrombosis (as well as stroke).
- Raised serum lipids (high levels of serum cholesterol and low levels of high-density lipoproteins) are strongly associated with arteriosclerosis.
- Cigarette smoking is an important risk factor; several studies have shown a marked increase in coronary thrombosis and other manifestations of arteriosclerosis in those who smoke cigarettes compared with those who do not.
- Diabetes mellitus is well recognized as a risk factor in arteriosclerosis.
- Hormonal levels have a role. There is little doubt that up to about age 45 females are at much lower risk of arteriosclerosis and coronary thrombosis than males, but after menopause the differences narrow or disappear.

Although it has not been proved, oestrogen appears to protect from coronary heart disease and testosterone may increase the risk.

- Lack of exercise is a factor. Sedentary people are more likely than active individuals to get arteriosclerosis.
- A genetic predisposition for the disease is a possibility; certain persons seem at greater risk, probably because of genetic influences or a family predisposition.

Of all the causative or risk factors that can be realistically manipulated to reduce arteriosclerosis, nutritional factors and smoking stand out as deserving of action. In experiments in animals dietary manipulation has been the easiest way to stimulate arteriosclerosis.

Mean levels of blood lipids and serum cholesterol in humans differ greatly between countries with high rates of heart disease mortality and those with low rates. Lipoproteins are classified as very low density lipoprotein (VLDL), low density lipoprotein (LDL) and high density lipoprotein (HDL). HDL is often termed "good cholesterol" and LDL "bad cholesterol". Increased rates of heart disease are associated with high levels of LDL, so high LDL levels indicate increased risk. In contrast, HDL may be protective against arteriosclerosis and low HDL levels increase risk. An LDL/HDL ratio above 3.5 indicates a high risk.

Total cholesterol concentration below 5.2 mmol/litre is interpreted as low risk of coronary heart disease, between 5.2 and 6.2 mmol/litre as moderate risk and above 6.2 mmol/litre as high risk. However, risk is also influenced by other risk factors, such as smoking.

Prevention

In general, people could take the following dietary and related steps to reduce the likelihood of getting coronary thrombosis.

- Ensure that energy obtained from fat constitutes less than 30 percent of total energy intake (35 percent if the person is active) and that less than 10 percent of energy comes from saturated fat; increase the proportion of fat coming from polyunsaturated fat.
- Consume less than 300 mg of dietary cholesterol per day.
- Consume food that provides energy in appropriate amounts to ensure desirable body weight while undertaking a healthy level of physical activity.
- Consume less than 10 g of salt per day. (This step is likely to help reduce hypertension – a condition associated with arteriosclerosis – among salt-sensitive individuals.)
- Avoid cigarette smoking.
- Maintain optimum body weight, and if obese lose weight.
- Treat and control diabetes if present.
- Maintain blood pressure in the normal range.

Some scientists also recommend a high intake of antioxidant vitamins, particularly vitamin C and beta-carotene but also vitamin E, to reduce the risk of arteriosclerosis and some cancers.

In view of the above, the practical dietary guidance would be to maintain energy balance and to ensure adequate intake of fruits, vegetables, legumes and grains.

In recent years several industrialized countries have reported that deaths from coronary heart disease have decreased parallel with dietary changes, particularly reduced intakes of certain fats and oils and increased consumption of fruit, vegetables and fibre. The changes have partly come about because the public has been educated and informed about diets and other lifestyle factors that may contribute to heart disease and because as a result the food industry has changed certain practices in response to consumer demand. Thirty years ago low-fat milk was hardly used in the United States; now milk that is skimmed or 1 or 2 percent fat is widely available, and the majority of Americans use non-fat or low-fat rather than whole-fat milk.

OBESITY

Obesity is often considered a condition of affluence. Certainly in affluent nations such as the United States obesity is highly prevalent, and in most poor African countries it is much less common. However, obesity or overweight is common in both adults and children even among the poor in some non-industrialized countries, particularly the middle-income nations. In several Caribbean countries over 20 percent of women are classified as obese.

Obesity, especially severe obesity, is associated with high risks of coronary heart disease, diabetes, hypertension, eclampsia during pregnancy, orthopaedic problems and other diseases. Obesity has been found to be associated with excess mortality.

Causes

When over a prolonged period more energy is ingested in food than is expended by physical exercise, work and basal metabolism, weight will be gained and obesity will result. Metabolic studies show that diets high in fat are more likely to induce body fat accumulation than diets high in carbohydrate. There is no evidence that simple sugars differ from complex sugars in this regard. High intake of dietary fat is positively associated with indexes of obesity.

Obesity is only rarely due to endocrine (glandular) dysfunction. A very small amount of food energy consumption above energy expenditure is enough to lead to obesity a few years later. Consuming 100 kcal more than needed per day (one slice of bread and butter, 100 g of maize porridge, 220 g of beer, 26 g or a little more than two tablespoonfuls of sugar) would lead to a gain of 3 kg per year, or 15 kg in five years.

While obesity is due to an imbalance between energy intake and energy expenditure, other underlying causes – a metabolic condition, endocrine disorders or genetic factors – may certainly contribute.

Among affluent people obesity may be in part due to a tendency to take less exercise and do less energetic physical work than less affluent people. Poor rural people who engage in agriculture and walk long distances burn up much energy because of their high exercise level. When rural people move to urban areas and become more affluent they may have less need to exert energy or to do heavy physical work, and they may have access to more food and more energy-dense food, which may contribute to obesity. Obesity may become a vicious cycle, because an obese person may have more problems than others in walking long distances or in doing heavy physical work.

Obesity is common in children as well as adults. Obese children generally become overweight adults. Infants who are bottle-fed with infant formula are more likely to become obese than babies who are breast-fed.

Manifestations

It has been stated that in the United States over 30 percent of adults are at least 20 percent above their desirable weight and thus by definition obese. It is possible, however, to be overweight in relation to height but not obese. Some athletes with major muscle build-up are overweight but not obese. Accumulation of fluid in the form of oedema or ascites may make a person overweight for his or her height without being obese.

Obesity refers to the excess accumulation of body fat or adipose tissue. Overweight is usually judged on the basis of the weight of the person in relation to height, taking into consideration the person's gender and age group. Tables showing the percentage above normal weight for height are published. Overweight can also be judged using standard deviations, or Z scores. Estimates of subcutaneous fat based on measurements of skinfold thickness using skinfold callipers are also used for diagnosing obesity. Common sites are the triceps and subscapular areas (see Chapter 12).

Recently weight for height has often been judged using what is called the body mass index (BMI). BMI is calculated as follows:

BMI = weight (kg) ÷ [height (m)]^2.

For example, for a woman who weighs 40 kg and has a height of 150 cm,

BMI = 40 ÷ $(1.5)^2$ = 17.78.

For a second woman, who weighs 65 kg and has a height of 160 cm,

BMI = 65 ÷ $(1.6)^2$ = 33.7.

BMI is often used in judging nutritional status (Table 31). Thus in the examples above, the first woman is possibly undernourished and the second woman is obese. Obesity has also sometimes been further classified as Grade I (BMI 25 to 29.9), Grade II (BMI 30 to 40) and Grade III (BMI above 40).

There are other more complex and more expensive ways to measure body fat, body density, body water and body composition. They include underwater weighing, bioelectric impedance analysis (BIA) and various ultrasonic measurements. These procedures are not generally possible in ordinary health facilities in developing countries. They are described in specialized textbooks.

The attitude to fat or relatively obese people varies from society to society and from one generation to the next. In many Northern countries thinness has been regarded as rather desirable for women, and many young females have aimed for the "twiggy" look. In contrast, in much of Africa a slightly overweight woman is considered more attractive than a very slim

TABLE 31

Nutritional status indicated by body mass index (BMI)

BMI	Nutritional status
<16	Undernourished
16-18.5	Possibly undernourished
18.5-25	Probably well-nourished
25-30	Possibly obese
>30	Obese

woman. In fact, at the turn of the century the wives of Ugandan royalty were mainly very obese women. In Uganda awareness of the wasting effects of acquired immunodeficiency syndrome (AIDS), locally called "slim disease", has led to the sometimes totally mistaken belief that a plump prostitute is safer than a thin one.

Obesity and health problems

Various health risks are associated with obesity or overweight.

- *Diabetes.* Obesity undoubtedly contributes to Type II diabetes, also known as non-insulin-dependent or adult-onset diabetes. Loss of weight can sometimes improve glucose tolerance.
- *Hypertension and cardiovascular disease.* Much evidence indicates that there is a relationship between excess body weight and hypertension and that weight reduction often leads to a lowering of blood pressure. Obesity increases resistance in the arteries, thus increasing blood pressure. It also puts an additional load on the heart which may lead to heart enlargement. These conditions may contribute to arteriosclerotic heart disease, to coronary thrombosis and to congestive cardiac failure.
- *Disease of the gall bladder.* Middle-aged females are especially at increased

risk of gall bladder disease if they are overweight.

- *Arthritis.* Arthritis is probably aggravated by excess body weight, if not caused by it. Joints can be stressed by having to bear extra weight.
- *Psychological disturbances.* Particular cultural and societal views on obesity and the overweight person's own body image will influence whether obese persons suffer psychologically. Serious mental disturbances are widely reported in obese children and adults, often more in females than in males.

Control of obesity

Because the treatment of obesity is difficult and often fails, prevention of overweight is preferable to treating the problem after it has developed. Nutrition education, starting in schools, can provide persons with the information, and perhaps the motivation, always to balance energy intake with energy expenditure. Maintaining a high level of activity is helpful. In developing countries, especially in rural areas, there is no need to institute programmes of jogging or aerobic exercises. Rather it is important to value physical work and to encourage all people of all ages to do an appropriate amount of physical work, be it labouring in the fields, chopping wood in the home or public service activity; to walk where feasible rather than use alternative transport for short-distance journeys; and, if desired and feasible, to indulge in sport.

Some health professionals would recommend that treatment is warranted only for Grade II and Grade III obesity. People with BMI between 25 and 29.9, if it remains in that range, do not have much added risk of disease or reduced life expectancy. Nevertheless, all obese people have passed through Grade I to reach Grade II and Grade III. Thus for Grade I subjects aggressive treatment is not called for but

prevention is; these people should take steps not to become more obese.

The only logical way to treat obesity is to reduce energy intake and increase its expenditure. Energy intake can be lowered by reducing the size of servings at each meal; energy expenditure can be raised by increasing the amount of exercise taken. However simple this may sound, long-term maintenance of lowered weight is very difficult for people who have been obese.

Recent studies suggest that energy balance is maintained under free living conditions if a balance between intake and oxidation is also reached for each macronutrient (carbohydrate, protein and fat). In the cases of protein and carbohydrate, oxidation normally matches intake. Fluctuations in energy balance are therefore mainly governed by variations in fat balance. In the context of weight reduction this means that to induce a negative fat balance, daily fat oxidation must exceed daily fat intake. Regular prolonged exercise and reduced intake of fat would thus result in substantial weight and fat loss. In the end a new fat balance is achieved by the human body at a reduced body fat mass. Therefore, the best way to reduce the energy intake of the diet for weight reduction is to cut down fat intake and increase the intake of vegetables and fruits.

There is no prophylactic treatment that will of itself induce weight loss. The use of amphetamines, thyroid extracts and other drugs in the treatment of obesity is in general to be condemned and at best should be carefully supervised by an experienced doctor. Similarly, most of the highly advertised rapid-reducing diets, of which some are even promoted by physicians, have been found to be ineffective and sometimes dangerous.

HIGH BLOOD PRESSURE OR HYPERTENSION

Hypertension is a very prevalent condition in most industrialized countries and has varied prevalence in developing countries. In North America and Western Europe approximately 25 percent of persons over 55 years of age have raised blood pressure. Hypertension rates in Japan are higher.

High blood pressure is very strongly associated with a greatly increased incidence of stroke and coronary heart disease. These conditions are both major causes of death in industrialized countries and are now also becoming important in developing countries, particularly in the emerging countries in Asia and Latin America and in affluent and westernized people in the poor developing countries, including those in Africa.

The most common type of high blood pressure is termed essential hypertension; it is distinguished from hypertension that is secondary to a disease condition.

Blood pressure is measured using a sphygmomanometer which gives two readings, the systolic (the higher) and the diastolic. The measurement is in millimetres of mercury. A normal reading is around 120/80 mm. The upper limit of normal is about 140/90 mm in adults. A slightly higher systolic reading in older subjects is not of serious concern but still is not normal.

Causes

The actual cause of essential hypertension is not known, but obesity and psychological factors are two of the important risk factors. It is likely that genetic factors predispose certain people to high blood pressure. The main dietary factor related to essential hypertension is sodium intake, although it is probably a factor only in those who have a sensitivity to salt which is genetically determined. This subject is still unsettled. As there is currently no reliable genetic marker to identify those persons at risk, most public health recommendations dictate that universal salt restriction is prudent. Although extreme

differences in sodium intake are associated with differences in blood pressure, there are no prospective randomized data to support the widely held belief that restriction of sodium intake in normotensive subjects (i.e. people with blood pressure that is typical for their age group and community) prevents subsequent appearance of hypertension.

Most people obtain the greatest part of their sodium from salt, sodium chloride, which can be added in cooking, added at the table or added in processing (as in tinned fish, ham or pretzels). In some Asian societies, however, monosodium glutamate (MSG), a commonly added condiment, may be the major source of sodium. People also get sodium from simple medicines such as aspirin or certain antacids. It is not uncommon for people to consume more than 50 g of salt per day, which is five times more than is necessary or recommended.

Manifestations

Essential hypertension can be present for a long time and blood pressure can be quite high without any symptoms before untoward complications arise. However, many symptoms, including headache, tiredness and dizziness, are often reported by hypertensives. These symptoms can also have other causes.

Complications include arteriosclerotic heart disease; cerebro-vascular insufficiency, which can entail cerebral haemorrhage and narrowing or thrombosis of blood vessels in the brain (often called stroke); kidney failure; and eye problems, such as retinal haemorrhages.

The severity of hypertension is usually judged by the level of the blood pressure and especially by how far the diastolic pressure exceeds normal levels. Viewing the retina or back of the eye using an ophthalmoscope also provides useful evidence. A skilled examiner can view the retinal vessels and the optic disc and classify the degree of changes which are related to the seriousness of the disease.

Control

Reducing salt intake in those with hypertension will often result in lower blood pressure. Sometimes salt reduction is the only treatment needed. Other nutritional factors in hypertension and stroke are obesity and alcoholism. There is strong evidence that the blood pressure of people who are overweight is often lowered by reducing body weight. In general, vegetarians have lower blood pressure than non-vegetarians.

Hypertension that does not respond to dietary regimes or to weight loss may require specific medicines. These are described in textbooks of medicine.

DIABETES MELLITUS

Diabetes mellitus is a chronic metabolic disorder in which blood glucose levels are raised because of a deficiency or diminished effectiveness of insulin. The disease is not curable, and it may lead to a variety of complications, some of them serious. Treatment can reduce the complications. Diabetes is occasionally secondary to other diseases, especially those that affect the pancreas, the organ that produces insulin.

There are different classifications of diabetes, but most cases can be divided as follows:

- Type 1 or insulin-dependent diabetes, which is also called juvenile-onset diabetes because it often begins early in life, commonly at age 8 to 14 years;
- Type 2 or non-insulin-dependent diabetes, which is far more common and usually begins much later in life.

Causes and prevalence

For a long time it has been known that diabetes occurs in families, and that

therefore there are genetic factors involved. However, families also usually share an environment, eat similar foods and have a common pattern of activity. Dietary factors and activity pattern have a role, and in Type 2 diabetes obesity is a frequent precursor. Obese diabetics who lose weight improve their condition. There is no evidence that large intakes of sugar increase the likelihood of diabetes or that diets high in fibre and complex carbohydrates reduce the likelihood of diabetes except insofar as they displace fat in the diet and lower the risk of obesity. Type 1 diabetes in some cases appears to be associated with early viral infections.

The report of the International Conference on Nutrition (FAO/WHO, 1992a) suggests that an "apparent epidemic of diabetes is occurring in adults 30 to 62 years of age throughout the world" and that the trend is "strongly related to lifestyle and socio-economic change". The trend concerns mainly non-insulin-dependent or Type 2 diabetes. For this age group levels of diabetes are moderate, between 3 and 6 percent, in Europe and North America and in some developing countries. A high prevalence (10 to 20 percent) is seen in some urban Indian and Chinese societies and in immigrants (sometimes second or third generation) from the Indian subcontinent who have settled in the Caribbean, Fiji, Mauritius, Singapore and South Africa. Diabetes is uncommon in many communities in the developing world where traditional diets and activity patterns are maintained.

It is not absolutely clear why particular migrant groups or others changing their lifestyles from traditional to sedentary seem to be at special risk for diabetes. It seems highly likely, however, that dietary changes, sometimes including excess alcohol intake, are a major factor. The dietary changes are also accompanied by an altered way of life, from rural to urban;

from hard physical work to a sedentary life; and possibly from rural poverty to somewhat greater affluence.

From a nutritional point of view diabetes is related to obesity, to cardiovascular disease and to alcoholism.

Manifestations

The disease is characterized by abnormally high levels of glucose in the blood. The first evidence of diabetes is often a urine test that is found to contain glucose. The diagnosis is confirmed by an elevated level of blood glucose: either a random blood glucose level above 11 mmol/litre (200 mg/dl) or a fasting level above 7 mmol/litre (120 mg/dl). An abnormal glucose tolerance test further confirms the diagnosis and provides more information.

Complications include, among others, arteriosclerotic heart disease, cataracts in the eyes, renal problems, impotence in men, neurological abnormalities and poor circulation, which sometimes leads to gangrene of the extremities.

Treatment and control

The aim of treatment is to maintain health and to avoid complications. This is achieved by trying to get blood glucose levels as close to normal as possible for as much of the time as possible, and by so doing to reduce the amount of glucose spilling into the urine. Control is greatly assisted by reduction of weight in obese diabetics and by maintenance of a healthy body weight in all diabetics.

There are three cardinal principles in the treatment and control of diabetes: discipline, diet and drugs. Diabetics must organize a regular and disciplined lifestyle, with timely eating, work, recreation, exercise and sleep. They must regulate their food intake to meet their diabetic requirements and use drugs as a recourse only when this regimen fails to control the condition. Control requires good coope-

ration between the sufferer and the health worker and an understanding that there is no cure but that often good health can be maintained into old age. Most Type 2 diabetes can be controlled by discipline and diet. Many young Type 1 diabetics and a few more serious Type 2 diabetics may need insulin or other drug therapy under close medical supervision. Elderly diabetics are often overweight, and their diets need to be adjusted to help them achieve desirable weight. This is feasible but not easy.

There is still debate and disagreement about the best dietary treatment for diabetes. Readers should consult comprehensive textbooks of nutrition or internal medicine for detailed advice. Many physicians now recommend a diet in which 55 to 65 percent of the energy comes from carbohydrate, 10 to 20 percent from protein and 20 to 30 percent from fat. The diet should be mixed and varied, containing cereals, legumes or root crops, fruits and vegetables. Foods high in fibre are desirable.

What is important is that feeding be regular. The diabetic should eat modest amounts frequently and avoid either bingeing or going for long periods without eating. Dietitians often find it useful to provide exchange lists which inform the diabetic about groups of foods or dishes that contain similar amounts of carbohydrate, protein, fat and energy.

Diabetics may need special attention during illness, especially infections; during pregnancy and delivery; or if they require surgery. Alcohol is not totally forbidden, but it should be consumed only in very modest amounts. Diabetics should be aware of possible complications so that they can seek early treatment.

CANCER

In the industrialized countries of the North various cancers are among the leading causes of death. There is increasing evidence that several different kinds of cancer are associated with certain diets and antinutritional factors. As with arterio-sclerotic heart disease, hypertension, obesity and diabetes, epidemiological evidence suggests that some cancers may be less common in people who regularly consume cereals, legumes, fruits and vegetables.

Cancers of the colon, the prostate and the breast, which are highly prevalent in industrialized countries, are in general much less common in developing countries. Many believe that these cancers become common as diets change to include less fruits, vegetables and fibre and more fat. Certainly colon cancer seems to be influenced by these types of diets. In contrast, vegetable-based diets in which the main foods are relatively unmilled cereals, legumes, fruits and vegetables seem to be protective against colon and perhaps other cancers. These traditional diets are high in fibre, and high-fibre diets increase the transit time of food from the stomach to excretion in the stools.

The question is still open as to whether vitamin C, vitamin E and beta-carotene (antioxidant vitamins) or other non-nutrient compounds which come mainly from fruits and vegetables are protective against these or other cancers, including those of the gastro-intestinal tract. A high consumption of alcohol appears to result in higher rates of cancer of the liver and stomach. Mothers who breastfeed their babies appear to have lower rates of breast cancer than mothers who have not breastfed.

In some developing countries, especially in Africa and Southeast Asia, primary liver cancer is much more prevalent than in the industrialized countries of the North. In some African countries this type of cancer, also called hepatoma, is the most common cancer. Research now shows that the high prevalence rates are the result of hepatitis earlier in life, caused by the hepatitis B virus. Some liver cancers, as well as some other liver diseases, may be related to consumption of hepatotoxins (liver toxins) in food. The most commonly mentioned is aflatoxin.

OSTEOPOROSIS

Osteoporosis is a chronic disease that is now very common in older people, particularly women, in industrialized countries. The disease is characterized by excessive demineralization of the bones of the skeleton. In general, reduction in the calcium content of the bones has been considered a normal ageing process. Particularly in post-menopausal women in industrialized countries, however, the loss of bone density is accelerated.

Osteoporosis greatly increases the risk of fractured bones, even from falls or minor trauma. Fractures of the neck of the femur (near the hip joint) are almost epidemic in female senior citizens in North America and Europe, and these people also frequently have fractured vertebrae. They may become shorter, have bent backs and suffer excruciating pain.

The cause of osteoporosis is not known. Almost certainly in females it is due in part to lower levels of female hormones (such as oestrogen) after the menopause and to taking little exercise. Some believe that low calcium intakes have an important role, and many millions of people take medicinal calcium with the belief that it will reduce their chances of getting osteoporosis. However, dietary intakes of calcium are much higher in North America, where osteoporosis is prevalent, than in many countries in Asia and Africa where osteoporosis is uncommon. High protein intakes increase the need for calcium, so Western people consuming high-protein diets do have increased calcium requirements.

There is some evidence that increasing

intakes of fluoride helps to maintain bone density, and fluoride in the past was tried in osteoporosis treatment, but it is not now widely recommended. Many women in industrialized countries now take oestrogen after the menopause, and this probably reduces the demineralization leading to osteoporosis. Regular relatively strenuous exercise also reduces the loss of bone density. Rural women in Africa, Asia and Latin America, who as long as they are fit work in the fields, carry wood and water, walk long distances to the market and in general are highly active, seem to do what is needed to lessen their likelihood of developing osteoporosis. Immobilized humans, be they fracture patients confined to bed or astronauts in space, definitely lose calcium from their bones.

In North America and Europe increasing intake of calcium may reduce the likelihood of developing osteoporosis. In the United States and the United Kingdom milk provides 30 to 50 percent of the dietary calcium consumed. Whole milk, if consumed in the quantities often recommended to prevent osteoporosis, will also markedly increase, possibly to unhealthy levels, intakes of total fat, saturated fat and energy. Calcium supplements are often recommended. Recent experimental evidence in humans suggests that treatment with parathyroid hormones may be effective in some cases of osteoporosis.

OTHER CHRONIC DISEASES WITH NUTRITIONAL IMPLICATIONS

Dental caries, or tooth decay, is the most prevalent disease of humans worldwide. This condition and the role of diet in its aetiology are described in detail in Chapter 21.

Excess alcohol intake, which may be sporadic, or alcoholism, which is a chronic dependence or addiction to alcohol, are both common problems in many countries both North and South. Alcohol provides energy (about 7 kcal per gram of ethanol), and in a person maintaining optimal weight the energy consumed from alcohol may reduce the energy consumed from food by 30, 50 or even 70 percent. A person who consumes only 50 percent of the food that other persons of the same age and size consume gets only half the essential minerals and vitamins provided by a normal diet. Thus deficiency diseases and conditions are common in alcoholics. One serious disease, Wernicke-Korsakoff syndrome, due to thiamine deficiency, is common in alcoholics (see Chapter 16). Alcoholics often develop cirrhosis of the liver, a condition that often progresses to cause death in the sufferer.

Chronic alcohol addiction may lead to serious family and social consequences, and these in turn may have nutritional implications. Money that could be spent to purchase food or family essentials may be expended on alcohol. An alcoholic spouse or parent may be a bad spouse or parent and may have increasing difficulty obtaining the family's livelihood. Alcoholism in society causes many problems, including, for example, deaths on the road and increased violence.

There is no evidence that moderate consumption of alcohol is harmful, provided that it remains moderate. There is even some evidence that one glass of red wine with the main meal, as part of a "Mediterranean diet", may reduce risk of heart disease.

Other chronic diseases that have nutritional implications include diseases of the kidneys and urinary system; of the gastrointestinal tract, including the stomach; of the gall-bladder; and of the liver. These are described in medical textbooks.

NUTRITIONAL PROBLEMS OF POVERTY AND AFFLUENCE – A CONTRAST

As described in several chapters in this book, many of the main deficiency diseases prevalent in developing countries are associated with food insecurity, poverty, infectious diseases, inadequate care and related factors. It has been clearly shown that so-called economic development, especially development that goes hand in hand with poverty alleviation, leads quite rapidly to major reductions in malnutrition and infections. Examples of countries where this has been the case include Costa Rica and Cuba in Latin America; Malaysia and Thailand in Asia; and Mauritius in Africa. The major reductions in malnutrition, in prevalence of communicable diseases and in infant and child mortality rates are probably usually a result of improved education and reduction in illiteracy, greater household food security, better hygiene and water supplies and wider access to reasonably good health services.

In most countries as the rates of protein-energy malnutrition and of infections such as gastro-enteritis and intestinal parasites go down, there is often an increase in the incidence of arteriosclerotic heart disease, obesity, certain cancers, diabetes and stroke. The transition and the changing health profile are often first evident in the most affluent and in urban rather than rural populations.

Reliable morbidity data are frequently not available, but in many countries mortality data are published. These data clearly show that in many of the better-off developing countries deaths from infections and malnutrition have markedly declined and infant mortality rates have greatly improved. However, the mortality rates from what are termed "diet-related non-communicable diseases" have increased in these nations. These diseases include malignant neoplasms, diabetes, obesity, circulatory system diseases (excluding rheumatic fever), chronic liver disease and cirrhosis, cholelithiasis and cholecystitis. World Health Organization

(WHO) statistics for 42 countries which had good mortality data for 1991 to 1992 (WHO, 1993d) show that in some industrialized countries such as Australia, Japan, the United Kingdom and the United States the mortality rates from these causes decreased from 1960 to 1990, while in more affluent developing countries such as Ecuador, Mauritius and Thailand the death rates from these causes markedly increased over the same period. In many of these middle-level developing countries the death rates from these diseases in persons 45 to 54 years of age were very similar to those of industrialized countries for the period from 1985 to 1989. It is likely that the significant decreases in the industrialized countries are due to educational efforts and public health messages that influence people to reduce their dietary intake of harmful dietary components and to change behaviours that increased the risk of dying from these disorders. Certainly non-nutritional behaviour changes, for example reduced cigarette smoking, also contribute to these reductions. The dietary change usually believed to be most important is a reduction in the consumption of certain fats.

An increase in the diet-related non-communicable diseases in rapidly developing countries is likely first to affect more affluent people, often productive well-educated persons in important positions in both the public and private sectors. These diseases then may reduce the productivity of these people, and their treatment may also begin to absorb a larger and larger segment of the health care budget. The challenge for nutritionists and others is to help emerging developing countries avoid the transition from a high prevalence of preventable infections and malnutrition to increasing rates of partly avoidable chronic diseases of affluence.

The developing countries, especially those that are rapidly industrializing and witnessing rapid increases in incomes, are in a position to take action before major increases in these diseases occur. This is a challenge that should be grasped and not ignored. Perhaps measures to reduce cigarette smoking are even more important than those to prevent harmful changes in food intake, but actions to prevent harmful dietary practices deserve priority. China is one country that is at least considering these problems and appropriate actions. Its attention to these problems is particularly important because China is the world's most populous country and has transformed itself in 50 years from a country with much extreme poverty, severe food shortages and many deaths from infections to a nation with a booming economy, food security and a health service that has controlled many preventable infections. The Chinese Government has a good deal more control over its citizens than do many other governments, and it could take steps to reduce the already rising rates of nutrition-related and cigarette-related chronic diseases. In so doing, China could set an example for other countries.

In the mid-1990s concern is now focused on the emerging problem of cardio-vascular disease in the countries of Eastern Europe and the former Soviet Union. The increasing incidence of chronic diseases in the developing countries deserves attention.

DIETARY GUIDELINES

Guidance in nutrition can have various purposes. It can be provided for the setting of national priorities in the health sector, or to facilitate the planning of national economies (dietary goals, dietary/nutritional targets); or it can address individuals (recommended nutrient intakes, dietary guidelines). All these forms of guidance have in common the goal of helping populations achieve a state of optimal nutrition which is conducive to good health.

Since human beings everywhere have rather similar nutrient requirements relative to their age, gender and body size, nutritional guidance can be prepared in a global perspective to some extent. Strategies for achieving nutritional goals, however, will vary from one population to another; they will need to take into account the biological and physical environment of the population, as well as economic and relevant socio-cultural factors. These aspects should be reflected in dietary guidelines.

Dietary guidelines are sets of advisory statements providing principles and criteria of good dietary practices to promote overall nutritional well-being for the general public. They are intended for use by individuals.

Dietary guidelines are primarily based on the current scientific knowledge regarding nutritional requirements and also, indirectly but strongly, on the types of diet-related diseases prevalent in the given society. The guidelines take into account the customary dietary pattern and indicate the modifications that should be made to contribute to the reduction of these diseases. They represent the practical way to reach the overall nutritional goals for a population.

Until recently, dietary guidelines have usually been expressed in technical nutritional terms. Now, however, food-based dietary guidelines, which express the principles of good dietary practice in terms of foods, are increasingly common. Where they cannot be expressed entirely in terms of foods they are written in ordinary language. These guidelines avoid as far as possible the technical terms of nutrition science. Food-based dietary guidelines vary among population groups. Hence it is important that each region or country recognize that more than one dietary pattern is consistent with health and develop food-based strategies that are appropriate for the local region.

Food and diet are not the only components of a healthy lifestyle. Therefore, organizations developing dietary guidelines are encouraged to integrate diet-related messages with other policies related to health (e.g. smoking, physical activity, alcohol consumption).

The following key points should be considered in the formulation of dietary guidelines:

- Public health issues should determine the direction and relevance of dietary guidelines.
- Dietary guidelines address a specific socio-cultural context and therefore need to reflect the relevant social, economic, agricultural and environmental factors affecting food availability and eating patterns.
- Dietary guidelines need to reflect food patterns rather than quantitative goals.
- Dietary guidelines need to be positive and should encourage enjoyment of appropriate dietary intakes.
- Various dietary patterns can be consistent with good health.

To address better the issues of optimal nutrient intakes for the development of food-based dietary guidelines, the recent FAO/WHO Consultation on Preparation and Use of Food-Based Dietary guidelines (1995) advocated the concept of nutrient density applied to total diet – i.e. the amount of essential nutrients provided per 1 000 kcal of energy provided by the diet – as an alternative to the traditional focus on recommended dietary allowances (RDAs) for specific nutrients. Reference nutrient densities for selected nutrients are given in Annex 4, with relevant public health implications of using the approach for developing and evaluating dietary guidelines.

GET THE BEST FROM YOUR FOOD – AN FAO INITIATIVE FOSTERING THE DEVELOPMENT OF PRACTICAL DIETARY GUIDELINES

FAO has recently produced a set of nutrition education materials which are based on the above considerations and can facilitate the development of practical dietary guidelines. The package, entitled *Get the best from your food*, is based on the recognition that food has value and significance well beyond the supplying of nutrients. Eating is among the most natural and pleasurable activities known, and within society food, and especially the sharing and securing of food, has considerable social significance. The multiple roles of food and eating behaviours need to be recognized and appreciated in the development of dietary guidelines.

The FAO initiative is based on four principles:

- The human body is a very adaptable organism, and a wide variety of dietary patterns and food intakes can lead to good health and nutritional well-being.
- From a nutritional perspective, a given food can neither be required nor proscribed. There are no good or bad foods, *per se*, only good and bad diets.
- Diets, in themselves, can only be judged good or bad in relation to a number of other variables, ranging from an individual's physiological status to physical activity levels, lifestyle choices and environmental conditions. Helping consumers understand what these variables are and how they can be modified beneficially is a major objective of dietary guidance.
- Dietary intake, except in extreme situations, is primarily a matter of choice, and dietary guidance can be most effective in helping people make good food choices through positive, non-coercive messages.

Four messages of positive dietary guidance

The *Get the best from your food* initiative is based on four messages that can be used to develop not only dietary guidelines, but also educational programmes for public information, schools and other training settings. The concept and messages are positive, simple and direct. They are intended to promote healthful and realistic consumption patterns among all age groups and to encourage sound, practical approaches to food and nutrition.

Enjoy a variety of food. This message embodies two concepts. The first is that food, eating and dietary guidance need to be seen in a positive light. This idea is especially important given the negative messages often associated with dietary guidance, especially in more affluent societies.

The second concept is that dietary adequacy must be based on dietary diversity. This message stresses that the consumption of a wide variety of foods is necessary and that all types of food can be enjoyed as part of a wholesome diet. Recognizing the benefits of mixed and varied diets is especially important in light of the still incomplete understanding of nutritional requirements, nutrient and non-nutrient interactions and diet-health relationships.

Eat to meet your needs. This message emphasizes the changing nutritional needs throughout the life cycle and how those needs can best be met from locally available foods. Attention is drawn to energy and nutrient requirements during high-risk periods (pregnancy, lactation, infancy, illness, old age) and in difficult situations such as times of low food availability. This message also permits problems associated with overconsumption and unbalanced dietary intakes to be addressed.

Protect the quality and safety of your food. This concept is often overlooked by those providing dietary guidance, yet it is of great importance in both developed and developing countries. In many developing countries malnutrition is often caused by the poor state of water and food sanitation, and in all countries the consumption of poor-quality, contaminated foods is a major health risk. Vigorous efforts to protect the quality and safety of food supplies need to be made within households, schools and other institutions and at village-level and commercial processing and storage facilities.

Keep active and stay fit. This message emphasizes that nutritional well-being is not just a matter of eating properly. Human bodies need exercise to function well and stay healthy. Many of the diet-related chronic diseases are closely linked to activity patterns, and efforts to improve nutritional well-being need to consider this fact.

Chapter 24
Famine, starvation and refugees

Famines are usually considered to be severe shortages of food often affecting either a large geographic area or a significant number of people. The consequence is often death from starvation in groups of the population, preceded by severe undernutrition or malnutrition. Starvation is a pathological condition in which lack of food consumption threatens, or causes, death. Refugees are persons who have been displaced from their normal homes across borders into other countries; displaced persons are those who have moved from their homes but still remain within the borders of their own country. These three conditions are described in this chapter because they are closely related.

There is very extensive literature, both historic and more recent, on famines, their causes, how they were dealt with and their consequences. In many of the publications starvation as a form of malnutrition is described, although this topic has not been very well studied. Fewer books describe refugee problems in detail or provide a complete picture of a particular refugee situation. However, there are millions of pages of reports on refugees. Many of these have been provided to or produced by the Office of the United Nations High Commissioner for Refugees (UNHCR) or the World Food Programme (WFP), two organizations much involved in refugee relief. Other literature, some of it very poignant, has been produced by numerous non-governmental organizations (NGOs) that work with refugees.

This book can only outline the important aspects of famine and refugees. Readers wanting more information are advised to consult other publications, a few of which are listed in the Bibliography.

STARVATION

Humans may die of extreme cold after six to 12 hours of exposure; of thirst after a few days if they consume no water or fluids; but of hunger only after a few weeks if they are in normal health when they are first deprived of food.

A healthy man weighing 70 kg has about 15 kg of adipose tissue or fat. This fat is his main usable store of energy which is used when he is in negative energy balance, when he receives inadequate food or when he is starving. The 15 kg of fat would theoretically yield approximately 135 000 kcal. This would not be exactly the amount of energy that a starving man would obtain from his fat; however, 15 kg of fat could provide about 1 350 kcal per day for 100 days, or 2 700 kcal per day for 50 days. Starving individuals can also burn up some protein, mainly from their muscles.

The average weight of an Asian or African man might be 55 kg rather than 70 kg, and that of a woman perhaps 45 kg, so their energy stores from fat and muscle might be considerably lower. It should also be appreciated that many persons who as a result of famine or displacement are threatened with starvation may be poor persons who prior to the crisis were not well nourished, were relatively thin and had only modest deposits of body fat. In these situations it is young children who may be the most vulnerable, in part because they may already be malnourished but also because they have relatively greater nutritional needs than adults because they are growing. However, young children are often protected as much as possible by their families. Another vulnerable group may be women of child-bearing age, who have increased nutrient needs because of pregnancy, lactation or menstruation. Old people, although they have somewhat lower energy needs than young people, may also be particularly vulnerable to starvation, in part because they cannot compete well for food or for social reasons have poorer access to food.

The classic images of starvation for most people are the emaciated, severely under-nourished adults released from concentration camps in Germany at the end of the Second World War and more recently the starving children in Bosnia, Rwanda or Somalia. A condition almost identical with the starvation that results from famine is the serious wasting of the body that results from acquired immunodeficiency syndrome (AIDS), tuberculosis, cancer, anorexia nervosa and some other diseases. This chapter considers starvation in groups of individuals caused by lack of availability of food. In such circumstances the degree of undernutrition ranges widely, from mild to fatal. A healthy adult can afford to lose one-quarter or a little more of his or her body weight, or can lose weight until the body mass index (BMI) (see Chapter 23) reaches 16. If much more is lost the person becomes ill and life may be threatened.

For example, an average adult African male weighing 55 kg may be forced to reduce his energy intake drastically during a famine year. Lacking food, he burns up body reserves. He loses fat, his muscles diminish in size and he becomes thin. At the same time he has a natural inclination to reduce his energy output. He is less energetic, and he rests and sleeps more. The energy expenditure of this average African male doing no exercise is about 1 300 kcal per day. If the food situation improves, for example with the new harvest, he is able to eat more food and hence increase his energy intake. His appetite also increases, and he regains his weight without having done his body any real harm. Many people have gone for ten days or more without any solid food at all (but with drinks of water or fluids). Under these conditions loss of weight occurs without permanent damage. People have been on hunger strikes for as long as 30 days and have fully recovered. If a person loses most of his or her body fat and some muscle and continues on a grossly energy-deficient diet, then definite signs and symptoms of starvation will develop.

Clinical features of starvation

In starvation the subject first becomes thin, the skin becomes dry and hangs loosely and the muscles become wasted. The hair loses its lustre, the pulse slows and the blood pressure is reduced. Hormonal disturbances cause amenorrhoea in women and impotence in males. If the woman is pregnant she may have a spontaneous abortion or miscarriage.

Oedema, sometimes called famine oedema, is a frequent feature of severe undernutrition. The bedridden patient looks puffy, and the ambulant person has swelling of the dependent parts of the body such as the feet and legs. Anaemia commonly develops. Diarrhoea is nearly always present. It may start early on in starvation or it may be a terminal event.

Preschool-age children are often severely affected (Photos 41 and 42). They develop nutritional marasmus and sometimes kwashiorkor, often accompanied by intractable diarrhoea, which may, in the very weakened child, lead to prolapse of the rectum.

The starving person usually has psychological and mental disturbances. The personality may change, and the ability to concentrate may be lost, but the person usually remains rational.

Concurrent with these signs and symptoms there may be evidence of deficiencies of vitamins and other nutrients. In Africa the mouth lesions of riboflavin deficiency and tropical ulcers commonly occur; in prisoners of war in East Asia during the Second World War the burning feet syndrome (intense burning of the soles) was a marked feature, but almost any symptom of deficiency disease may arise, depending in each case on the diet.

Untreated starvation often leads to intractable diarrhoea, vascular collapse or heart failure and death. More commonly, however, the severely malnourished individual develops an infection and dies of pneumonia, tuberculosis or some other infectious disease.

Treatment

The basis for treatment is to provide adequate food in a form that can be utilized by the individual and to treat any specific conditions in the manner appropriate to them. Refeeding should be introduced progressively. In a famine area a person suffering mild undernutrition but showing few signs of starvation will often recover simply by eating whatever food becomes available at the end of the famine.

In severe starvation institutional treatment may be necessary. The patient may have a huge appetite, but the disturbed digestive tract can seldom cope with a large intake of varied rich foods. Milk, bland foods and limited roughage form the basis for successful treatment. Treatment of the young child is similar to that described for kwashiorkor and nutritional marasmus (see Chapter 12).

FAMINE

Famines can be defined as severe food shortages that cover a large geographic area or affect a large number of people.

They are often divided into those that are natural and those that are caused by human actions. Natural causes include most commonly inadequate rainfall, which is termed drought, and less frequently flooding, earthquakes, volcanoes, insect plagues that destroy crops or widespread plant disease. Human actions that can cause famine include most commonly war, either between nations or within a country (civil war), but also sieges, civil disturbance or deliberate food crop destruction. Widespread chronic hunger and malnutrition, although not usually termed famine, not uncommonly result from other causes, for example:

• an increase in an area's population that is disproportionate to the ability of the people to produce, purchase or acquire sufficient food;

• widespread poverty;

• gross inequity in a poor country;

• inefficient or disrupted food transportation or distribution.

Even if the term famine is not generally used in these cases, the effects on people are the same.

The topic of famine and famine relief is very important for nutritionists and others. It is a broad subject and much has been written about it. Those who wish to know more or participate in famine relief should refer to relevant publications listed in the Bibliography.

Some past famines

Both small and large famines have occurred throughout recorded history, some of them resulting in many millions of deaths from starvation and related causes. Among the best known and best described is the great famine in Ireland in the 1840s, which resulted from a disease that reduced the potato yields in that country, where potatoes had become the staple food. Over 1.6 million Irish people emigrated, most of them to the United States.

Colonial India, prior to independence, had severe famines, for example in 1769/70 when it is believed that 10 million persons died (some one-third of the population). In 1943 another disastrous famine in Bengal killed over 1 million people (more than the total British and American war dead from the Second World War), affected 60 million people and made many destitute. A severe famine in Bihar in 1966/67, after Indian independence, has been much described; the government's handling of that famine provides lessons of how appropriate measures can greatly reduce suffering and deaths.

China has also witnessed many famines, but the more recent ones have not been very well documented. Some authorities believe that between 1958 and 1961 over 15 million persons died in China from starvation resulting from droughts and floods but much aggravated by the economic and political chaos resulting from the industrialization programme termed the "Great Leap Forward". In Europe the Second World War saw serious famine in the Netherlands because of the German occupation and the withholding of food from the civilian population and in Leningrad (now Saint Petersburg) because of the German siege of that city. In Africa there was the Sahel famine which became known throughout the world between 1968 and 1973 [especially in Chad, Mali, Mauritania, the Niger, Senegal and Upper Volta (now Burkina Faso)] (Photo 43), and a few years later serious famine and much starvation in Ethiopia. These were both weather-related famines, and there are not accurate figures of the numbers who died. North and South America and Australia have been relatively free of large-scale famines.

The decade of the 1990s has seen famine and starvation in many countries because of crises caused by humans. Civil war in

former Yugoslavia has led to serious food shortages in Bosnia; in Somalia clan strife and poor rainfall in 1992/93 brought about severe starvation and many deaths; and in Angola, Liberia, Mozambique and the southern Sudan civil unrest or the governments' loss of control of parts of these countries has caused widespread malnutrition and famine deaths. Strife in Rwanda has led to starvation deaths and to outbreaks of cholera and dysentery in refugees fleeing to Zaire in 1994.

In contrast, drought which greatly reduced food production in East Africa in 1984 and in southern Africa in 1992 saw practically no starvation deaths, because countries such as Kenya, the United Republic of Tanzania and Zimbabwe acted with speed, good planning and appropriate action to get food to those in need. It is likely that the Global Information and Early Warning System for Food and Agriculture (GIEWS) supported by FAO in southern Africa was of assistance; it permitted the governments to predict drought and low crop yields, to plan measures and obtain external assistance and to receive early help from WFP. This example illustrates that if there is no civil strife, if there is early warning, if there is a timely appeal for assistance and if governments make the political choice to deal with famine, malnutrition can be kept in check and famine deaths can be prevented.

Consequences of famine

An important consequence of famine is starvation, described above. Starvation has nutritional, health and psychological manifestations. The reader is also referred to Part II of this book, where several chapters describe the disorders of malnutrition. Many of these, such as protein-energy malnutrition (PEM), nutritional anaemias, vitamin A deficiency and several other micronutrient deficiencies, are common consequences of famine. In addition to these nutritional effects of famine, there are also important social and health-related repercussions.

One important result of famine, and also of wars or civil disturbances without famine, is population migration. The potato famine in Ireland led to substantial emigration, and recent civil wars have resulted in the creation of millions of refugees. The refugee problem is described below.

The progress of a famine is often judged by figures on deaths from starvation, but these are less a measure of the severity of the conditions causing the famine than a reflection on how the authorities have or have not coped with the famine.

Besides social disruption, population movement and sometimes civil disturbance, the next serious consequences of food shortages in famine are epidemics or increased rates and seriousness of infectious diseases. Throughout history famine and pestilence have occurred together. In past famines, serious epidemics of typhus, plague, smallpox and cholera killed many people who were affected by famine. In current famines markedly increased numbers of deaths, particularly in children, have resulted from diarrhoea (from cholera, dysentery or other causes), measles, tuberculosis and other respiratory infections. Typhus and plague can be controlled by insecticides, smallpox has been conquered, and cholera deaths are much reduced by oral rehydration as part of treatment.

Increased rates of infectious diseases and of other infections (including parasitic diseases such as malaria or intestinal worms) result often from a reduced ability of people to fight infections because of malnutrition. Other factors may include increased exposure to infections because of overcrowding in refugee camps, breakdown of water supplies and sanitation, lack of immunization for measles and other

diseases and poor housing. The 1994 deaths of Rwandan refugees in Zaire provide a good example.

Famines often result in marked increases in micronutrient deficiencies as well as PEM or deficiencies of intakes of carbohydrate, protein and fat. Recent famines have seen increased rates of nutritional anaemias, xerophthalmia and ariboflavinosis as well as outbreaks of pellagra and scurvy in populations where these deficiency diseases had not been seen. The lesson to be learned is that food relief must go beyond providing only sufficient calories or energy; it must also include adequate micronutrients (vitamins and minerals) and be accompanied by immunizations, adequate water supplies and sanitation.

Famine prevention

Natural disasters and droughts usually cannot be prevented, but it is possible to prevent these conditions from turning into famines. The ultimate preventive measure, of course, is a diversified economy and a well-developed food and agriculture sector. India experienced a severe drought in 1967, yet the country was able to prevent famine because of its spectacular progress in basic food production arising from the adoption of new agricultural technologies, coupled with an effective food reserve and disaster management plan. Famine is generally the result of a series of agricultural, economic and political failures. Effective interventions at a number of points can prevent an emergency or food crisis from becoming a famine. Crop losses from pests or plant diseases can sometimes be markedly reduced or even avoided. For example, efforts led by FAO and other organizations to destroy locust breeding sites help prevent damage in the Near East before locust swarms move south to devastate crops in Africa. Some plant diseases can be controlled or cured.

Famines arising from natural causes are the ones in which starvation and deaths related to starvation can most easily be prevented. Government and political choice are required for action to prevent starvation. A system of early warning and an established contingency plan with clearly defined responsibilities are critical elements of famine prevention. Actions or programmes to prevent famine must be sensitive to the social and cultural mores of the people in the affected areas. Poor countries such as India, Botswana, Kenya, Tanzania and Zimbabwe have proved that famine can and should be prevented in this way.

Famines that are caused by human actions are of course totally preventable. If humans chose not to undertake these actions, then these famines and starvation would not occur.

The World Declaration on Nutrition approved by over 150 nations at the International Conference on Nutrition in Rome in 1992 contains these words:

> We reaffirm our obligations as nations and as an international community to protect and respect the needs for nutritionally adequate food and medical supplies for civilian populations situated in the zones of conflict. We affirm in the context of international humanitarian law that food must never be used as a tool for political pressure. Food aid must not be denied because of political affiliation, geographic location, gender, age, ethnic, tribal or religious identity.

If all nations honoured these words the number of people starving in the 1990s would be markedly reduced. A ban on the use of food as a weapon of war has been solicited for years. Germ warfare and gas warfare have been banned, and most countries have accepted this ban. Nonetheless food continues to be used as a weapon of war and for political purposes. Whenever and wherever food has been used as a weapon the worst effects have been on the civilian population, particularly on women, children and the elderly. Seldom are combatants, politicians or senior government officials made hungry, and they certainly do not starve when there are blockades or food wars. In the mid-1990s there have been dozens of armed conflicts, many of which include food wars or situations where an adequate diet as well as access to adequate health and care are compromised. Such situations have occurred in Afghanistan, Angola, Cambodia, Haiti, Iraq, Liberia, Mozambique, Rwanda, Somalia, the Sudan, former Yugoslavia and other countries. Because adequate food and good nutrition are considered basic human rights, these common infringements are violations of human rights. The United Nations and member countries could help reduce famine deaths by acting to ban or even markedly reduce human actions and political decisions that cause malnutrition and starvation deaths, and by taking any action that can promote peace and reduce armed conflicts. More attention needs to be given to this issue in the years ahead.

Famine relief

The first and most important action in famine and pre-famine conditions is to procure and make available enough food to prevent starvation and malnutrition, to maintain the good nutritional status of those who are well nourished and to rehabilitate those who are undernourished. However, famine and disaster relief will be successful and deaths will be prevented only if certain conditions are present nationally and locally. Some famines are confined to one part of a country and therefore require local actions, perhaps supported by the national government, international agencies and NGOs.

Famine conditions occur repeatedly, yet when they happen a country is often not ready to deal with the problem. Some nations do not have a plan, and those placed in charge of famine relief may have little knowledge of how other countries have acted and little experience in famine relief strategy. As a result the wheel gets reinvented and mistakes are made, mistakes that could easily be avoided. Clearly a smoothly running government, a good civil service, a sound infrastructure and well-established and well-run social and health services are all helpful. The participation of NGOs that are well run and know the country is another asset. A good relationship between the country and food donor nations is also helpful.

The authorities need to obtain, transport, store safely and finally distribute fairly sufficient food for those in the famine area who are threatened with starvation (Photo 44). It is important to provide foods that participants like and understand how to prepare and that are culturally acceptable to all or nearly all people.

There is some difference in dealing with food emergencies that are short-term, for example those caused by earthquakes, volcanoes and floods, and those that are long-term, for example those resulting from crop failures from drought or prolonged civil strife. In short-term food emergencies attention to micronutrient deficiencies is less important than in long-term famines.

There are several different ways of making food available when famine is threatened or exists. Decisions should be made only with local consultation and knowledge of the situation and the people affected, and they should preferably be based on the best information available. If the situation is stable (for example, no warfare, no mass movement of people) and there is simply a food shortage, for example because poor rains have reduced food production, then the simplest means of avoiding famine-related malnutrition and

deaths is to ensure that food is available through normal market mechanisms. Food shortages in nations with a free-market economy often result very soon in marked increases in food prices and in food hoarding. One means of preventing this or reducing it is for the government, possibly with international assistance, to move foods in short supply, particularly cereal staples, into the area; a second means is to introduce price controls. Food shortages and increased food prices will have an especially negative impact on the poor, so attention needs to be addressed to poor families if food prices rise. Often a crisis results not so much because food itself is in short supply, but rather because incomes and markets have collapsed. Efforts to stimulate the local economy and to replace lost income through public works programmes have been very effective in many countries.

In more serious situations, or if the preceding approach is not feasible, emergency food needs to be provided. Such assistance usually entails providing foods for people to prepare themselves. Occasionally – in very severe emergencies, in certain camps or institutions for displaced persons or in medical units that have admitted seriously malnourished persons – the assistance can entail on-site feeding of prepared meals.

The first goal of emergency feeding is to ensure that all people, but especially the poorest families, have enough food to meet their energy and other nutritional needs. They must also be in a position to prepare and cook the food. Beyond these needs it is important that treatment be available for those who are malnourished, since famines often occur where chronic hunger and some degree of malnutrition were prevalent prior to the emergency. In some situations it is appropriate to target the food to those considered most in need. This is often difficult to do and requires special arrangements. Emergency feeding plus attention to health care needs should help to prevent large numbers of people from migrating from their normal places of residence. Those providing food should keep in mind the need to prevent long-term dependency on free or subsidized foods. Action to encourage and assist food production should be initiated soon after other steps have been taken and while famine deaths are being prevented.

If take-home rations are provided, local consultation or, better, local decision-making about the types of food and methods of food distribution is important. Certain important principles are almost universal:

- If at all possible the foods should be those normally consumed in the area. For example, the main food provided should be maize in maize-eating areas and rice in rice-eating areas.
- Distribution sites should be as close to where people live as possible. Locating sites many kilometres from where people live causes hardship and en- courages people to migrate and to camp near the distribution sites.
- The population should be informed about the progress of the famine, how food is being made available, ways to prepare the food and all other relevant matters. Information provided to the people can be extraordinarily helpful but is often ignored.
- It must be ensured that a reasonable level of primary health care is available, that health and nutrition education is provided, that people are immunized and that breastfeeding is protected, supported and promoted.
- Some form of monitoring should be established to assemble data on food available, food distributed (at the community and family levels) and deaths, especially those caused by malnutrition or common infections. It

is very helpful to monitor nutritional status if possible, especially for vul- nerable groups such as children. This may be done, if feasible, by measuring weights and heights and possibly by also plotting weights on growth moni- toring cards. If weighing is not feasible, measurement of mid-upper-arm cir- cumference (MUAC) may be used if it is done by a well-trained person.

Many publications, including FAO's *Food and nutrition in the management of group feeding programmes* (FAO, 1993b), state that the same ration should be given to each person irrespective of age and that the minimum average individual energy content of the ration should be 1 900 kcal. This is the daily amount, and must exclude food losses due to any cause. The standard requirement of 1 900 kcal is based on a typical demographic distribution of the population in which 20 percent would be children under five years of age; 35 percent children five to 14 years; 20 percent females aged 15 to 44 (with 40 percent of these either pregnant or breastfeeding); 10 per- cent males aged 15 to 44; and 15 percent males and females over 44 years of age. It should be appreciated that 1 900 kcal is the very minimum. It is suggested that in the ration protein should supply 8 to 12 percent and fat at least 10 percent of the energy. This ration of 1 900 kcal has to be complemented by other locally available foods, and the recommendation assumes that beneficiaries have access to them. In some instances insufficient local foods are accessible or the age or gender distribution of the assisted population is different from the normal distribution. In these cases the ration needs to differ from the standard. [Readers wanting more detailed infor- mation on emergency rations should consult the WFP publication *Food aid in emergencies* (WFP, 1991).]

In the past, with concentration on the energy content of the ration, the micronutrient content of emergency foods has been relatively ignored. This should never happen. Rations should provide at least the recommended dietary allowances for micronutrients. The nutrient content of the ration and of other foods available should be appraised, and consideration should be given to adding to the ration other foods with high levels of particular micro-nutrients or insisting that only fortified cereals or other foods be used. Some foods, such as groundnuts, in relatively small quantities will help increase the nutrient content of the diet. In longer-term famines production of fruits, vegetables and small animals can be promoted. Seldom in localized famines are funds made available to purchase the cheapest and most nutri-tious fruits and vegetables available in a neighbouring district and transport them into the famine-affected area, but this action should be encouraged.

Table 32 shows three examples of rations that provide 1 900 kcal. Each of these rations provides at least 10 percent of energy as fat and about 12 percent as protein. Wheat flour, maize or rice appears as the major item in all three diets, and as mentioned earlier, the preferred local cereal should be provided as far as possible. Ration 2 provides 30 g of a fortified cereal blend to add micronutrients while reducing pulses or legumes. Ration 3 also reduces pulses and adds canned fish or meat.

Additional guidelines include the fol-lowing:
- Ensure that adequate fuel and cooking utensils are available.
- Foods should be distributed weekly if possible, or every two weeks.
- Bottle-feeding or breastmilk substitutes should be strongly discouraged, and breastfeeding encouraged.
- Dried skimmed milk or other milk products, if included, should be mixed with the cereal if possible so that such

TABLE 32
Examples of typical 1 900 kcal rations [a]

Food item	Quantity (g)		
	Ration 1	Ration 2	Ration 3
Wheat flour/ maize meal/rice	400	400	400
Pulses	60	20	40
Oils/fats	25	25	25
Fortified cereal blend [b]	–	30	–
Canned fish/meat	–	–	20
Sugar	15	20	20
Salt	5	5	5

Source: WFP, 1991.
[a] Each of these rations provides approximately 1 930 kcal, 45 g protein and 45 g fat.
[b] Examples: Maize-soybean blend, wheat-soybean blend, *likuni phala, faffa.*

products cannot be used for bottle-feeding. (An exception might be made where fluid milk is an important part of the traditional diet.)
- Some means of providing vitamin A and vitamin C needs to be found when fruits and vegetables are not available. The means might be fortification or, if necessary, medicinal supplementation.
- If at all possible, it is very important to try to add to the rations certain items that are valued by the society or that enhance their palatability, such as curry powder or other spices, tea, extra sugar or concentrated flavourings such as beef-flavoured cubes. If these extras are not included beneficiaries may sell some of the cereals or pulses on the market to earn money to purchase them, and energy intakes may be compromised.

In many famines additional supple-mentary feeding targeted to certain vulnerable groups of the population may be very helpful. There has been a tendency to confine supplementary feeding to children who already have moderate or serious malnutrition, perhaps those below three standard deviations of the standard weight for height. Such supplementation constitutes a treatment, an action to rehabilitate these children. However, it is better to take a preventive approach and to find some way to provide extra feeding to children and others at risk before they have serious malnutrition. The supplement might provide an extra 300 to 500 kcal per day plus other nutrients and might be in an energy-dense form. It is often a cereal-based blended food.

In other famine situations where the people have general access to food or where the government is reducing food shortages by instituting price policies, putting food on the market or subsidizing the price of staple foods, supplementary feeding may be introduced when a general ration is not provided. Again supplements should be provided for prevention of malnutrition as well as rehabilitation. Criteria may be established for selection of recipients and then for discharge from supplementary feeding.

In some instances rather than providing rations to be taken home or food for people to prepare and feed themselves, special circumstances may make it necessary to provide on-site meals. This option generally involves the establishment of feeding centres. Communal feeding is necessary when many people do not have the facilities or ability to cook their own food. For example, in a refugee camp in Kenya most of the population comprises unaccompanied minors, mainly young boys. In other instances where people are displaced from their homes, they may have no utensils or facilities and at least at first require cooked food. However, most refugees do cook their own rations in refugee camps.

Under optimal conditions on-site meals should consist of dishes that are palatable and culturally appropriate to the people being fed and should provide all the nutrients necessary for health and perhaps rehabilitation. High standards of food hygiene must be maintained if at all possible. In many famines major donors and national governments arrange to have non-governmental private voluntary organizations run the feeding centres. These centres need to be set up near where people live, otherwise people will move or camp near them. An alternative which is often more expensive is to use mobile kitchens or mobile canteens.

Other actions which might be considered by those involved in famine relief are discussed in detail in other publications (see Bibliography). These include:
- rationing, which has occasionally been very successful (as in Britain from 1942 to 1947) but has often failed;
- price controls, which can prevent food from being priced out of the market for the poor but can also create problems;
- means to reduce or prevent food hoarding;
- estimating food needs in various ways;
- monitoring, surveillance and evaluation in famines.

In any major famine a system of weekly reporting is highly desirable.

Food-for-work

In some famine situations food is provided to some people only in exchange for work. Food-for-work is often used by WFP and other organizations in non-famine situations. If it is decided that food will be given as a payment for work, then meaningful work has to be organized for large numbers of people, within relatively easy access of where they live. Work has often been arranged in large public works projects, for example in road building or tree planting.

Food-for-work can be successful, but before it is implemented all the pros and cons need to be examined. An advantage of food-for-work over free food is that taking food in lieu of a stipend for work gives dignity to the beneficiary. It often helps prevent the recipients from acquiring the mentality of assisted people. Often both free food donations and food-for-work are implemented together. Sometimes where this is possible there can be a phasing out of free distribution and a phasing in of food-for-work as the situation improves. Some disadvantages of food-for-work are that hard work increases energy needs and therefore the food needs of those working; that the public works involved are sometimes quickly and badly planned and serve little purpose; and that many of those most in need of food, such as children, the elderly, pregnant women and women with young children, may not be able to work or work adequately and may then not receive food.

Health actions in famines

Although providing food is the first essential in a famine, the provision of health services is also important and is often neglected. As mentioned, famines and pestilence go hand in hand, and often more people die of infections and related disease than of starvation. Prevalence and severity of infections are increased, and not infrequently epidemics sweep through famine areas and refugee camps. Therefore it is highly necessary to institute public health measures to prevent disease and to establish treatment centres where needed therapy, immunizations, health education and other health actions can be provided. Very important preventive measures include actions to ensure good sanitation, potable water, personal hygiene and safe feeding.

Assessments and monitoring of the health situation, followed by analysis and interpretation of the situation and likely interventions, can result in action to control epidemics; to distribute medicines and supplies; to immunize children; to improve sanitation and water supplies; to ensure primary health care; and where needed to introduce specific measures to control specific diseases. Nutrition and health education, especially for women, deserves a high priority. Continuous monitoring and refinement of the interventions are needed.

In famines information is needed on both nutrition and health. Without reasonable information, famine relief can often be inefficient, inappropriate and / or seriously flawed. Data are needed regarding both healthy and diseased people.

REFUGEES

There are estimated to be close to 35 million refugees in the world today. The United Nations assigns the main responsibility for dealing with refugees to UNHCR, but that agency is assisted by other United Nations organizations such as FAO, WFP, the United Nations Children's Fund (UNICEF) and the World Health Organization (WHO). In addition, many NGOs are much involved in refugee relief, most notably the International Red Cross, based in Geneva, Switzerland.

UNHCR defines a refugee as:
any person who owing to a well founded fear of being persecuted for reasons of race, religion, nationality, membership of a particular social group or political opinion is outside the country of his nationality and is unable, or because of fear is unwilling to avail himself of the protection of that country; or who not having a nationality and being outside the country of his former habitual residence, is unable, or having such fear is unwilling, to return to it.

According to this definition the term "refugee" refers to true political refugees but not to those termed economic refugees, i.e. those who flee their country and enter another country not for the reasons defined above but because they see better economic advantages in the country to which they have fled. The definition also excludes internally displaced persons, i.e. people who have left their homes but not their country. UNHCR is mandated to address the needs of refugees but not internally displaced persons. The definition should not be seen as suggesting that refugees are all male.

Refugees may live in refugee camps or settlements or reside freely away from their homes. What follows deals more with communities of refugees than with individual refugees or refugee families who move into the general population in an area away from their home.

This chapter briefly considers the nutrition and health of refugees, and not other refugee problems. Many books and reports have dealt with refugees, and some are included in the Bibliography.

Nutrition in refugee camps and settlements

Much in this book concerning the causes, clinical aspects, treatment and control of malnutrition is relevant to the problem of refugees. In fact there has recently been major concern that a wide variety of micronutrient deficiencies have been diagnosed in refugee camps, some of them camps where the refugees have received food for many weeks. The food provided may have provided sufficient energy but did not nearly meet the nutritional requirements for certain essential nutrients. Thus scurvy, pellagra and beriberi have been seen in countries where these are rare diseases. Beriberi resulting from thiamine deficiency has been reported in Cambodian refugees in Thailand; pellagra in Mozambican refugees in Malawi; and scurvy in Somali refugees in Ethiopia. In some refugees moderately prevalent conditions such as PEM, vitamin A deficiency and anaemias

have worsened, rather than lessened. Similarly there have been serious outbreaks of preventable diseases such as measles and whooping cough in refugee camps. In the mid-1990s these problems should not occur. The world has the resources, and it should have the compassion, to ensure that the nutritional status and health of refugees improves rather than deteriorates once they are in camps or settlements and receiving UN assistance and care from NGOs (Photos 45 and 46).

Micronutrient deficiencies are likely to occur where few foods are provided (often less than three), where other foods are relatively inaccessible or unavailable to refugees and where there is very little diversity in the daily food pattern. Examples of solutions to recognized problems include replacement of beans with groundnuts, which was done in Malawi to control pellagra, and fortification of flour or other foods.

Much of what has been written about starvation and famine above applies also to refugees and displaced persons. Displaced persons arriving in a new area of their own country or refugees arriving in a new nation may be dying of starvation or related diseases, and they often have been or are still in famine areas. The first needs are for safe and adequate water and for shelter against the elements, most importantly against cold, because cold can kill more quickly than lack of food. Provision of adequate water and protection against cold are easier to supply, however, than the next needs, which are for food and for health services, including medical treatment and preventive measures. The health and nutritional status of refugees in camps or settlements should from time to time be appraised in an organized and regular way. As described in Chapter 1, good nutrition is dependent on adequate food, health and care. This dictate applies profoundly also to refugees, and especially to refugee children. Almost all refugees are vulnerable and usually very poor, with few resources. They have often fled with no or little money, few possessions and none of the tools or instruments needed to make a living except their minds, their bodies and their strength. Peasant farmers who have fled do not have tools to cultivate; tailors do not have their sewing-machines; and so on.

Refugees, like all people, have a human right to good nutrition, and because they are temporarily under the care of the United Nations and NGOs it is an international obligation to provide good nutrition, adequate health services, sufficient food providing all essential nutrients and care. The basic essentials are simply described:

- adequate food to satisfy both energy needs (and perhaps wants) and micro-nutrient requirements, provided in acceptable forms (described in the previous section on famines);
- water of adequate quality and sufficient quantity;
- latrines that help prevent the spread of diseases caused by faecal contamination;
- shelter – tents, temporary structures or existing buildings such as schools or churches – that ensures protection from the weather (heat, cold, rain, etc.), that averts overcrowding and that is secure, safe and vermin free, or at least does not promote the spread of disease;
- health services that provide a reasonable level of primary health care including appropriate treatment for common diseases and preventive services including, for example, immunizations, nutrition and health education and other public health measures;
- safety from human depredation and other dangers;
- an environment that is made as socially

and psychologically stimulating as possible, in which cultural and religious beliefs and practices are respected.

Refugees who are likely to be in a settlement for more than a few weeks should be given assistance and encouragement to be active, to run the affairs of the camp and to use their skills where appropriate. From a nutritional viewpoint, this means that displaced farmers should be helped to begin gardening, especially to produce foods that supplement the rations and that yield a harvest within a short time after planting. Possible choices include vegetables such as amaranth and other green leafy vegetables, tomatoes and carrots and legumes such as various beans and peas, especially those that are locally familiar, perhaps chickpeas, pigeon peas or kidney beans. Production of small animals should be encouraged, not only poultry, but also perhaps pigeons, rabbits, guinea-pigs or others that are culturally appropriate. Any persons with health training should be recruited to work in the dispensary or health post, those with secretarial experience in the camp records office, and so on.

Refugees who spend more than a few weeks as displaced persons in a camp or other mass location will usually very quickly enter into various forms of trade and attempt to acquire money to purchase a variety of needed items, both perceived food wants (for greater dietary variety) and non-food needs or wants such as clothes or items to improve the level of living. Part of the rations described in the previous section on famines, which provide 1 900 kcal mainly in the form of a staple cereal and legumes, may soon be sold by refugees to obtain cash. Their intake of energy and other nutrients is then reduced, and this may be a reason for deteriorating nutritional status. Foods provided in rations are often bartered rather than sold.

Those running refugee camps or determining what is provided to refugees need to consider the economic desires and needs of the refugees and to provide them with assistance or a means to help meet these economic desires. Although donor organizations are in general opposed to providing cash to refugees, and their rules may not allow it, under certain circumstances provision of cash could be advantageous, allowing refugees to purchase food and other commodities on the open market. This would only be feasible if the market system in the area had sufficient food and other commodities.

Food rations could also be formulated to provide not only for the purely nutritional requirements but also for the economic desires of the refugees. The total amount of food provided might well be somewhat above the base amount supplying 1 900 kcal; the ration might include foods besides those in Table 32, for example more sugar and animal protein foods, spices, condiments, vegetables and fruits, in other words any additional food that seems acceptable, desired and nutritionally sensible.

The authorities need also to consider whether it is wise to condemn or to try to prevent the sale of food rations. As the refugees begin to become more self-sufficient, either by raising money or by growing their own foods, the rations can sometimes be reduced below the standard 1 900 kcal per person per day.

Prevention of micronutrient deficiencies

Elsewhere in this book descriptions are provided of the most important micronutrient deficiencies and their prevention. Much of the discussion applies also to refugees. It is a duty of those involved in feeding refugees to ensure that outbreaks of micronutrient deficiencies do not occur. Consideration needs to be given in refugee camps especially to the three micronutrient deficiencies most important in developing countries, namely those of iron, iodine and vitamin A (see Chapters 13, 14 and 15). Ideally the rations consumed by refugees should contain adequate quantities of these three micronutrients. If they do not, then some fortification can be provided in a fortified cereal blend, most commonly a maize-soybean blend. Such cereal blends should always provide good quantities of minerals and vitamins.

When it is not possible for rations to provide sufficient micronutrients for any reason, or when there is a reasonable belief that significant numbers of refugees may be at risk of micronutrient deficiencies, then a means of preventing specific deficiencies should be established.

Vitamin A deficiency. Supplements should be given where risk is present, for example when refugees show signs of this deficiency or are known to come from areas with a known vitamin A public health problem, or when rations provide less than 2 500 IU (750 RE) of vitamin A per day. It is recommended that high doses of vitamin A be provided orally: 400 000 IU (120 000 RE) for all children one to five years of age and 200 000 IU (60 000 RE) for infants from age six to 12 months, given every four months. It is not generally recommended that infants under six months receive this dose. Lactating mothers should be given 200 000 IU of vitamin A soon after parturition. Treatment of cases of xerophthalmia should follow the recommendations in Chapter 15.

Anaemia. As described in Chapter 13, iron deficiency is the most important nutritional anaemia, but folate deficiency is not uncommon. Women of child-bearing age are most at risk, but anaemia occurs at all ages and in both females and males. Iron, perhaps folate and vitamin C supplements should be given to refugees when the ration contains inadequate amounts of these micronutrients or if anaemia rates are high. Corn (maize)/soybean/milk (CSM) supplements, if used, provide additional iron. Ferrous sulphate and perhaps folate should be provided, as described in Chapter 13, to pregnant and breastfeeding women in refugee camps. If there is a way to provide a good level of vitamin C intake using the food basket, this may help reduce anaemia by assisting with utilization of dietary iron.

Other micronutrient deficiencies. Where there are cases of iodine deficiency disorders (IDD), pellagra, scurvy, beriberi or other micronutrient deficiencies, then the treatment and preventive measures recommended in the preceding chapters should be implemented. It is recommended that only iodized salt be used in food rations and supplementary feeding in refugee camps.

Health services for refugees

As mentioned above, a reasonable level of both curative and preventive health services is a necessity in refugee camps and other places where refugees are living. These services, like health services everywhere, are designed to reduce deaths, to cure disease and, most importantly, to prevent disease as far as possible.

Mortality. Usually the causes of death in refugees are similar to those reported in the areas from which the refugees emanated. In the poor developing countries important causes are infections, almost always made worse by underlying malnutrition. Common infections include diarrhoea and acute respiratory infections (both having a number of possible causes such as bacteria, viruses and parasites), measles and malaria. In the more industrialized and less poor countries such as those of former Yugoslavia and Eastern Europe, the causes may be different. As discussed in Chapter 3, high mortality rates from infections are often the result of the interaction of malnutrition with the infection, so if refugee diets can improve general nutritional status, mortality and case fatality rates from infections may fall significantly.

Very high rates of starvation deaths in refugee camps early in an emergency are often the result of severe PEM, especially nutritional marasmus but also not infrequently kwashiorkor. In refugee camps in many African countries and elsewhere, measles has been an important cause of mortality although it is relatively easy to prevent. Deaths attributed to measles or diarrhoea are nearly always associated with PEM and could just as accurately be termed malnutrition deaths.

Morbidity. Causes of serious morbidity usually mirror the causes of mortality. They include gastro-enteritis (diarrhoea), acute respiratory infections, malnutrition, measles and often malaria. Other diseases may also be common and are particularly important for health personnel to treat. For example, tuberculosis requires attention because it is insidious and requires long, difficult treatment. Intestinal helminthic infections may cause anaemia, reduce growth and cause complications such as intestinal obstruction; these infections may be extremely prevalent but are easily treatable. The wide range of treatable conditions also includes, for example, scabies and conjunctivitis. In particular refugee camps and in specific situations, serious outbreaks of cholera, dysentery, meningitis and hepatitis have needed special attention.

The dispensary, clinic or first-aid post in a refugee camp will also need to be able to treat injuries. In certain situations many of those arriving in the camps have war- or violence-related injuries, and in some there are high rates of physical disabilities. Facilities are needed to provide special attention for women during pregnancy, childbirth and lactation. In some camps it may be important to ensure that sexually transmitted diseases can be treated and that measures to reduce transmission of human immunodeficiency virus (HIV) can be taken. The situation differs from country to country and from camp to camp. In some instances refugees in camps benefit from better health services and better diets than are available to the local population in the areas surrounding the camps.

Health programmes. It is highly desirable that a system be established for surveillance of health, including nutrition (discussed below). Data need to be collected on mortality, morbidity, nutritional status and health actions [for example, staff activities, immunizations, health education and maternal and child health (MCH) activities]. When many persons arrive in an area over a short length of time and are admitted to a camp or other facility, it is helpful if a rapid health assessment can be carried out; this provides baseline data for later evaluations.

A set of actions to prevent diarrhoea deaths and to control diarrhoea is important. Diarrhoea is usually treated using oral rehydration therapy, often based on oral rehydration solution from packets or commonly used fluids and foods. This therapy is life saving when there is dehydration. For diarrhoea without dehydration, foods and fluids prepared at home, plus continuing breastfeeding in the young breastfed child, may be what is needed. More difficult, but of great importance, is prevention of diarrhoea through provision of good latrines, safe water, improved personal and food hygiene and health education. The health personnel should have the training and

ability to suspect cholera, and if they find this disease they should be prepared to deal with it.

Many infectious diseases can be prevented by immunizations. These include measles, diphtheria, whooping cough, tetanus, poliomyelitis and meningitis. BCG (bacillus Calmette-Gu rin) vaccine reduces tuberculosis. It is now generally recognized that a very high priority should be given to measles immunization, and that it should be a very early action in a new emergency. Only then should other immunizations be planned including oral polio vaccine and diphtheria, pertussis, tetanus (DPT) vaccine.

Nutritional surveillance

As soon as a camp for refugees is established, or as early as possible, the nutritional status of all should be assessed, and then it should be followed. A system to assess the nutritional status of all new arrivals should be initiated.

Nutritional status assessment usually means the use of anthropometric measurements to assess PEM in children or undernutrition or relative thinness and wasting in adults. Chapter 12 describes the use of anthropometry in assessing PEM. The method should be decided on the basis of what is feasible. Assessment of the extent of low weight for height and surveillance of the changes would be ideal. However, in a refugee situation it may not be possible to weigh and measure all children. If it is not feasible to obtain length or height measurements, then serial weight measurements are useful for surveillance, although they are less useful for assessment of the initial nutritional status of the refugees. MUAC is a simpler measurement because it needs only a tape-measure and not a scale. This method should be used mainly during emergencies for screening purposes, not for surveys or monitoring.

Initial examinations plus follow-up

assessment should also seek to find clinical signs of malnutrition, such as oedema which may be evidence of kwashiorkor, eye signs of xerophthalmia and skin lesions of pellagra.

If it is clear that newly arrived refugees come from areas where xerophthalmia is a problem, then at the time of the first nutritional assessment a dose of vitamin A (400 000 IU or 120 000 RE for children over one year of age) and measles immunization are recommended. Information could be collected on night blindness rates as reported by mothers.

The nutrition surveillance system must funnel data to a person who has the ability to analyse and interpret them and to initiate needed action. If the rates of children who have wasting, low MUAC, clinical evidence of severe PEM, xerophthalmia or other deficiencies remain high, then action should be triggered. If the evidence comes from anthropometric data,

it may indicate either defects in the food distribution system (perhaps children do not receive their fair share or families are not receiving their ration) or an adverse influence of disease morbidity (diarrhoea, intestinal parasites, malaria, etc.) on nutritional status.

Regular collection of data is invaluable if there is to be assurance that the feeding is fulfilling its objectives, which should be to improve the nutritional status of the refugee population and to prevent malnutrition. Special surveillance of micronutrient deficiencies (for example, following haemoglobin levels in at-risk groups) may be needed and would follow the lines discussed in Chapters 13, 14 and 15. Surveillance should also include monitoring of the feeding programmes and perhaps obtaining data on dietary intake in subgroups of the population, especially vulnerable groups.

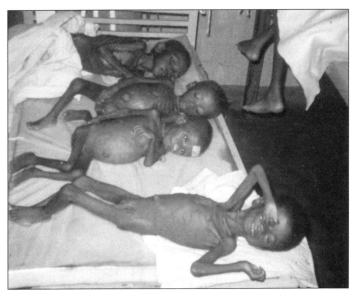

PHOTO 41
Starving, severely malnourished children during the Nigerian civil war

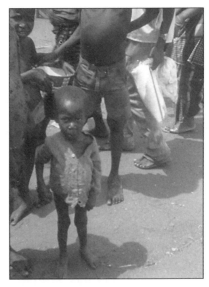

PHOTO 42
Starving child lining up to get relief food

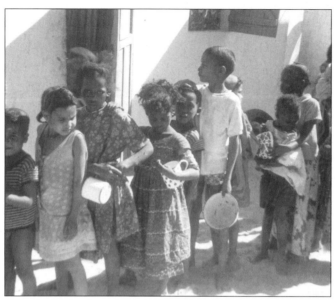

PHOTO 43
Children in Mauritania waiting for food during the Sahel famine

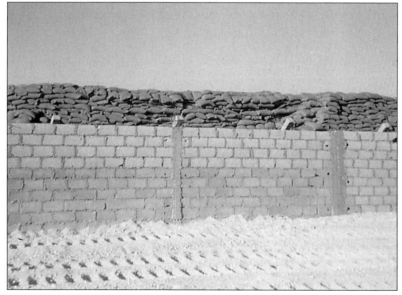

PHOTO 44
Famine relief maize in storage

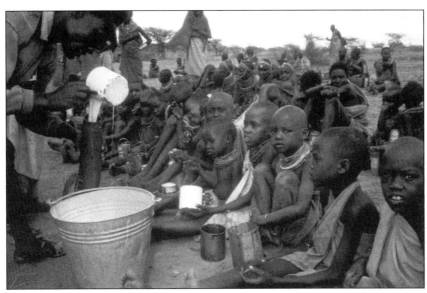

PHOTO 45
Refugee feeding by the World Food Programme in Africa

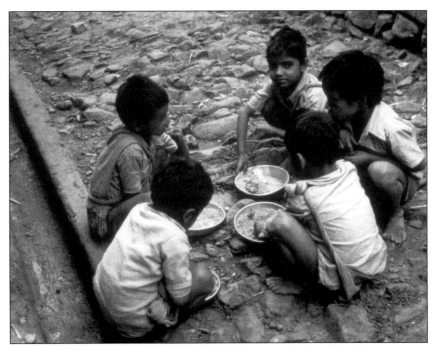

PHOTO 46
Children in Bhutan consume bulgur wheat from the World Food Programme

Part IV
Foods

Chapter 25

Food composition tables, nutrient requirements and food balance sheets

Different tools are used to assess the nutritional situation of groups of people, including families, communities and nations. Food composition tables provide a means to estimate the nutrient content of foods consumed by the population being studied. Tables of nutrient requirements or of recommended dietary allowances (RDAs) indicate either the suggested daily requirements of each important nutrient judged necessary to maintain satisfactory nutritional status or allowances intended to serve as goals for intakes of nutrients. These allowances often afford a margin of sufficiency; except for the energy allowance they are usually set somewhat above the physiological requirements of individuals. In general both suggested requirements and RDAs are designed for use by groups of persons, not by an individual subject. Assessment of the nutritional status of an individual needs to be based on determination of food consumption (translated into daily nutrient consumption using food composition tables), clinical examination, biochemical assessment, anthropometry and perhaps other tests.

Food balance sheets are used to provide data on food available nationally for the whole population. FAO assists many countries in assembling data on estimates of food production, imports, exports and other food uses to provide an estimate of food that was available in a particular year for the population of the country. If the population figures are available, then mean available foods can be calculated. Through the use of food composition tables, these can then be translated into mean nutrient availability [for example, the daily (or annual) availability of energy, protein and each of the important micronutrients] per head of population.

Thus food composition tables, estimates of nutrient requirements or dietary allowances and food balance sheets are tools used in different ways and for different purposes by persons wishing to assess the nutritional situation of groups of persons or of nations.

FOOD COMPOSITION TABLES

A food composition table usually consists of a list of selected foods with figures for the content of selected nutrients in each food. Annex 3 provides a very limited table of the nutrient content of foods that are known to be quite widely used in developing countries. The annex is included in this publication so that using one volume the professional reader can, for example, estimate the nutrient consumption of certain groups of people or calculate the nutrient content of diets that are used or recommended, for instance for institutional feeding or emergency rations.

Many books provide much more comprehensive data on food composition and are appropriate for use in research or for nutrition surveys. These include the United States Department of Agriculture's massive *Composition of foods – raw, processed and prepared*, in several volumes, first published as USDA Handbook No. 8 in 1963 and revised in 1984; the various editions of and supplements to McCance and Widdowson's *The composition of foods*; food composition books concerning either certain geographic areas (some published by FAO) or particular developing countries; and others that deal with only certain nutrients.

The food composition table in Annex 3, taken from the recent FAO publication *Food and nutrition in the management of group feeding programmes* (FAO, 1993b), provides the content of nutrients per 100 g edible portion of each food. The nutrients included, which have been selected as the most important for developing countries, are energy, protein, fat, calcium, iron, vitamin A, thiamine, riboflavin, niacin, folate and vitamin C. Readers wishing to know the content of other nutrients, for example zinc, selenium or biotin, in a food will have to refer to more detailed food composition tables.

Some tables list the nutrient content per "normal serving size" rather than by weight, and some provide data on the nutrients in various prepared foods rather than, as in this book, the raw food. Although the table in Annex 3 gives the nutrient content of both wheat flour and a prepared product, bread, in general most prepared foods are not included. Thus the nutrient content of maize is given but not that of the tortillas eaten in Central America or that of *ugali*, a maize-based dish consumed in East Africa. The foods, for simplicity, are listed in categories to allow easy use of the table.

A word of caution is needed for those using any food composition tables. The figures given for the content of a particular nutrient in a particular food are based on analyses of samples of that food. However, foods often vary in their nutrient content depending on the country and climate where they are grown, the type of food analysed, how the food is prepared before consumption (which varies among different cultural groups) and many other factors. It should also be recognized that analyses conducted even in very sophisticated laboratories have a margin of error, which is larger for some nutrients than for others. For example, tomatoes come in many different varieties, are grown in different soils in both tropical and temperate climates and can be picked green or ripe; therefore there is a wide variation in the amount of carotene (which can be converted to vitamin A in the body) in 100 g of tomatoes consumed. The table in Annex 3 shows that a 100-g edible portion of tomato contains 113 µg of vitamin A. Some tomatoes have much higher and others much lower content of vitamin A. Food composition tables are useful but must be used judiciously.

NUTRIENT REQUIREMENTS AND RECOMMENDED DIETARY ALLOWANCES

A great deal of research has been conducted to determine the needs or requirements of human beings for different nutrients. Nutrient requirements of course vary in certain groups of people, for example in children because they have added needs for growth and in women during pregnancy and lactation. Large comprehensive textbooks discuss in detail the research leading to the best estimates of the requirements of different individuals for each nutrient.

Many countries provide recommendations regarding the amounts of each of the important nutrients that should be consumed by their populations. In many cases these provide for levels of safety and take account of variations in requirements; often, therefore, the figures are somewhat higher than minimum requirements for health.

Generally recommended dietary allowances for a country provide only guidelines for the evaluation and development of good diets for the population. It is important to understand clearly that the values presented are not requirements, since many individuals are known to consume smaller amounts than those listed and still enjoy good health. On the other hand, it is recognized that the actual requirement for any nutrient is not precisely known. Recommended dietary allowances therefore must not be considered requirements but rather levels of intake that should be entirely adequate for essentially all members of the population. This kind of dietary guidance seems appropriate in affluent countries such as the United States. It may not be appropriate in many parts of the world where there are more urgent problems and where food and money are more limiting factors for many people.

For the purposes of this book Annex 1 provides recommended intakes of nutrients and "safe levels of intake", which apply to groups of persons and not to individuals. They pertain to healthy, not diseased people. These tables are designed to recommend, based on current knowledge, intakes of selected macronutrients and micronutrients that will maintain health, prevent deficiency diseases and allow adequate stores of nutrients in normal circumstances. The recommendations for children are for amounts of nutrients that allow proper growth, and those for women of child-bearing age take into account their special needs, including those of pregnancy and lactation.

Research workers and policy-makers in the developing countries should use, where available, tables of recommended dietary intakes or allowances that have been adopted in their own countries or geographic regions. Over 40 countries have such tables. They should all be used critically, and often in conjunction with publications from international organizations such as FAO, the World Health Organization (WHO) and the International Union of Nutritional Sciences (IUNS).

FOOD BALANCE SHEETS

Many developing countries, using their own resources or with assistance from FAO or other organizations, have from time to time published food balance sheets, which are the best estimates that can be made from existing data of the total amount of food available for consumption by the human population in a particular year (or other period). Usually these estimates are based on the total quantities of food produced in the country, the foods imported and the changes up and down of food reserves or food stocks for the period. Deductions are made for foods such as cereals or legumes used as seeds rather than for consumption, for those used for livestock consumption (termed "animal feeds"), for those used for industrial non-food purposes (for example, fats or oils used for production of soap or for ethanol fuels) and for a waste factor. The final figures deduced are construed to represent the amount of food potentially available for consumption by the population of the country.

These figures then can be divided by the total mid-year population of the country to derive average per caput availability of food for the year, which can in turn be translated into per caput availability of nutrients using food composition tables. Total availability of energy and of other nutrients for the nation can also be calculated. These figures can then be compared with the calculated nutrient needs of the country to assess the adequacy of food availability. Most important, the data provide information on the dietary energy supply (DES), which combined with information about the distribution of food supplies allows an estimate of the number of people whose energy intakes are too low. The main limitation of DES is that it is not a direct assessment of food consumption. Food balance sheets also do not take into account age and gender factors, internal distribution differences within a country or seasonal variations in food availability.

Food balance sheets are often used to indicate a country's sufficiency and/or deficiency of food or particular nutrients. When prepared over successive years, they show trends in the country's food availability, indicating whether it is improving or declining and thereby allowing the country to institute appropriate policy to safeguard national food security and to channel agricultural production. The tables may also help the country to devise appropriate crop diversification policy to improve both agricultural income and production of nutritionally desirable foods. In addition the data indicate how much a country depends on its own food production relative to food importation and could thus contribute to the design of national food importation policy.

Food balance sheets for most poor developing countries are only very rough estimates of the food situation. The accuracy of the data used in the preparation of food balance sheets varies widely depending on the availability of good-quality data and the level of development of agrostatistics services. Generally they are much better in developed than in developing countries. Accurate census data on population are not available in many developing countries. Therefore the limitations of food balance sheets should be examined critically before the information is used in designing important agricultural, food security or economic policies in a particular country.

Chapter 26
Cereals, starchy roots and other mainly carbohydrate foods

Early peoples lived mainly on foods obtained by hunting and gathering. Among the first crops to be planted and harvested were the cereal grains. Ancient civilizations flourished partly because of their abilities to produce, store and distribute these cereal grains: maize in the Americas before the arrival of Europeans; rice in the great Asian civilizations; and barley in Ethiopia and northeast Africa.

Foods with a predominantly carbohydrate content are important because they form the basis of most diets, especially for poorer people in the developing world. In the developing countries these foods usually provide 70 percent or more of the energy intake of the population. In contrast, in the United States and Europe often less than 40 percent of energy comes from carbohydrates.

CEREALS
Through the ages many plants from the family of grasses have been cultivated for their edible seeds; these are the cereal grains. Cereals form an important part of the diet of many people. They include maize, sorghum, millets, wheat, rice, barley, oats, teff and quinoa. A new cereal of considerable interest is triticale, a cross between wheat and rye.

Although the shape and size of the seed may be different, all cereal grains have a fairly similar structure and nutritive value; 100 g of whole grain provides about 350 kcal, 8 to 12 g of protein and useful amounts of calcium, iron (though phytic acid may hinder absorption) and the B vitamins (see

Table 33). In their dry state cereal grains are completely lacking in vitamin C and, except for yellow maize, contain no carotene (provitamin A). For a balanced diet, cereals should be supplemented with foods rich in protein, minerals and vitamins A and C. (Vitamin D can be obtained through exposure of the skin to sunlight.)

The structure of all cereal grains (Figure 15) consists of:
- the husk of cellulose, which has no nutritive value for humans;
- the pericarp and testa, two rather fibrous layers containing few nutrients;
- the aleurone layer, which is rich in protein, vitamins and minerals;
- the nutrient-rich embryo or germ,

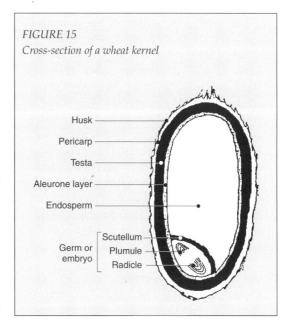

FIGURE 15
Cross-section of a wheat kernel

Husk
Pericarp
Testa
Aleurone layer
Endosperm
Germ or embryo — Scutellum / Plumule / Radicle

TABLE 33
Content of certain nutrients in 100 g of selected cereals

Food	Energy (kcal)	Protein (g)	Fat (g)	Calcium (mg)	Iron (mg)	Thiamine (mg)	Riboflavin (mg)	Niacin (mg)
Maize flour, whole	353	9.3	3.8	10	2.5	0.30	0.10	1.8
Maize flour, refined	368	9.4	1.0	3	1.3	0.26	0.08	1.0
Rice, polished	361	6.5	1.0	4	0.5	0.08	0.02	1.5
Rice, parboiled	364	6.7	1.0	7	1.2	0.20	0.08	2.6
Wheat, whole	323	12.6	1.8	36	4.0	0.30	0.07	5.0
Wheat flour, white	341	9.4	1.3	15	1.5	0.10	0.03	0.7
Millet, bulrush	341	10.4	4.0	22	3.0	0.30	0.22	1.7
Sorghum	345	10.7	3.2	26	4.5	0.34	0.15	3.3

consisting of the plumule and radicle attached to the grain by the scutellum;
• the endosperm, comprising more than half of the grain and consisting mainly of starch.

The embryo is the part of the grain that sprouts if the grain is planted or soaked in water. It is very rich in nutrients. Although small in size, the embryo often contains 50 percent of the thiamine, 30 percent of the riboflavin and 30 percent of the niacin of the whole grain. The aleurone and other outer coats contain 50 percent of the niacin and 35 percent of the riboflavin. The endosperm, although by far the largest part of the grain, often contains only one-third or less of the B vitamins. Compared with other parts, it is also poorer in protein and minerals, but it is the main source of energy, in the form of a complex carbohydrate, starch.

Processing

Cereal grains are subjected to many different processes during their prepara-

tion for human consumption. All of the processes have in common that they are designed to remove the fibrous layers of the grain. Some processes, however, are also intended to produce a highly refined white product consisting mainly of endosperm. Another common characteristic shared by all the processes is that they reduce the nutritional value of the grain.

Traditional methods of processing, involving the use of a pestle and mortar or stones, usually produce a cereal grain that has lost some of its outer coats but retains at least part of the germ, including the scutellum. Although very careful and prolonged processing using traditional methods can yield a highly refined product, such preparation is unusual. Light milling, similar to home pounding, also produces a product that retains most of the nutrients. Mechanization of this type has the additional advantage of taking a great burden off the woman of the household, as it is usually the woman who is responsible for pounding grain.

Heavy milling to produce a highly refined product is undesirable from a nutritional point of view. Highly milled cereals such as white maize flour, polished rice and white wheat flour have lost most of the germ and outer layers and with them most of the B vitamins and some of the protein and minerals. Millers are, however, servants of the public, and the public increasingly demands products that are pure white, have a bland, neutral taste and are easily digestible. These demands led, in the first half of the twentieth century, to a vast increase in the production of highly refined cereal flours and white rice. The millers have responded to public demand by devising "improved" milling machinery that separates more and more of the nutritious parts from the grain, leaving the white endosperm.

The percentage of the original grain that remains in the flour after milling is termed the extraction rate. Thus an 85 percent extraction flour contains 85 percent (by weight) of the whole grain, 15 percent having been removed. Therefore, a high-extraction flour has lost little of the nutrients in the outer coats and germ, whereas a low-extraction flour has lost much. The advantages of low-extraction flours over high-extraction flours from the trade point of view are that they are whiter, and so more popular; they have less fat, and hence less tendency to become rancid; they have less phytic acid, which possibly means that minerals from associated foods are absorbed better; and they have better baking qualities. The disadvantages of low-extraction flours to the consumer are that they contain less B vitamins, minerals, protein and fibre than high-extraction flours.

In many countries food fashions begin among the wealthier people. As long as the new food fashion remains confined to those with a high income, it need not do much harm, for they can afford a better all-round diet which compensates for the nutrients lost to fashion. However, the white-flour fashion has spread to all levels of society, rich and poor, in many countries. In addition, highly milled rice spread across Asia quite rapidly over 80 years ago.

Where preference for white flour or highly milled rice leads to the consumption of a staple cereal rendered deficient by milling, widespread ill health could be, and has been, the result among those who do not include in their diet other foods that make up for this deficiency. Much misery, suffering and death resulted directly from the introduction of milled cereals to the people of Asia around the beginning of the twentieth century, when the disease beriberi became highly prevalent (see Chapter 16).

Increasing industrialization and urbanization in developing countries have brought with them a much greater use of bread because of its convenience for workers eating away from home.

Manufactured cereal products are being increasingly sold as baby and breakfast foods. In developing countries these products are mainly imported. They may be convenient but they are relatively expensive and have no inherent advantage, from a nutritional point of view, over local cereals prepared in a traditional manner. However, they may be highly advertised, considered as prestige foods and falsely regarded as more nutritious than local foods. Their use should be discouraged for those who cannot really afford them.

Legislation requiring millers to put additional vitamins into cereal flours exists in some countries and can be effective. This procedure does not work as well with rice because it is most commonly bought and eaten in its granular form, whereas maize and wheat and most other cereals are more often bought as flour. Attempts have been made in Asia to add vitamins in a concentrated form to a few artificial granules and then to mix these with rice. This method has not proved entirely successful, partly because one of the B vitamins, riboflavin, is yellow and lends a colour unacceptable to those who want a uniformly white product.

Maize

Maize (*Zea mays*) is a very important food in the Americas and much of Africa. It was first cultivated in the Americas, and it was an important food of the great Aztec and Mayan civilizations long before the arrival of Columbus and the colonizers. Seeds were brought to Europe and later to Africa, where maize is now the most important part of the diet in many areas (Photo 47). Maize is popular because it gives a high yield per unit area, it grows in warm and fairly dry areas (much drier than those needed for rice, although not as dry as those where sorghum and millet can be raised), it matures rapidly and it has a natural resistance to bird damage. The United States is the largest producer of maize, but much of what is grown there is used to feed domestic animals.

Nutrient content. Maize grains contain about the same amount of protein as other cereals (8 to 10 percent), but much of it is in the form of zein, a poor-quality protein containing only small amounts of lysine and tryptophan. The association noted between maize consumption and pellagra (see Chapter 17) may be due in part to a deficiency of these amino acids. Whole-grain maize contains 2 mg niacin per 100 g, which is less than that in wheat or rice and about the same as the amount in oats. The niacin in maize is in a bound form and not entirely available to humans. In Mexico and some other countries maize is treated with an alkaline solution of lime which

releases the niacin and helps prevent pellagra; maize treated with lime is used for making tortillas, an important food in Mexico.

New varieties of maize, for example opaque-2 maize, have now been developed with an improved amino acid pattern.

Processing. Milling reduces the nutritive value of maize just as it does that of other cereals. The increased popularity and use of highly milled maize meal as opposed to traditionally ground or lightly milled maize in Africa could create a problem, since the highly milled product is deficient in B vitamins (Table 34); it is necessary to eat 600 g of highly milled maize to obtain the amount of thiamine present in 100 g of lightly milled maize. The vitamin B constituents lost in milling may be replaced in maize meal, as in other cereal flours, by fortification. Enrichment of this kind has been effective in many countries. Legislation to ensure an adequate level of B vitamins in cereal flours may be feasible and worthwhile for more countries to adopt.

Rice

Rice, like other cereals, is a domesticated grass (Photo 48); wild varieties have existed for centuries in both Asia (*Oryza sativa*) and Africa (*Oryza glaberina*). Rice is a particularly important food for much of the population of China and for many other countries in Asia, where close to half the population of the world lives. It is also important in the diets of some peoples in the Near East, Africa and to a lesser extent the Americas. Much of the rice is produced in small irrigated fields or paddies in Asia, but some is grown in rain-fed areas without irrigation.

Nutrient content. The outer layers and the germ together contain nearly 80 percent of the thiamine in the rice grain. The endosperm, though constituting 90 percent of

TABLE 34
Effect of milling on vitamin B content of maize (mg per 100 g)

Level of processing of maize	Thiamine	Riboflavin	Niacin
Whole grain	0.35	0.13	2.0
Lightly milled	0.30	0.13	1.5
Highly milled (65 percent extraction)	0.05	0.03	0.6

the weight of the grain, contains less than 10 percent of the thiamine. Lysine and threonine are the limiting amino acids in rice.

Processing. After harvesting, the rice seeds or grains are subjected to different milling methods. The traditional home method of pounding rice in a wooden mortar and winnowing it in a shallow tray usually results in the loss of about half of the outer layers and germ, leaving a product containing about 0.25 mg thiamine per 100 g. The procedure of milling and subsequently polishing rice, which produces the highly esteemed white rice on sale in many shops, removes nearly all the outer layers and germ and leaves a product containing only about 0.06 mg thiamine per 100 g. This amount is grossly deficient. In Asia, many poor people have a diet consisting mainly of rice for much of the year. A person eating 500 g of highly milled polished rice per day would get only 0.3 mg thiamine. The same quantity of home-pounded or lightly milled rice would provide approximately 1.25 mg thiamine, which is about the normal requirement for an average man.

Fortification is one method of adding micronutrients. Another way of providing highly milled rice that is reasonably white and yet contains adequate quantities of B vitamins is by parboiling. This process is usually done in the mill, but it can be done in the home. The paddy, or unhusked rice, is usually steamed, so that water is absorbed by the whole grain, including the endosperm. The B vitamins, which are water soluble, become evenly distributed throughout the whole grain (Figure 16). The paddy is dried and dehusked, and it is then ready for milling in the ordinary way. Even if it is highly milled and polished, the parboiled grain still retains the major part of its thiamine and other B vitamins.

The solubility of the B vitamins has its disadvantages. Rice that is washed too thoroughly in water loses some of the B vitamins, which are dissolved out. Similarly if rice is boiled in excess water, a considerable proportion of the B vitamins is likely to be discarded with the water after cooking. Rice should therefore be cooked in just the amount of water it will absorb. If any water is left over it should be used in a soup or stew, since it will contain valuable B vitamins which should not be wasted.

Wheat

Wheat (genus *Triticum*) is the most widely cultivated cereal in the world and its products are very important in human nutrition. In many parts of the world where wheat cannot be grown it is imported and is becoming an increasingly important part of the diet, especially for the urban population. However, importation of wheat, like that of all products, must be offset by adequate exports to prevent a drain on a country's foreign exchange.

Bread, usually made from wheat flour, is a popular convenience food. When purchased, it saves time and fuel for poor families. Pasta is also becoming increasingly popular in some developing countries.

Nutrient content. Wheat provides a little more protein than does rice or maize, about 11 g per 100 g. The limiting amino acid is lysine. In many industrialized countries

FIGURE 16

Effects of milling and parboiling on thiamine in rice

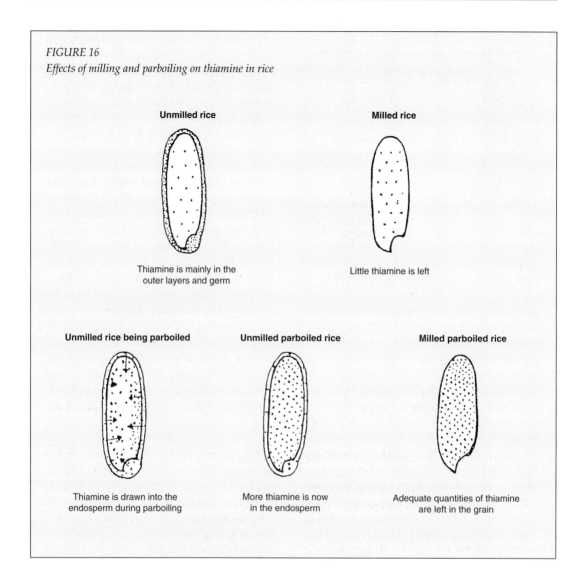

Unmilled rice

Thiamine is mainly in the
outer layers and germ

Milled rice

Little thiamine is left

Unmilled rice being parboiled

Thiamine is drawn into the
endosperm during parboiling

Unmilled parboiled rice

More thiamine is now
in the endosperm

Milled parboiled rice

Adequate quantities of thiamine
are left in the grain

wheat flour is fortified with B vitamins and sometimes iron and other nutrients.

Processing. Wheat is usually ground and made into flour. As with other milled cereals, the nutrient content depends on the degree of milling, i.e. the extraction rate. Low-extraction flours have lost much of their nutrients. In some developing countries where wheat is being increasingly used, the bakers have encouraged the trend towards highly refined products because white wheat flour has better baking qualities. Traders also prefer the highly milled product because it stores better. Its low fat content reduces the chances of rancidity, and its low vitamin content makes it less attractive to insects and other pests.

Millets and sorghum

Millets and sorghum are cereal grains widely grown in Africa and in some countries in Asia and Latin America.

Although less widely grown than maize, rice and wheat, they are important foods. They survive drought conditions better than maize and other cereals, so they are commonly grown in areas where rainfall is low or unpredictable. They are valuable food crops because they nearly all contain a higher percentage of protein than maize and the protein is also of better quality, with a fairly high content of tryptophan. These cereals are also rich in calcium and iron. Because they tend to be ground at home and not in the mill, they are less frequently subjected to vitamin, mineral and protein losses. However, in many areas of Africa, they are being replaced by rice and maize, although they usually continue to be grown for making beer. In some parts of Asia millets are regarded as low-class foods for poor people.

Many millet and sorghum varieties have the disadvantages of susceptibility to attack by small birds and a tendency to shed their grain. Losses are often high. In some countries millets and sorghum are used mainly to feed animals.

Sorghum (*Sorghum vulgare* or *Sorghum bicolor*) is believed to have originated in Africa but is now cultivated in many countries. It is also called guinea corn or durra, and in India it is known as *jowar*. There are many varieties of sorghum; most grow tall and have a large inflorescence, but there are also dwarf varieties. The grain is usually large but varies in colour and shape with the type. Sorghum requires more moisture than millets but less than maize. Sorghum is a nutritious food and many varieties have a higher protein content than other cereals.

There are several species of millet. The most important in Africa are bulrush millet (*Pennisetum glaucum*), also called pearl millet, and finger millet (*Eleusine coracana*). The former, as the name implies, looks rather like a bulrush, but the inflorescence may be much longer and thicker, some-

times 1×8 cm (Photo 49). The inflorescence of finger millet is shaped like a rather flaccid hand. The seeds are smaller than those of bulrush millet. It is very commonly used for making beer.

Other cereals

Oats. Oats are not important in the diets of most developing countries. The crop is grown in a few cold highland areas, where it is locally prepared and not usually milled. Oats are a good cereal containing rather more protein than maize, rice or wheat, but they also contain a considerable quantity of phytic acid which may hinder absorption of iron and calcium. Oatmeal is imported for use in porridge and is used in some manufactured infant foods.

Rye. Rye is little grown in Africa, Asia and Latin America, and even in Europe it is not an important item of the diet. It has nutritive properties similar to those of other cereals and is sometimes added to bread.

Barley. Barley is grown in some of the wheat-growing districts of Africa and in highland areas of Asia and South America. In these places it is usually consumed as a stiff porridge after home preparation. In Europe it is now used mainly for animal feeding and in the preparation of alcoholic beverages such as beer and whisky.

Triticale. This new cereal (Photo 50) is a cross between wheat and rye. It has promise of high yields and good nutritive value. It is particularly suited to temperate climates.

Teff. Teff (*Eragrostis tef*) is an important cereal in Ethiopia, where it is held in special regard although it gives a relatively low yield per unit area. It is usually ground into a flour, cooked and eaten as *injera*, a type of baked pancake. The nutritive value of teff is similar to that of other cereal grains, except that it is richer in iron and calcium. The high consumption of teff in parts of Ethiopia may be an important reason why iron deficiency anaemia is rarely reported there.

Quinoa. Quinoa is a millet-like cereal grain which is grown in South America in the Andes, particularly in the altiplano. It grows well even where rainfall is low, soil is not very fertile and nights are very cold. As a food it has a special place in the diets of some Andean peoples.

STARCHES AND STARCHY ROOTS

A number of edible tubers, roots and corms form an important part of the diet of many peoples in different parts of the world. In tropical countries cassava, sweet potatoes, taro (cocoyam), yams and arrowroot are the most important foods in this class. In the cooler parts of the world the common potato is also widely grown.

These food crops are usually relatively easy to cultivate and give high yields per hectare. They contain large quantities of starch and are therefore a fairly easily obtainable source of food energy. As staple foodstuffs, however, they are inferior to cereals because they consist of about two-thirds water and have much less protein, as well as lower contents of minerals and vitamins. They usually contain less than 2 percent protein, whereas cereals contain about 10 percent. Taro and yams, however, contain up to 6 percent good-quality protein.

Cassava

Although cassava (*Manihot esculenta*), also known as yuca or manioc, originated in South America, it is now widely grown in many parts of Asia and Africa, mainly for its starchy tuberous roots which may grow to an enormous size. Readily established from cuttings, it will grow in poor soil,

requires relatively little attention, withstands adverse weather conditions and until recently was not greatly afflicted by pests or disease. However, in some parts of Africa, notably Malawi, cassava plants in the fields have been attacked and destroyed by mealy bug.

Energy yields per hectare from cassava roots are often very high, potentially much higher than from cereals. The leaves of the plant are eaten by some societies and are nutritious. However, cassava has the great disadvantage of containing little but carbohydrate. It is especially unsuitable as the main source of energy for the infant or young child because of its low protein content. It should therefore be supplemented liberally with cereals and also with legumes or other protein-rich foods. However, in non-arid areas where the main food and nutrition problems arise from shortage of total food and deficient energy intake, cassava should be encouraged because of its high yields and other agricultural advantages.

Cassava contains less than 1 percent protein, significantly less than the 10 percent in maize and other cereals (Photo 51). It is not surprising, therefore, that kwashiorkor resulting from protein deficiency is much more common in young children weaned on to cassava than in those weaned on to millet or maize. Cassava also has considerably less iron and B vitamins than the cereal grains.

Cassava, particularly bitter varieties, sometimes contains a cyanogenic glucoside. This poisonous substance is present mainly near the outer coat of the tuber, so peeling cassava helps reduce the cyanide. Cassava that is soaked in water or boiled in water that is then discarded also has reduced cyanide levels. In addition, toxicity can be reduced by pounding, grating and fermentation of the cassava roots. Toxic effects tend to occur where these practices are not used. Cassava consumption has also been linked with goitre and iodine deficiency disorders (see Chapter 14).

Cassava leaves are frequently used as a green vegetable. Their nutritive value is similar to that of other dark green leaves. They are an extremely valuable source of carotene (vitamin A), vitamin C, iron and calcium. The leaves also contain some protein. To preserve the maximum quantity of vitamin C in the leaves, they should not be cooked for longer than about 20 minutes.

Cassava tubers may be eaten roasted or boiled, but more often they are sun-dried after soaking and then made into a powdery white flour. In some countries cassava is milled commercially. In some of this processing the end product is tapioca, which is mainly cassava starch. In West Africa cassava is used to make *fufu* (a boiled, mashed product). In some countries, for example Indonesia, cassava is regarded as a poor persons' food, and in others as a famine food.

Sweet potatoes

Sweet potatoes originated in the Americas and are now widely grown also in tropical Africa and Asia, usually from stem cuttings. Like cassava, the irregularly shaped, variously sized tubers contain little protein. They contain some vitamin C, and the coloured varieties, especially the yellow ones, provide useful quantities of carotene (provitamin A). Sweet-potato leaves are often eaten and have properties very similar to those of cassava leaves. However, the leaves should not be picked to excess since, as with other tuber crops, this may reduce the yield of tubers.

Yams

There are innumerable varieties of yams (genus *Dioscorea*), some of which are indigenous to Africa, Asia and the Americas. They vary in shape, colour and size as well as in cooking quality, leaf structure and palatability. Besides the many domesticated varieties a number of wild varieties are eaten.

Yams are more extensively grown in West Africa than in East Africa. In Nigeria, for example, yams are still an important root crop despite an increase in the popularity of cassava. Yams require a warm, humid climate and soil rich in organic matter; these requirements limit their cultivation.

The proper cultivation of yams entails initial deep digging and subsequent staking of the twining vine-like plant. The work involved is more arduous than for cassava, and the yields, though high, are usually a little lower than cassava yields. Yams usually contain about twice as much protein (2 percent) as cassava, although very much less than cereals.

Taro or cocoyams

Taro (*Colocasia* sp.) originated in Asia but is quite extensively grown in areas where there is fairly high rainfall spread over much of the year. It is widely grown and consumed in the Pacific islands. In Africa, taro is common in forest areas (e.g. in the Ashanti country of Ghana) and on mountain slopes where precipitation is high (e.g. Mount Kilimanjaro). Taro is often grown in association with bananas or plantains (e.g. by the Buganda) or together with oil-palms. The plant has large "elephant ear" leaves. Both the tubers and the leaves are eaten. The nutritive value of taro is similar to that of cassava. In some areas taro is being replaced by tania or new cocoyam (*Xanthosoma* sp.), a somewhat similar but more robust plant originally from South America, which outyields taro.

Potatoes

Potatoes were first taken to Europe from South America and became a cheap, useful, high-yielding alternative to the existing main staples, just as cassava replaced millet in parts of Africa and Asia. However, the mistake of relying almost entirely on one crop was emphasized by the great Irish potato famine of the nineteenth century: when the potato crop failed because of a blight, over one million people died and even larger numbers emigrated. Potatoes remain a very important food of people living in the Andean countries of South America. Much research on this crop has been conducted in Peru. From Europe, potatoes travelled to Africa and Asia, where they are grown in higher cool areas (Photo 52). If well cultivated in the right soil and climate, they can give a very high yield per hectare.

Like other starchy tubers, potatoes contain only about 2 percent protein, but the protein is of reasonably good quality. Potatoes also provide small quantities of B vitamins and minerals. They contain about 15 mg vitamin C per 100 g, but this amount is reduced in storage. The keeping quality of potatoes is not good, unless they are stored carefully.

Arrowroot

Arrowroot, which is grown in areas with adequate rainfall, is liked by certain peoples in Africa and Oceania. The nutritive value of arrowroot is similar to that of potatoes. The roots are eaten in a variety of ways, often roasted or boiled.

OTHER PREDOMINANTLY CARBOHYDRATE FOODS
Bananas and plantains

Strictly speaking, bananas and plantains should be discussed with fruits; from the nutritional point of view, however, they are more appropriately considered under starchy foods. It is difficult to differentiate among the many varieties of plantain and of banana. For the purposes of this book, plantains may be described as bananas that are picked green and are cooked before eating. Plantains contain more starch and less sugar than bananas, which are usually eaten raw like other fruits.

Bananas and plantains originally grew wild in damp, warm forest areas. They have probably been used as food by humans since earliest times. Bananas and plantains are now cultivated extensively in many of the humid tropical areas. Some peoples such as the Buganda in Uganda and the Wachagga in the United Republic of Tanzania depend on plantains as their main food.

A 100-g portion of green bananas or plantains provides 32 g carbohydrate (mainly as starch), 1.2 g protein, 0.3 g fat and 135 kcal. Plantains also have a high water content. Their very low protein content explains why kwashiorkor commonly occurs in young children weaned on to a mainly plantain diet. Bananas usually contain about 20 mg vitamin C and 120 mg vitamin A (as beta-carotene equivalent) per 100 g. For this reason fresh fruits and vegetables are much less important in the diet for those whose staple food is banana than for those whose staple is a cereal or root. Bananas are, however, low in their content of calcium, iron and B vitamins. As bananas supply only 80 kcal per 100 g, about 2 kg must be eaten to provide 1 500 kcal.

Plantains are usually picked while they are still green. The skin is peeled off and they are then either roasted and eaten, or, more commonly, cut up, boiled and eaten with meat, beans or other foods. Plantains are frequently sun-dried and made into a flour.

Sago

Sago (*Metroxylon* sp.) is almost pure starch and comes from various forms of the sago palm. The trees are widely grown in Indonesia, but sago as a food is particularly popular in certain Pacific islands. Sago has low protein content.

Sugar

Sugar, as sold in shops, is almost 100 percent sucrose and is essentially pure carbohydrate. In Africa, Asia and Latin America nearly all locally produced sugar comes from sugar cane, while in Europe and North America some comes from sugar beet.

In areas where much sugar cane is grown, the consumption of sugar or sugar-cane juice (chewed cane) is often high. In other parts of the world the consumption of sugar tends to rise with economic advancement. In the United States and the United Kingdom in 1995 about 18 percent of energy consumed came from sugar (sucrose), mainly in sweetened foods. In contrast, in many African countries less than 5 percent of energy comes from sucrose. Sugar is a good and often inexpensive source of energy and can be a valuable addition to bulky energy-deficient diets. Contrary to popular belief, customary consumption of sugar is not related to obesity, diabetes, hypertension or any other non-communicable disease. Frequent sugar consumption can be associated with dental caries when coupled with poor oral hygiene, but sucrose is no more cariogenic than other fermentable sugars.

White sugar contains no vitamins, protein, fat or minerals. Many people find that its sweet taste adds to the enjoyment of eating. The yields of energy per hectare of land are very high on productive sugar estates.

Honey

From time immemorial honey has been extensively gathered in developing countries from wild hives. Now more and more hives are being kept, often in hollowed and suspended pieces of tree-trunk or in other more managed ways. The incentive to keep bees tends to be the high price of beeswax rather than just the honey.

Honey has gained the false reputation of being of special nutritive value. In fact it contains only sugar (carbohydrate), water and minute traces of other nutrients. Although merely a source of energy, it has sensory value as a pleasant food for humans.

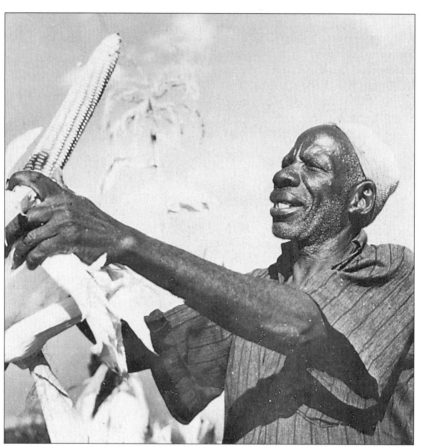

PHOTO 47
A farmer inspects his maize crop

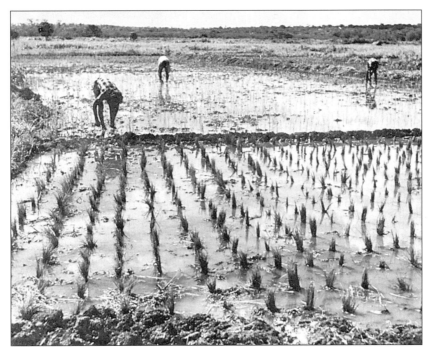

PHOTO 48
Growing rice

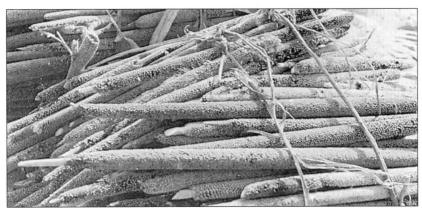

PHOTO 49
Bundles of bulrush millet

PHOTO 50
Triticale

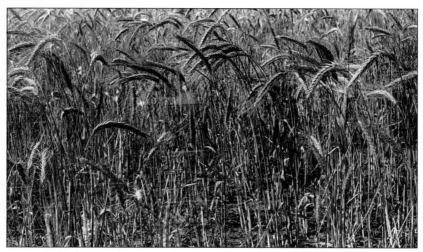

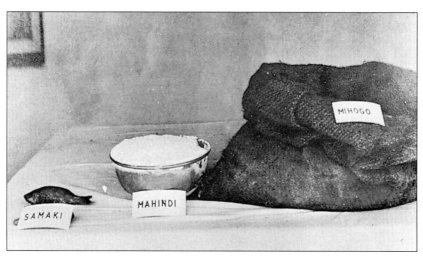

PHOTO 51
One small dried fish (samaki) *weighing 150 g or 1.4 kg maize meal*
(mahindi) *contains the same quantity of protein as 6.8 kg cassava* (mihogo)

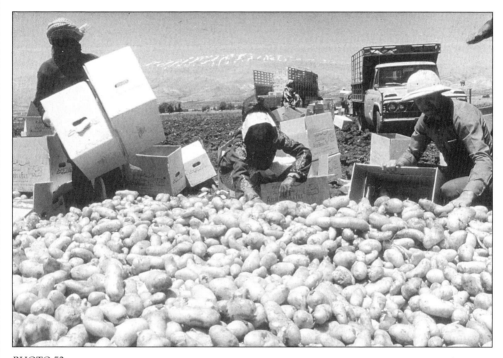

PHOTO 52
Potatoes in Lebanon

Chapter 27
Legumes, nuts and oilseeds

LEGUMES OR PULSES

Beans, peas, lentils, groundnuts and their like belong to the botanical family of Leguminosae. Their edible seeds are called legumes or pulses. Agriculturally the plants of this group have the advantage of being able to obtain nitrogen from the air and also add some to the soil, whereas most other plants take nitrogen from the soil and do not replace it. Legumes usually thrive best when they can get water early in their growth and then have a warm dry spell for ripening. They are therefore often planted at the end of the rains to ripen early in the dry season.

In Africa, Asia and Latin America the seeds are usually left on the plant to reach full maturity and are then harvested and dried. Some may be picked earlier and eaten while partly green, as in Europe and North America.

The dried seeds can be kept and stored in much the same way as cereals.

Some varieties are susceptible to attack by weevils; spending a small amount of money on insecticides to prevent this is definitely economically sound. However, care must be taken to ensure that an excess of insecticide is not applied, that the insecticide is relatively safe and that the beans are well washed before cooking.

The legumes are very important from a nutritional point of view because they are a widely available vegetable food containing good quantities of protein and B vitamins in addition to carbohydrate. Some legumes, such as groundnuts and soybeans, are also rich in oil. They usually supplement very well the predominantly carbohydrate diet based on cereals. Most legumes contain more protein than meat, but the protein is of slightly lower quality because it has less methionine. However, when pulses and cereals are eaten together at one meal they supply a protein mixture containing good quantities of all the amino acids, which improves the protein value of the diet. Legumes also contain some carotene (provitamin A) and ascorbic acid if eaten green. Similarly, dried legumes allowed to sprout before eating have good quantities of ascorbic acid. Some legumes contain antivitamins or toxins (see Chapter 34).

Unless there is a very good reason for introducing a new crop such as soybeans, it is more sensible to encourage increased production and consumption of whatever legume is already grown and popular in any area. The local people will have a taste for it, and agricultural conditions are usually suitable. It is also highly important to try to introduce beans (and other pulses) into the diet of children at an early age. Children are just as able as adults to digest beans easily.

Beans, peas, lentils and grams

A wide variety of beans, peas, lentils, grams, etc. are grown and are important in the diet of people in Asia, Africa and Latin America (Photo 53). All three regions have indigenous legume varieties but also grow varieties that originated on other continents.

There are many kinds of beans. Haricot or kidney beans (*Phaseolus vulgaris*) were originally from the Americas but are now widely grown in Asia and Africa. Broad beans (*Vicia faba*) are more common in temperate areas. Lima beans (*Phaseolus lunatus*) originated from Peru but are eaten all over the tropics and subtropics. Mung beans (*Phaseolus aureus*), indigenous to the Indian subcontinent, are small seeds but very popular. Scarlet runner beans (*Phaseolus multiflorus*) are popular as a fresh vegetable in Europe and North America, but the large mature seeds are eaten dried in many countries.

Lentils (*Lens esculenta*) and some similar legumes often known as grams are very important in the diets of people in many developing countries. Lentils have been cultivated for food by humans for thousands of years. The plants are of small size, as are the seeds. Grams include the important pigeon pea (*Cajanus cajan*), chickpea (*Cicer arietinum*) and green gram or mung bean (*Phaseolus aureus*). In many South Asian countries various dhals made from these legumes form a significant part of the diet, providing important nutrients to supplement the staple food, which may be rice or wheat. In many parts of Africa both cowpeas and pigeon peas are grown and consumed. The pigeon pea is perennial and relatively drought resistant. *Lathyrus sativus*, another drought-resistant legume, is grown widely in India, but consumption of large amounts can lead to the severe toxic condition called lathyrism (see Chapter 34). Winged bean (*Psophocarpus tetragonolobus*) is another important legume with a very high protein content (35 percent), but it is not yet widely grown.

Peas are commonly consumed as a green vegetable (fresh, canned or frozen) in Europe and North America and by more affluent people elsewhere. In developing countries the seeds are allowed to mature and are dried and consumed in the same manner as other legumes.

These legumes (excluding soybean) all have a somewhat similar nutritive value, but the mature beans are eaten in a variety of ways and have different flavours and other culinary qualities. Most legume seeds usually contain about 22 percent protein (as opposed to 1 percent in cassava roots and 10 percent in maize) and good quantities of thiamine, riboflavin and niacin; in addition they are richer in iron and calcium than most of the cereals.

The large number of other legume seeds of various shapes, colours and sizes on sale at food shops or marketplaces in almost any village or town in tropical countries is evidence of an appreciation of dietary variety and culinary finesse. Culture and local taste importantly determine how these foods are eaten.

Soybean

Soybean (*Glycine max*) originated in Asia, but now the main producers are the United States and Brazil. However, the soybeans produced by these countries are mainly used commercially for oil and as animal feeds. Asia still produces much of the soybeans for direct human consumption. They are not widely grown in Africa or Latin America.

Soybeans contain up to 40 percent protein, 18 percent fat and 20 percent carbohydrate. The protein is of a higher biological quality than that from other plant sources.

Soybeans, used in a wide variety of ways, are very important in the diets of the Chinese and in those of some other Asian countries. In China soybeans are made into a variety of tasty dishes which supplement the staple food of rice or other cereal. Soy products such as tofu (soybean curd) and tempeh (a fermented product) are important in Indonesian cuisine and popular elsewhere. Soybeans have not become a popular food in Africa or Latin America, where there is little local knowledge of the best methods of preparing them. People lacking experience with soybeans find them difficult to prepare and cook.

Where soybeans are grown they can be

locally processed for use in the country as an enrichment of cereal flours, as an infant food or for institutional and school-feeding purposes. The oil can be exported and the protein-rich residue cake can be utilized in the country.

Groundnuts (peanuts, monkey-nuts)

The term "groundnut" is a misnomer since, although botanically a nut, the groundnut (*Arachis hypogaea*) is a true pulse, a member of the Leguminosae family. It originated in Brazil but is now extensively grown in warm climates around the world. It is an unusual plant in that the flower stalk bearing the ovary burrows into the ground, where a nut containing the seed or seeds develops (Photo 54).

Groundnuts contain much more fat than other legumes, often 45 percent, and also much more niacin (18 mg per 100 g) and thiamine, but relatively little carbohydrate (12 percent). The protein content is a little higher than that of most other pulses (27 percent). Groundnuts are an unusually nutritious food with more protein than animal meat. They are energy dense because of their oil, and they are rich in vitamins and minerals. As suggested in Chapter 9, if every child, woman and man in Africa ate a handful of groundnuts per day in addition to their normal diet, Africa would be rid of most existing malnutrition.

Groundnuts are fairly widely grown in the tropics. Farmers should produce them for home consumption as well as for cash crops, since they form a very useful addition to the primarily cereal or root diets of many poor families. They supply much-needed fat, which is high in energy and assists in the absorption of carotene as well as serving other functions. In predominantly maize diets, relatively small quantities of groundnuts, with their high content of niacin and also of protein (including the amino acid tryptophan), can prevent pellagra. When groundnuts are added to children's diets, their high protein and energy content serves to prevent protein-energy malnutrition.

However, groundnuts are often grown mainly as a cash crop even in developing countries. The world's largest producer is the United States. Groundnuts are usually utilized for oil extraction, and the residue, groundnut cake, is used for animal feed. In the United States a good proportion is consumed as peanut butter. In many countries groundnuts are consumed roasted, boiled or cooked in other ways.

Groundnuts, if damaged during harvesting or if poorly stored in damp conditions, may be attacked by the mould *Aspergillus flavus*. This fungus produces a poisonous toxin known as aflatoxin, which has been shown to cause liver damage in animals and to kill poultry fed on infected groundnuts. It may be toxic also for humans and may be a cause of liver cancer (see Chapter 34).

Bambara groundnut

The bambara groundnut (*Voandzeia subterranea*) originated in Africa and is grown widely. It resembles the groundnut physically but is not nutritionally similar, having only 6 percent fat. Its protein content of 18 percent is a little lower than that of most other pulses, but it has about the same mineral and vitamin content as beans. Because of the lower fat content the crop is not in great demand for oil production. Therefore, instead of being sold as a cash crop, it is more often used locally for food.

TREE NUTS
Coconut

Coconut (Photo 55) is the most important nut crop in Africa. Its origins are uncertain. The nut, being light and impervious to water, no doubt drifted across many seas to germinate on a new shore. It is now extensively cultivated. The tree that bears it is a picturesque and highly useful plant, apart from the food it provides for humans. When it is green, the nut contains about half a litre of water; this is a very refreshing and hygienic drink, but apart from a little calcium and carbohydrate, it has no nutritive value. The white flesh, however, is rich in fat.

The flesh of the coconut is usually sun-dried into copra. The oil from copra is used both for cooking and for making soap. Copra itself is used in the tropics and elsewhere as an addition to many dishes. It is an important ingredient in a variety of cuisines from Thailand to Saudi Arabia. Coconut oil has the disadvantage of containing a relatively high proportion of saturated fatty acids. The coconut sap in many countries is fermented to yield alcoholic beverages.

Cashew nut

The cashew nut is produced on a small tree that originated in dry areas of the Americas. It is widely grown in the tropics, and the nuts are mainly exported. They are rich in fat (45 percent) and contain 20 percent protein and 26 percent carbo-hydrate. The edible swollen stalk of the nut contains good quantities of vitamin C. Cashew nuts are a useful local food but too expensive for most people.

OILSEEDS
Sesame

Sesame, or simsim (benniseed in West Africa), is grown fairly widely throughout the world and is largely used for oil extraction. The seeds, which are of various colours, contain about 50 percent fat and 20 percent protein. They are also rich in calcium and contain useful quantities of carotene, iron and B vitamins. Sesame seeds can form a nutritious addition to the diet.

Sunflower seeds

Sunflowers are grown mainly as a cash crop, but some of the seeds and some of the oil are eaten locally. The oil has the advantage of being relatively high in polyunsaturated fatty acids. The seeds contain about 36 percent oil (less than sesame), 23 percent protein and some calcium, iron, carotene and B vitamins.

Red palm oil

The product from oil-palm (*Elaeis guineensis*) is discussed in Chapter 30 with other oils and fats.

Other oilseeds

A number of other oil-rich seeds are eaten or used for oil extraction. These include pumpkin seeds, melon seeds, oyster nut (*Telfairia pedata*) and cottonseed. The last is a major source of oil in the cotton-growing areas of Asia, Africa and Latin America. In West Africa and elsewhere, shea butter (*Butyrospermum parkii*), butternut and several other oilseeds are used in the diet. Most of these grow on indigenous trees.

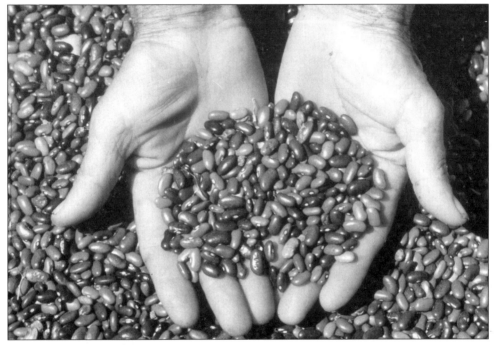

PHOTO 53
Beans harvested in Honduras

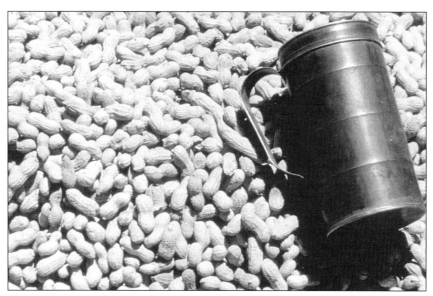

PHOTO 54
Groundnuts produced in Mexico

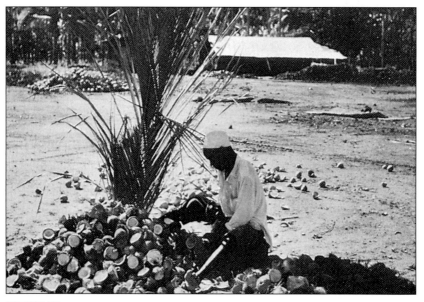

PHOTO 55
*The coconut: its trees provide shade; its husks fuel; its juice refreshment; its copra
oil, food and money; and its leaves roofing for houses*

Chapter 28
Vegetables and fruits

VEGETABLES

The foods called vegetables (Photos 56 to 59) include some fruits (e.g. tomatoes and pumpkins), leaves (e.g. amaranth and cabbage), roots (e.g. carrots and turnips) and even stalks (e.g. celery) and flowers (e.g. cauliflower). Many of the plants from which these various edible parts are taken are unrelated botanically. However, "vegetable" is a useful term both in nutrition and in domestic terminology.

In developing countries, nearly all types of vegetables are eaten soon after they are harvested; unlike cereals, tubers, starchy roots, pulses and nuts, they are rarely stored for long periods (with a few exceptions such as pumpkins and other gourds).

It is not uncommon for rural people in parts of Asia, Latin America and Africa to forage for an important proportion of the vegetables they consume. With increasing population, however, the availability of wild fruits and vegetables is decreasing. Therefore vegetables are obtained from the farm or the household garden or from the marketplace, neighbours or small stalls along the roadside. When rural families with low income move to an urban environment they may resent having to purchase vegetables, because they are used to being able to gather wild ones or grow their own. They may therefore spend relatively little on this component of the diet. In any case, vegetables are rarely a prestige food, and in few societies are they high on the list of food preferences.

Vegetables are a very important part of the diet. They are nearly all rich in carotene and vitamin C and contain significant amounts of calcium, iron and other minerals. Their content of B vitamins is frequently small. They usually provide only a little energy and very little protein. A large proportion of their content consists of indigestible residue, which adds bulk or fibre to the faeces.

In many tropical diets the dark green leaves are the most valuable vegetables because they contain far more carotene and vitamin C, as well as more protein, calcium and iron, than pale green leaves and other vegetables. Thus amaranth is much superior to cabbage or lettuce. Leaves from pumpkin, sweet potato and cassava plants, as well as many wild edible leaves, are also excellent.

An increase in the consumption of green leaves and other vegetables could play a major part in reducing vitamin A deficiency, which is often prevalent in children, and could contribute to lessening the prevalence of iron deficiency anaemia in all segments of the population but especially in women of child-bearing age. Increased vegetable consumption would also supply additional calcium and vitamin C which would prevent the rare disease scurvy and perhaps also assist the healing of ulcers and wounds. Vitamin C also enhances iron absorption.

It is not possible here to describe the individual properties of the many vegetables commonly eaten in developing countries. A few, such as pumpkins, can be stored for several months with little loss of nutritive value; others, such as leaves and even tomatoes, are frequently sun-dried, but with considerable loss of vitamin content. The vitamin C content of vegetables is also lowered by prolonged cooking.

Vegetables grown in home and school gardens could be a valuable source of food for the family and the school and could make an important nutritional contribution, particularly to micronutrient intake. Home gardens can be raised with spare family labour and the participation of women and children. It is therefore important for most rural households and virtually every school to devote more time to growing vegetables. A community garden near the village source of water is often a useful adjunct to the villagers' own backyard gardens. In towns, even the smallest piece of land behind a house could, with the assistance of waste water, yield a valuable supply of vegetables all year round. The allocation of allotment plots for vegetable growing deserves serious consideration by town councils and other urban authorities. Even people living in flats can grow certain varieties in pots kept on their verandas.

FRUITS

A wide variety of fruits grow wild or are cultivated in tropical countries (Photo 60). The varieties available at any one time in a given area depend on the climate, the local tastes for fruit, the species cultivated and the season.

The main nutritive value of fruits is their content of vitamin C, which is often high. Some fruits also contain useful quantities of carotene. Fruits (except the avocado and a few others) contain very little fat or protein and usually no starch. The carbohydrate is present in the form of various sugars. Fruits, like vegetables, contain much unabsorbable residue, mainly cellulose. The citrus fruits, such as oranges, lemons, grapefruits, tangerines and limes, contain good quantities of vitamin C but little carotene. In contrast, papayas, mangoes and Cape gooseberries (*Physalis peruviana*) contain both carotene and vitamin C.

Papayas (Photo 61) are a useful fruit, especially for those who cultivate a piece of land for a few years and then move on to new land. The papaya grows rapidly and may yield fruit after one or two years. The mango, on the other hand, grows slowly, but once established (and it may establish itself) needs no care and yields fruit for half a century. Guavas, which are quite widely grown, contain five times as much vitamin C as most citrus fruits, as well as useful amounts of carotene.

The avocado requires special mention because, unlike other fruits, it is rich in fat, a substance that is lacking in many tropical diets. It could with benefit be much more widely grown and eaten and fed to children.

Bananas are widely grown and eaten in tropical countries. They contain fair quantities of carotene and vitamin C, and they are rich in potassium. In East Africa plantains or bananas are commonly picked when green. Cooked and eaten as a mainly starchy food, they form the staple diet of many people. When bananas are ripe their starch is converted into other sugars.

A few fruit-trees would be a useful addition to all households, both urban and rural.

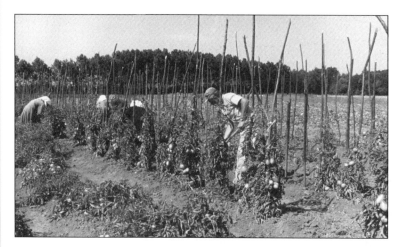

PHOTO 56
Tomatoes being grown in Turkey

PHOTO 57
Growing vegetables in Saudi Arabia

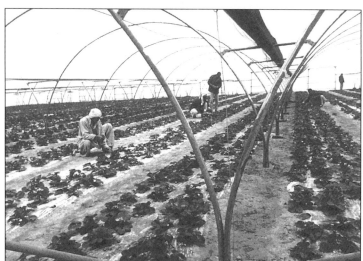

PHOTO 58
Cabbages growing in Laos

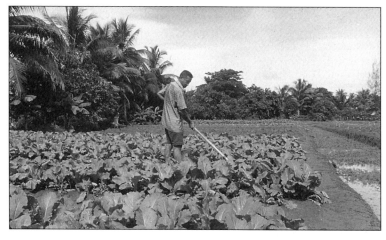

PHOTO 59
Vegetables are often rich in carotene, vitamin C, iron, calcium and other micronutrients

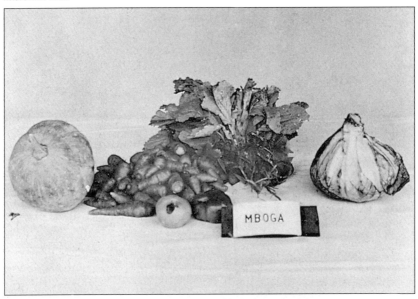

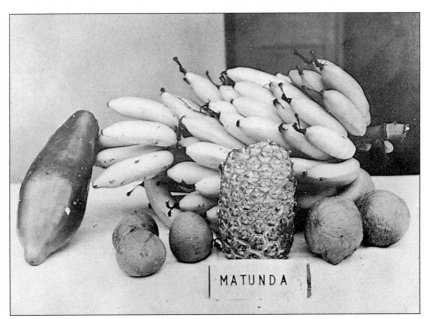

PHOTO 60
Fruits are a good source of vitamin C, and many are also rich in carotene

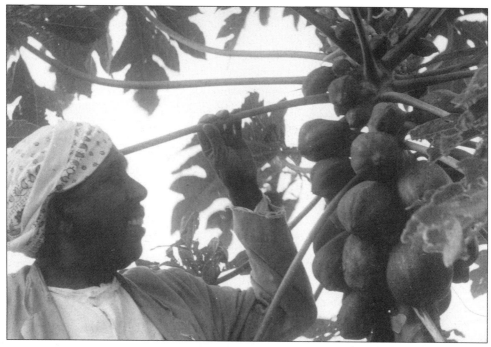

PHOTO 61
Papaya tree in Mauritius

Chapter 29
Meat, fish, eggs, milk and their products

Foods of animal origin are not essential for an adequate diet, but they are a useful complement to most diets, especially to those in developing countries that are based mainly on a carbohydrate-rich staple food such as a cereal or root crop. Meat, fish, eggs, milk and dairy products all provide protein of high biological value, which is often a good complement to the limiting amino acids in plant foods consumed. These products are also rich in other nutrients. The iron provided by meat and fish is easily absorbed and enhances the absorption of iron from common staple foods such as rice, wheat or maize. However, foods of animal origin are usually relatively expensive and not within the purchasing power of poorer families. Some wealthier people in both developing and industrialized countries consume large quantities of these foods; in consequence their intake of fat, especially saturated fat, may become excessive, increasing the risks of heart disease and obesity. Americans consume about 80 kg of meat per person per year – almost 0.25 kg per day.

MEAT AND MEAT PRODUCTS

Meat (Photo 62) is usually defined as the flesh (mainly muscles) and organs (for example, liver and kidneys) of animals (mammals, reptiles and amphibians) and birds (particularly poultry). Meat is some-times subdivided into red meat (from cattle, goats, sheep, pigs, etc.) and white meat (mainly from poultry). The animals providing meat may be domesticated or wild. The amount of meat consumed often depends mainly on cultural factors, on the price of meat in relation to incomes and on availability.

Meat contains about 19 percent protein of excellent quality and iron that is well absorbed. The amount of fat depends on the animal that the meat comes from and the cut. The energy value of meat rises with the fat content. The fat in meat is fairly high in its content of saturated fatty acids and cholesterol. Meat also provides useful amounts of riboflavin and niacin, a little thiamine and small quantities of iron, zinc and vitamins A and C. Offal (the internal organs), particularly liver, contains larger quantities. Offal has a relatively high amount of cholesterol. In general all animals – wild and domestic, large and small, birds, reptiles and mammals – provide meat of rather similar nutritional value. The main variable is the fat content.

Worldwide, a vast range and variety of animal products are eaten. Not all of them are popular everywhere, of course. Certain foods that are popular in some parts of the tropics and East Asia – such as locusts, grasshoppers, termites, flying ants, lake flies, caterpillars and other insects; baboons and monkeys; snakes and snails; rats and other rodents; and cats and dogs – are not found in European or North American diets. Similarly, the French liking for frogs' legs and horse meat and the English and Japanese taste for eels and raw oysters are not shared by many people living else-where. Liked or disliked, however, all these foods are nutritious and contain protein of high biological value.

Contaminated meat can lead to disease. There is a need for improvements in conditions associated with production of meat both for local or family consumption and more importantly for commercial sale. For meat to be safe for human consumption, hygienic practices are essential at all levels, from the farm, through the slaughterhouse, to the retailer and into the kitchen. Most countries have regulations governing meat hygiene and authorities responsible for applying the regulations, but their effectiveness varies widely.

FISH AND SEAFOODS

Fish and seafoods, like meat, are valuable in the diet because they provide a good quantity (usually 17 percent or more) of protein of high biological value, particularly sulphur-containing amino acids. They are especially good as a complement to a cassava diet, which provides little protein.

Fish varies in fat content but generally has less fat than meat. Fish also provides thiamine, riboflavin, niacin, vitamin A, iron and calcium. It contains a small quantity of vitamin C if eaten fresh. Small fish from the sea and lakes such as sardines and sprats (*dagaa* in the United Republic of Tanzania, *kapenta* in Zambia) are consumed whole, bones and all, thus providing much calcium and fluorine. Dried *dagaa*, for instance, may contain 2 500 mg calcium per 100 g. Fish offal is not usually consumed as part of any diet anywhere. However, fish liver and fish oils are very rich sources of the fat-soluble vitamins A and D. The amount varies, usually with the age and species of fish.

Wherever water is available, fish provide a simple way of increasing protein consumption. The stocking of dams, the construction of fish ponds (Photo 63) and better and more widespread fishing in rivers, lakes and the sea should all be given greater encouragement.

There is much regional variation in the variety of sea creatures people will eat. Encouraging children in coastal districts to collect sea urchins, sea slugs, limpets and the numerous other edible sea creatures, just as inland children collect locusts and lake flies, would considerably improve poor diets. The introduction of swimming lessons in youth clubs and as a community development activity would encourage development of this pastime as well as fishing both for pleasure and for profit; fear of the water because of inability to swim is a deterrent to these activities, particularly among people who do not live beside water.

EGGS

The egg is one of the few foods containing no carbohydrate. Just as the foetus in the mother's uterus draws nutrients from the mother's blood in order to grow and develop into a human being, so the bird embryo draws all its nutrients from within the egg. It is not surprising therefore that eggs are highly nutritious. Each egg contains a high proportion of excellent protein, is rich in fat and contains good quantities of calcium, iron, vitamins A and D and also thiamine and riboflavin.

Eggs are an essential part of the reproductive cycle of birds, so it is hardly surprising that their consumption, particularly by females, is forbidden by taboos in many societies. The irony is that eggs are often more easily available than most other high-quality foods. In developing countries it is not often that a family can afford to kill a cow or even a goat for food, but eggs are small and frequently laid. They are also an easily prepared, easily digestible, protein-rich food suitable for children from the age of six months onward. Eggs do have a nutritional disadvantage: very high cholesterol content. The cholesterol is present in the yolk.

Production of eggs for family use should be encouraged wherever possible, even in the small garden or yard of an urban dwelling (Photo 64). Toddlers should be given priority in eating the eggs.

BLOOD

Cattle blood, which is regularly consumed raw by many pastoral peoples, particularly in Africa, is highly nutritious. It is rich in protein, has high biological value and contains many other nutrients. It is a particularly valuable source of iron. It is also a good source of nutrients in its processed form, usually a type of sausage.

MILK AND MILK PRODUCTS

Animal milks and other dairy products are highly nutritious and can play an important part in human diets for both children and adults. The composition of milk varies according to the animal from which it comes, providing the correct rate of growth and development for the young of that species. Thus, for human infants, human milk is better than cows' milk or any other milk product. Exclusive breast-feeding without other foods or liquids is the optimum means of feeding for the first six months of an infant's life (see Chapter 7). Continuing breastfeeding for many more months is of great value, while the baby is introduced to other foods. If breastmilk remains an important food for the child into the second or even third year of life, then animal milk is not necessary in the child's diet.

The composition of human and cows' milk is compared in Chapter 7 (Table 7). Except for certain vitamins, the composition of human breastmilk is fairly constant, regardless of the diet of the mother. Maternal malnutrition will not cause a mother to produce milk of markedly lower nutrient content, but it will reduce the quantity she can produce. A few nutrients such as thiamine and vitamin A may be low if mothers are deficient in these nutrients.

Caseinogen and lactalbumin, proteins of high biological value, are among the most important constituents of cows' milk. The carbohydrate in cows' milk is the disaccharide lactose. Fat is present as very fine globules, which on standing tend to coalesce and rise to the surface. The fat has a rather high content of saturated fatty acids. The calcium content of cows' milk (120 mg per 100 ml) is four times that of human milk (30 mg per 100 ml), because calves grow much more quickly and have a larger skeleton than human babies and therefore need more calcium. When a human infant is fed entirely on cows' milk the excess calcium does no good but causes no harm. It does not produce a rate of growth beyond the optimum. The excess is excreted in the urine.

Milk is also a very good source of riboflavin and vitamin A. It is a fair source of thiamine and vitamin C, but it is a poor source of iron and niacin. The mother usually provides her infant with a store of iron before birth. However, this store is exhausted by about the sixth month of life, and if feeding of milk alone is prolonged, iron deficiency anaemia may develop.

The amount of thiamine in human milk varies more than the other constituents and is largely dependent on the mother's intake of this vitamin. Infantile beriberi may occur in infants breastfed by thiamine-deficient mothers. The vitamin A content of human milk is to some extent dependent on the diet of the mother.

Despite the variation in the composition of milk from different animals, all milk is rich in protein and other nutrients and constitutes a good food for humans, especially children (Photo 65). Although most animal milk for human consumption comes from cows (Photo 66), in certain societies the milk of buffaloes, goats, sheep and camels is important. Some peoples have taboos against milk.

In many parts of the world, milk is more often consumed sour or curdled than fresh; in fact, some people dislike fresh milk. There is no need to alter this habit, for curdled milk keeps longer, retains its nutritive value and may be more digestible and more hygienic than fresh milk. However, it is much safer to drink milk that has been boiled and kept in a clean container, because milk can provide a vehicle for the transmission of some disease-causing organisms.

Pasteurization of milk carried out efficiently in a large, well-run dairy greatly reduces the risk of pathological organisms spreading, provided that the milk is placed in clean containers destined for direct delivery to the consumer. However, in many small towns where pasteurization is not well controlled, the milk may be insufficiently heated, the containers may not be well cleaned, and the milk may go from the plant into large churns for bottling elsewhere in insanitary surroundings. The consumer should not be overconfident in all milk labelled "pasteurized", since it is not necessarily free from pathological organisms.

In many countries where cows' milk is a normal item of the diet, it is customary to wean infants from breastmilk on to a diet in which cows' milk plays an important part. This is a valuable practice, for it helps ensure that the child will receive a balanced diet that provides all the requirements for growth, development and health.

Some people limit their milk consumption because of lactose intolerance, a condition resulting from low levels of the digestive enzyme lactase, which is responsible for digesting lactose, the main carbohydrate in milk. It is probably normal for human adults to have low levels of intestinal lactase, and the condition is very common in non-white peoples. Research shows that most lactose-intolerant persons can in fact consume milk in moderate quantities (perhaps three to five cups of milk per day) without developing symptoms.

Skimmed milk and dried skimmed milk

Skimmed milk is milk from which the fat has been removed, usually for making butter. In its dried form (DSM), it is a familiar product in many countries. It contains nearly all the protein of milk, as well as the carbohydrate, calcium and B vitamins. It is an excellent food, especially for those on predominantly carbohydrate diets and those who have extra needs for protein. In some places DSM is supplied to those with special needs through clinics and health centres. It is extensively used in hospitals and dispensaries as the basis for the treatment of protein-energy malnutrition (PEM). It is also issued at child-welfare clinics to prevent this most devastating form of malnutrition. Skimmed milk is an excellent food to add to any diet, but it is particularly useful in the diets of children and pregnant and lactating women. However, it is not a suitable substitute for whole milk for infants. It is sometimes added to dietary supplements such as, for example, corn (maize)/soybean/milk mixture (CSM).

Whole powdered milk

This product, as the name implies, is whole milk that has been dried. Unlike DSM, it contains fat. It is suitable for infants when no breastmilk is available.

Evaporated and condensed milks

These are milks that have had much of their water removed but that are still liquid. Condensed milk is sweetened by the addition of sugar, whereas evaporated milk does not contain added sugar. Many brands of condensed milk have vitamins added. These brands should be preferred to those that do not have vitamins added, especially if they are used in the diets of young children. They are not suitable as breastmilk substitutes for infants.

Yoghurt and soured or fermented milks

Many different organisms are used in the process of making yoghurt and fermented milks. These products are easy to prepare, are highly nutritious, have enhanced keeping quality and are a little less likely than fresh milk to harbour pathogenic organisms. Their use should be encouraged.

Casein

Casein is the protein from milk. It tends to be rather expensive. It is commonly mixed as part of a formula or mixture for treatment of children with PEM (see Chapter 12).

Cheese

The making of cheese no doubt arose from the desire of farm people to preserve some of the excess milk of the summer. Numerous processes are used, but essentially cheese is made by letting milk clot and subsequently removing some of the water. Salt and other flavourings may be added. Cheese-making is an excellent way of using any excess milk produced during the seasons when milk yields are high.

Butter and ghee

Butter and ghee are both milk products, but being mainly fat they are discussed in Chapter 30, "Oils and fats".

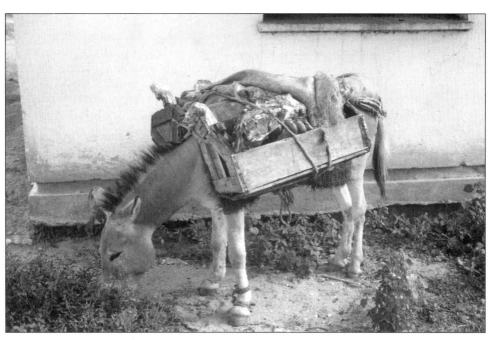

PHOTO 62
Meat, an important food in Somalia, being carried by donkey

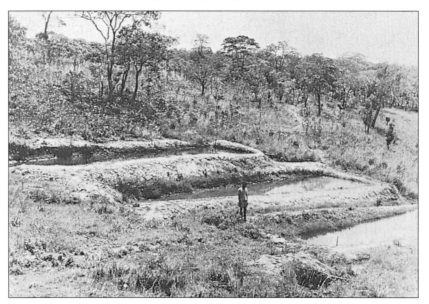

PHOTO 63
Construction of fish ponds should be encouraged wherever perennial water is available

PHOTO 64

Backyard poultry-keeping in Accra, Ghana provides eggs, an easily digestible, protein-rich food good for infants and toddlers

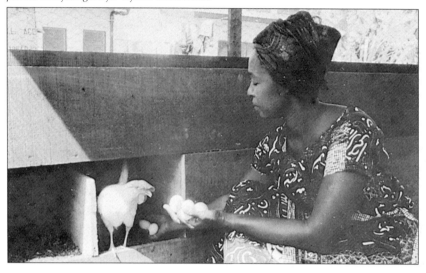

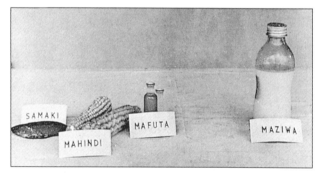

PHOTO 65

Milk (maziwa) contains protein as in fish (samaki), fat as in oil (maputa) and carbohydrate as in maize (mahindi)

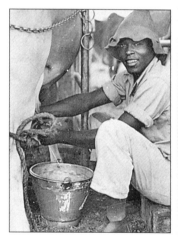

PHOTO 66

Milking a cow in Kenya

Chapter 30
Oils and fats

In general adults should consume at least 15 percent of their energy intake from dietary fats and oils, and women of child-bearing age should consume at least 20 percent. Active individuals who are not obese may consume up to 35 percent and sedentary individuals up to 30 percent of energy from fat as long as saturated fatty acids do not exceed 10 percent of the energy intake and cholesterol intake is limited to 300 mg per day. Annex 1 gives levels of fat intake for low-income countries calculated according to the recommended range (15 to 35 percent) of dietary energy from fat.

Infants fed human milk or formula usually receive 50 to 60 percent of their total energy from fat. Infants should receive breastmilk, but if they do not, the fatty acid composition of infant formula should correspond to the range found in the breastmilk from omnivorous women. During complementary feeding up to two years of age or beyond, the diet should provide 30 to 40 percent of energy from fat.

To achieve the recommended levels of fat intake, poor people, particularly in developing countries, would need to increase their intake of fat and oils. In contrast, most people living in rich industrialized countries would need to reduce their consumption of fat and oils, which now often provide 40 percent or more of the energy they consume.

The fat consumed in human diets is often divided into two categories: "visible" fat such as cooking oil and "invisible" fat such as the oil naturally present in cereals and legumes. Persons in developing countries who may get only 15 percent of their energy from fat will often obtain two-thirds as invisible fat and one-third as visible fat (or fat added to food). In contrast, in North America and Europe, where mean intakes of fats are high, some 70 percent may be visible fat and 30 percent invisible fat.

A diet very low in fat tends to be unpalatable and dull. It is difficult to cook a really good meal without any fat or oil, although the desired amount is largely a matter of habit and taste. However, like animal proteins, fats are relatively expensive, so the diet of poorer people is often short of fat. Fat is important because weight for weight it provides more than twice as much energy as carbohydrate or protein, thus reducing the bulk of the diet. Fats and oils may be good sources of fat-soluble vitamins, and they assist with the absorption of other nutrients. Recent work has established that certain unsaturated fatty acids are essential for pre- and postnatal development of the brain in children and are also essential for health in adults.

Fats contain a variety of fatty acids. Fats derived from land animals (e.g. butter and lard) usually contain a high proportion of saturated fatty acids and are solid at room temperature. Fats derived from vegetable products and marine animals (e.g. groundnut and cod-liver oils) contain more unsaturated fatty acids; they are usually liquid at room temperature and are termed oils. Coconut oil is an exception in that it contains mainly saturated fatty acids. A high intake of saturated fatty acids may contribute to raised serum cholesterol levels, which in turn may increase the risk of coronary heart disease.

BUTTER

Butter consists mainly of the fat from milk. It usually contains about 82 percent fat, with a trace of protein and carbohydrate; the rest is water. Butter is rich in vitamin A and has a small amount of vitamin D, but the content varies with the time of year and the diet of the cow from which it was derived. Usually about 800 mg of retinol and 50 IU of vitamin D are present in 100 g of butter. Butter and margarine are increasingly used in diets in developing countries as the use of bread increases.

MARGARINE

Developed as a substitute for butter, margarine is made from various vegetable oils that are partially hydrogenated to give a product with a consistency similar to that of butter. In most countries vitamins A and D are added so that the final product is nutritionally very similar to butter. If these vitamins have been added, they will usually be mentioned on the margarine container.

GHEE

Ghee is made by heating butter to precipitate the protein, which is then removed. Ghee contains 99 percent fat, no protein or carbohydrate, about 2 000 IU of vitamin A per 100 g and some vitamin D. It has good keeping qualities and is much used in tropical countries in place of butter, because butter soon goes rancid if kept unrefrigerated in warm temperatures.

LARD

Lard is collected during the heating of pork. Like other similar animal fats (e.g. drippings, suet), it consists of 99 percent fat and contains no carbohydrate, proteins, vitamins or minerals.

VEGETABLE OILS

Vegetable oils are the cooking fats most commonly used in Africa, Asia and Latin America, and there are many different kinds. Except for red palm oil, they have the disadvantage of containing no vitamins except vitamin E. They are mainly low in saturated fatty acids.

Commonly used vegetable oils are soybean, olive, maize, groundnut, sunflower, sesame, cottonseed and coconut oils. In their pure form, they are 100 percent fat and contain no water or other nutrients.

Red palm oil is widely produced in West Africa and in certain Asian countries (e.g. Malaysia). In West Africa it is important in human diets, but elsewhere it is exported for soap production and not much consumed locally. The oil contains large quantities of carotene, the precursor of vitamin A, commonly 12 000 µg per 100 g (with a range from 600 to 60 000 µg per 100 g). It is therefore a very valuable food wherever a shortage of vitamin A occurs in the diet. Vitamin A deficiency will not be a problem in areas where all members of the family consume even small quantities of red palm oil. Encouragement should be given to its wider cultivation and consumption.

Chapter 31
Beverages and condiments

BEVERAGES

It is essential that the human body receive water, yet the human taste prefers that much of this water be obtained in the form of beverages. These include beer, wine, spirits, fruit juices, tea, coffee, cocoa, synthetic sweetened soft drinks and aerated waters. Some of these beverages contain small amounts of drugs such as caffeine (tea, coffee and some colas) or alcohol in varying amounts (beer, wine and spirits), and some are sources of minerals and vitamins.

In most countries there are traditional beverages of great variety. In Africa many of these are made from cereal grains that have been soaked and sprouted. These beverages may or may not be alcoholic, and some are useful sources of B vitamins. In other parts of the world local beverages may be made from honey or coconut or any number of local products.

In the industrialized countries aerated soft drinks, often called "sodas", many with a cola base, are highly popular and consumed in huge quantities. In many parts of Africa, Asia, Latin America and the Near East, manufactured soft drinks and sodas are replacing traditional beverages. Most of these sodas provide no significant nutrients other than carbohydrates.

In contrast, fruit juices, either purchased or home-made from fresh fruit, usually contain useful amounts of vitamin C, and some provide carotene. They are good beverages, especially for children.

It is not uncommon to find mothers giving their babies and children orange squash or fruit-flavoured sodas because they were told at the clinic to give them fruit juice. These manufactured beverages are no substitute for fruit juice and will do the child no good; they are simply a waste of money.

Certain vitamin-rich proprietary beverages have been designed for infants and children. Their vitamin content is nearly always clearly stated on the label. They need to be used with caution, however. They are not necessary if the child is getting fresh fruit and vegetables, and they are often a very expensive way of providing vitamin C to a child. The advertising promoting them is pervasive, however, and can persuade mothers that they are useful.

Another major group of beverages comprises those usually consumed hot. Tea, which was probably first drunk in China, is now the favourite beverage of many people in Africa, the Near East and Europe. Coffee originated in Africa but is now drunk most in the Americas, Europe and the Near East. The two main types are Arabian, *Coffea arabica*, and robusta, *Coffea canephora*. In all regions of the world tea, coffee and to a lesser extent cocoa are popular beverages. All three provide small amounts of caffeine, which is a mild stimulant. None have any great nutritional significance. Tannin and polyphenols in tea may reduce iron absorption.

For thousands of years people from all continents have produced beverages that contain ethyl alcohol. Usually certain yeasts are used to ferment a local carbohydrate-rich food (for example, cereals or root crops), but fruits, palm sap, honey and other raw ingredients are also used. In the industrialized countries beer (often made from barley), wine (made from grapes) and various spirits (drinks with a relatively high alcohol content made by distillation) are very widely consumed, and this practice has spread to many countries of the South. Alcohol produces a good feeling for many who drink it, but it also impairs the senses, and it can be addictive. It can be claimed that alcohol consumed in moderation provides a sense of well-being and may improve social interaction; but alcohol in excess is a serious cause of automobile and other accidents, and alcoholism is a highly prevalent and very damaging disease in all continents of the world.

Animals and primitive men and women obtained most of their fluids in the form of water; then for thousands of years other beverages became the favourite drink for humans; and now there is almost a craze to drink "natural" or "spring" waters, either aerated or still. Many consumers believe that these waters, coming from springs, lakes, rivers or wells, have near-magical qualities and great nutritive value. This idea is false. Bottled water may contain small amounts of minerals such as calcium, magnesium and fluoride, but so does tap-water from many municipal water supplies. A study comparing popular brands of bottled water showed that they were in no way superior to New York tap-water. They have only the advantage of being safe in areas where tap-water may be contaminated. However, for low-income people bottled waters are very expensive, and boiling local water renders it safe at a much lower cost.

CONDIMENTS

Salt consists mainly of sodium chloride. It is the only mineral salt that humans customarily consume in a chemically pure form. The body has a definite need for sodium and chlorine. The amount of sodium chloride in the body is regulated by the kidneys. In hot countries a person doing heavy work may lose 15 g of sodium chloride in body sweat in one day. Urinary excretion ranges from 1 to 30 g or more per day. Despite this loss, salt is not essential in the human diet unless sweating is profuse, because sufficient sodium and chlorine can be obtained from food alone. Nevertheless, nearly all people use salt, obtaining it by digging, making or buying it, however small the income. Certainly a salt-free diet is unpalatable. Adults usually consume about 10 g of salt a day, but there are enormous variations. A high intake of salt may contribute to the development of hypertension or high blood pressure in some individuals.

Other spices and flavourings are of less physiological or nutritive importance. In all countries, in all ages, people have added such items to their food to improve and vary its taste. In Africa, Asia and Latin America a variety of wild leaves are used, partly for flavour, partly as vegetables *per se*; hot chilies, both red and green, are frequently used; and pepper and curry powder are popular additions to the sauce or stew accompanying the staple food. Few of these flavourings have much nutritional importance, but all serve to make the food more pleasing to the taste. They therefore both increase the appetite and assist digestion by stimulating the secretion of saliva and intestinal juices. With the march of so-called civilization, many of the traditional and natural condiments and herbs are being replaced by proprietary sauces and flavourings. Some of these are artificial chemical agents (for example, monosodium glutamate) and some are based on traditional spices (garlic, cloves, ginger, etc.).

Chapter 32
Food processing and fortification

Humans are unique in the animal kingdom in that they harvest, store and process food that they have grown. Almost all animals harvest food, and many animals store it for later consumption, but they do not grow it or process it. In their evolution from the apes humans learned to grow food for their own sustenance and then to develop many processes to preserve the food or to increase its desirable characteristics, sometimes thus decreasing or improving its nutritional value.

People seek to preserve food and to improve its quality using a variety of techniques such as drying, canning, pickling, adding chemical preservatives, refrigeration, freezing and irradiation. The main aim of these processes is to allow foods to remain in good edible condition, without serious deterioration, for longer than would be possible if these preservation methods were not used. The processes include cooking; adding substances to improve the taste or appearance of the food; taking measures to make the foods more nutritious, for instance adding micronutrients or germinating grains; and removing undesirable constituents, including toxins. Some food processing techniques have multiple effects. For example, milling of cereal grains may make them less nutritious, but it may also make them easier to cook and digest and less likely to deteriorate on storage.

Today food processing includes both traditional and some more industrial and modern techniques. Almost all aspects of food processing have some relevance to nutrition. The effects of various processes, including cooking, on the nutrient content of foods are summarized in Table 35. In addition to those effects, milling and cooking break down cell walls so that nutrients are digested more easily.

Research, teaching and extension regarding modern techniques of food processing are within the domain of food scientists rather than nutritionists. Food science is a very important subject which is advancing rapidly not only in academic institutions but also in the food industry, where large manufacturers often have advanced food science laboratories. Many books deal with food science, and some are included in the Bibliography.

This chapter and Chapter 34 discuss those aspects of food processing that have an impact on the nutritional quality of foods consumed in developing countries or that influence their safety. Fortification of foods with nutrients is an aspect of food processing directly aimed at reducing deficiency diseases.

COOKING

In ancient times and in traditional societies everywhere, cooking was and is the main food processing technique used. Humans learned to harness and make fire, and cooking their food became a way to improve the quality of their diets. Cooking techniques have changed much over the years in some societies and very little in others. Many people still cook over open fires and on traditional stoves, but in contrast now almost a majority of households in Western Europe and North America have a microwave oven in the kitchen, a relatively new invention. Similarly, industry uses both old and new cooking methods.

TABLE 35
How processing alters the nutrient content of foods

Nutrient	Processes that decrease the amount	Processes that increase the amount	Other effects of processing
Vitamin A	Drying, especially in the sun; Boiling for a long time in contact with air (without a lid on the pan); Frying for a long time or at high temperatures	Fortification	
Thiamine	Washing of rice		
Riboflavin	Leaving milk in daylight		
Folate	Cooking (for example, in green leaves 35 percent and in potatoes 25 percent of folate may be lost); Storage		
Vitamin C	Storage (except for citrus or baobab fruits), drying, canning and bottling, cooking and reheating of fresh roots, vegetables and fruits (for example, 40 percent of vitamin C in green leaves may be lost in cooking, as some passes into the water and some is destroyed by heat); Chopping the foods into small pieces, preparing them long before cooking and cooking them long before eating	Germinating of seeds (for example, of legumes)	
Minerals	Milling	Fortification (for example, salt may be fortified with iodine)	Fermentation and germination increase the absorption of non-haem iron and other minerals; Milling may remove some minerals but increase their absorption
Carbo-hydrate, fats and protein	Milling may reduce the amount of fat, protein and fibre	Milling may increase the proportion of starch; Bottling and canning may add sugar; Frying increases the fat content	Fermenting and malting alter the proportions of starch and sugar; Fermenting may add alcohol
Water	Drying foods		By decreasing water content, drying foods increases the concentration of other nutrients

Cooking is practised by almost every-body, everywhere. Except for fruits and some vegetables, most groups of foods are generally cooked before being eaten. In many African and Asian countries even vegetables are seldom eaten uncooked, and there is little tradition of eating salads. The practice of cooking vegetables probably helps protect consumers from diseases spread by faecal contamination including parasitic, bacterial and viral infections of the gastro-intestinal tract. Most tropical fruits are eaten raw, but the exposed peel is not consumed so they do not present the same risk of infections. Bananas, mangoes, papayas and citrus fruits, for example, are not dangerous because their peel is not eaten.

Cooking of food is a universal practice mainly because it improves the taste of food, makes inedible foods edible or makes foods more digestible. Cooking also kills organisms, including many disease-causing microorganisms in food. Cooking of high-starch foods including cereals (rice, wheat, maize, etc., which for most of humankind provide the bulk of the energy and even protein consumed) and also potatoes, yams and cassava makes these foods palatable and also more digestible. Cooking of some foods removes undesirable compounds such as antinutrients, for example trypsin inhibitors in soybeans and undesirable constituents in cassava.

There is more to cooking than merely roasting, baking, grilling, or boiling of foods as gathered or harvested. It usually also involves mixing of foods or perhaps more commonly adding food items to the main food being cooked, which may alter the nutritional value of the main food but is usually intended to make the food, dish or meal taste better. For example, fat is added in frying; salt, sugar, fruit and other products may be added to baked foods; and often the staple food such as potatoes may be cooked in a stew or soup with added onions, tomatoes and small quantities of meat. Cooking can be an art. It makes food tasty and desirable, and in most societies sharing a meal with family and friends is a pleasurable social occasion and is expected to do more than just fill the belly, assuage hunger and provide essential nutrients; it fuels feelings of mutuality and underpins the sense of community.

For all its good points, cooking can have some negative nutritional effects. Frying foods at very high temperatures can destroy some vitamins and can produce undesirable components such as carcinogens in the food. Smoking of food can also produce such substances. Boiling some items in water that is then discarded can remove water-soluble vitamins.

GERMINATION OF GRAINS

There is intense interest now in the use of traditional germinating methods to produce malted foods. For many years people in the United Republic of Tanzania and other countries have allowed sorghum, millet and other cereals to germinate by soaking the grains in water for some hours, then keeping them damp for two or three days, and finally drying them, often by spreading them in the sun. The dried cereal grains are then pounded using a traditional large pestle and mortar. The resulting flour is stored, and small amounts are used mainly for brewing local beer (*pombe*). The dried germinated flour, known as *kimea*, is also used to thin and sour traditional porridges made from maize for child feeding. The *kimea* thins the porridge because it produces the enzyme amylase, which breaks down the starch (see Chapter 6).

PRESERVATION OF FOOD
Physical methods

Cooling or freezing greatly prolongs the time it takes for many foods to spoil or become inedible. In this sense it is a very important method of food preservation. Refrigerators are now very common appliances in the homes of better-off people in developing countries and are found in the majority of houses in industrialized countries. Freezers are also widely used.

Other methods used traditionally, but also in industry, are drying and smoking of foods (Photos 68 and 69). Removal of water prevents or reduces the ability of organisms to grow and multiply on or in many foods. Organisms thus inhibited include moulds and their toxic products, such as aflatoxin, as well as microorganisms that spoil the food and produce undesirable odours and taste. Dry cereals store better, and dried fish remains edible for relatively long periods. Some foods, such as milk, are dried in factories so that the preserved product can be easily marketed, transported and made available for consumption.

Chemical methods

Food may be kept edible longer by the use of substances termed chemical preservatives. The most widely used in the home are salt (sodium chloride) and sugar, which most homemakers would not consider to be chemical preservatives. Foods with high levels of salt or sugar are less attacked by organisms and so are preserved. Industry also uses salt and sugar to preserve food.

Over 100 years ago chemicals not usually available in the home (as salt and sugar are) were introduced as food preservatives. Some of these are not now used because of fears of toxicity; others are deemed safe and are widely used. International meetings have discussed safety issues, and most industrialized countries have regulations which list permitted food preservatives and concentrations that can be used. Among the widely used preservatives are sulphur dioxide and benzoates, which are mainly effective in controlling moulds and yeasts, respectively. Baked goods such as bread are often preserved using propionic acid, which inhibits the attack and growth of moulds and then prolongs the time before spoilage. Meats, particularly salted meats such as bacon and ham, are further preserved with sodium nitrite and sometimes sodium nitrate.

Sterilization

Both in the home and in the factory, foods of almost all kinds are preserved by a process termed canning, although some are actually put in jars or bottles. In general the foods (vegetables, fruits, meat products and others) are sterilized by heating them to kill all living organisms and are sealed in a can or bottle while still hot. Sometimes salt and sugar are used as part of the process. Home canning or bottling of foods

of animal origin, particularly meat or fish of any kind, can be risky. Highly resistant bacteria such as *Clostridium botulinum* can survive, produce toxins and cause very serious disease (see Chapter 34).

Microbiological methods

Fermentation, which involves chemical breakdown of substances by microorganisms such as yeasts and bacteria, is used traditionally to preserve foods or to improve their palatability in many countries, as is the case with soy products in Indonesia. The process is also used commercially, for example in the manufacture of yoghurt or commercial alcoholic beverages.

Fermentation using yeasts and other organisms which act on the carbohydrate in the food produces alcohol. Humans almost all over the world, without food science classes, have discovered this mechanism and have found that alcohol consumption can be mood changing and pleasant. Thus with any carbohydrate they have, they use some to make alcoholic beverages. The carbohydrate may be a common cereal such as wheat, rice, barley or sorghum, or it may be honey, used to make mead in ancient Britain and modern Africa; coconut sap to make coconut wine in Oceania; or cassava or plantain to make strong drinks called *waragi* and *koinage* in Uganda.

Yeast also acts on sugars to produce carbon dioxide gas in food. This principle is used to make bread.

In some foods non-disease-causing organisms are encouraged to multiply to sour the food. Souring results when the microorganisms produce acid from the carbohydrate. Souring foods to some extent prevents pathogenic or harmful organisms from multiplying in the food, which keeps it safer and makes it last longer. Common soured foods are dairy products such as sour milk and yoghurt; fermented soy products such as tempeh; and fermented cereal porridges, consumed in much of sub-Saharan Africa. In some cases souring enhances the nutrient content of the food.

In many countries, including China, pickling is widely used to preserve vegetables and vegetable products.

Other methods

A purely industrial method of food preservation is irradiation. In this process the food is exposed to radiation, usually gamma rays, which kills microorganisms and fungal spores. The food is then sealed and is safe until opened. Irradiation can also be used to prevent or delay sprouting of certain cereals, legumes or other seeds and so to increase their shelf-life. Although irradiated foods are generally regarded as safe, there remains considerable debate about possible hazards of the irradiation process itself.

FORTIFICATION

Fortification is a form of food processing that is of special interest to nutritionists. When properly used it can be a strategy to control nutrient deficiencies. The terms "fortification" and "enrichment" are often used interchangeably. Fortification has been defined as the addition of one or more nutrients to a food to improve its quality for the people who consume it, usually with the goal of reducing or controlling a nutrient deficiency. This strategy may be applicable in nations or communities where there is a problem or a risk of a deficiency of the nutrient or nutrients concerned.

In some instances fortification may be the easiest, cheapest and best way to reduce a deficiency problem, but care needs to be taken to avoid its excessive promotion as a general panacea for controlling nutrient deficiencies. The pros and cons of fortification need to be weighed in each circumstance. Even so, as a strategy to control micronutrient deficiencies in developing countries fortification has often been underutilized, whereas in many industrialized countries it is generally overused. Ironically, it may add nutrients that are not generally lacking for consumers who are not at much risk of deficiency of those nutrients.

Outsiders should not rush into recommending fortification in a particular country. Local professionals need to be much involved in the planning, implementation and monitoring of a fortification programme. It is important to have a very clear picture of the local situation: nutrient deficiencies, food habits, food preparation practices, food processing facilities, marketing practices, etc. Food fortification is easier with one food, such as salt, and where there are very few manufacturers. Under other circumstances fortification is possible, could work and might have a major role in improving nutritional status and reducing the risk of deficiencies, even at the local level. In the past people have tried to find one ideal food to fortify with vitamin A or iron. Now it is recommended that countries consider fortifying several foods at the same time.

Two kinds of fortification that have been highly effective in many countries are the addition of iodine to salt (iodization) and the addition of fluorine to water (fluoridation). In the latter case (see Chapter 21) the fluoride in a municipal water supply is augmented to provide levels that are considered optimal (i.e. one part per million) in order to reduce the incidence of dental caries or tooth decay.

In industrialized countries, and to some extent in developing countries, fortification is used to adjust the nutrient content of processed foods so that nutrient levels are close to those of the food before processing. For example, highly milled cereals such as wheat flour may have nutrients added to replace those lost during the refining process. An alternative would be to insist, or even legislate, that cereals not be highly refined.

Micronutrients

Other chapters in this book describe the important micronutrient deficiencies and ways in which they have been, or can be, controlled. Food fortification offers an important strategy to help control, in particular, the three main micronutrient deficiencies, namely deficiencies of iodine, vitamin A and iron. In developing countries the greatest priority should be given to fortification with these nutrients. With iodine, fortification alone, in the form of salt iodization, is often the only strategy used. With vitamin A and iron, fortification should be used in combination with, not to the exclusion of, other interventions. Particular care needs to be given to possible toxic problems with vitamin A, especially in women who are pregnant or planning to conceive. The advantages of fortification over some of the other strategies for controlling vitamin A and iron deficiencies are often relatively ignored and deserve more attention.

As indicated elsewhere in the book, other micronutrient deficiencies are of some importance in some countries, and fortification may be a good strategy to reduce the prevalence of deficiencies of, for example, niacin, thiamine, riboflavin, folate, vitamin C, zinc and calcium.

Macronutrients

A somewhat different kind of fortification is the addition of macronutrients to enrich food. Enrichment could involve the addition of fat or oil to increase the energy density of a food; the addition of amino acids to cereal products to improve protein quality; or the addition of protein, sugar or oil (as well as micronutrients) to a formulated food, for example a manufactured weaning food, or to a food supple- ment such as corn (maize)/soybean/milk (CSM) for emergency feeding.

Criteria or principles for fortification

The following are some of the conditions, considerations and principles relevant for those planning to fortify one or more foods to improve nutritional status. They apply mainly to fortification as a strategy to tackle micronutrient deficiencies.

Known nutrient deficiency in the population. Dietary, clinical or biochemical data must show that a deficiency of the nutrient being considered exists to some degree in significant numbers of the population when they consume their usual diet, or that a risk exists.

Wide consumption of the food to be forti- fied among the at-risk population. The food or foods to be fortified must be consumed by significant numbers of the population who have a deficiency of the nutrient being considered for fortification. If the deficiency disease occurs only in the very poor but they seldom purchase the food that is fortified, then it will do little good. Thus, for example, fortifying a relatively expensive manufactured wean- ing food with vitamin A may not help the poor children who have the highest pre- valence of xerophthalmia if their parents cannot afford to purchase that food.

Suitability of the food and nutrient together. Adding the nutrient to the food must not create any serious organoleptic problems. The items must mix well and this mixing must not cause an undesirable chemical reaction, any disagreeable taste, colour or odour changes or any other unacceptable characteristics.

Technical feasibility. It must be technically feasible to add the nutrient to the food to satisfy the preceding condition.

Limited number of food manufacturers. It is very helpful in a national or even a local fortification programme if there are relatively few manufacturers or processors of the food being considered. For example, if there are hundreds of salt producers, an iodization programme will face major problems. Similarly, if there are many millers, fortifying cereals will be difficult.

No substantial increase in price of the food. It is important to consider the impact of fortification on the price of the food to be fortified. If adding a nutrient greatly increases the price of the food, consumption of the food may decline, particularly among poor people whose families are at special risk of the deficiency. If fortification does increase the price of the food, then it is possible to consider subsidizing the cost.

Range of consumption of the food. Attention should be given to the usual range of consumption of the food being considered for fortification. If there is a very wide range between the smallest amount consumed, perhaps by 25 percent of the population, and the greatest amount consumed, perhaps by another 25 percent of the population, it may be difficult to decide the nutrient level for fortification. If large numbers of people at risk of the nutrient deficiency consume very small amounts of the food, then they may not benefit much from fortification. If significant numbers of individuals consume so much of the food that they may get toxic amounts of the nutrient, then the food may be unsuitable. In general there is a range of consumption of salt, and mean intakes may be 20 g per day, but practically no one consumes 200 g per day, every day. It is important to avoid a situation where people receive undesirable amounts of added nutrients, particularly in the case of fat-soluble vitamins or nutrients known to be toxic in large amounts.

Legislation. When a government is moving in earnest to control a serious micronutrient deficiency using fortification, the appropriateness of legislation needs to be considered. Many industrialized countries have legislation to ensure that required minimum levels of B vitamins and sometimes also iron are present in wheat flour and some other cereal products. Many countries in the North and South have legislation to require that all salt sold is iodized, usually at a particular level. Fluoridation of water supplies to certain levels has been mandated legally, sometimes by municipalities (as in the United States) and sometimes nationally.

Monitoring and control of fortification. Monitoring to provide information on fortification of foods is useful. It is particularly important where fortification is legislated. In this case failure to fortify adequately could lead to prosecution and penalization of delinquent food manufacturers. Monitoring by governments is dependent on the availability of laboratory facilities and the trained personnel. Many countries lack adequate laboratory facilities to monitor salt iodization, and salt merchants are often aware that they can sell salt that is not iodized at all or at the level required by law. A good monitoring system needs to include testing, perhaps at sentinel sites all over the country. In the case of fluoridation, cities often monitor the fluoride content of their water. It is useful if a national laboratory also monitors the level of fluoride in municipal water provided to consumers.

Methods of fortification and suitable foods
The technology of fortification is a complex topic, discussed in many publications. Many different methods are used, and the choice of method depends on both the nutrient and the food.

A frequently used technique in a flour

or a fine-grained product involves adding a nutrient premix at a measured rate into the powdery food as it flows at some stage in the processing. Thorough mixing is necessary. This method is suitable for mills and large processing plants. For smaller processing facilities, or even at the village level, packages of premix are supplied. Instructions are given on the proportions to use (for example, one packet per 50 kg of food) and on methods to ensure a good mixture.

Difficulties have been encountered in fortifying rice because it is mainly eaten in a granular or whole-grain form. Therefore adding a powder, which is easy with wheat flour, is not possible with rice. At least two methods have been used. In one, rice grains are coated or impregnated with the nutrients to be used. In the second, artificial rice grains fortified with the desired nutrients are mixed with the rice. The artificial grains have to be well made so that they appear similar to ordinary rice grains. In the Philippines some decades ago it was reported that prior to cooking many housewives removed and threw away the fortified artificial rice grains because they had a yellowish colour from the added thiamine and riboflavin.

Some nutrients such as the B vitamins are relatively easy to add (although riboflavin has the disadvantage of being yellow). Although vitamin A deficiency is of great importance, vitamin A is less easily used than the B vitamins in fortification programmes, in part because it is fat soluble and not water soluble. It is also likely to become oxidized. The most simple means is to add vitamin A to cooking oils and margarine, but food technology has overcome the difficulties, and many different foods have been successfully fortified with vitamin A in both industrialized and non-industrialized countries.

For quite different reasons iron fortification of foods has presented serious challenges. Many different iron salts have been used. Often those that humans utilize best, such as ferrous sulphate, present the greatest difficulties and serious organoleptic problems. As discussed in Chapter 39, sodium iron EDTA is increasingly recommended.

Table 36 lists some nutrients that have been used and their food vehicles.

TABLE 36
Some types of food used as vehicles in fortification programmes[a]

Nutrient	Types of food	Comments
Ascorbic acid	Canned, frozen and dried fruit drinks, canned and dried milk products, dry cereal products	Ascorbic acid must be protected from air if in neutral solution.
Thiamine, riboflavin and niacin	Dry cereals, flour, bread, pasta, milk products	Rice and similar food grains may be impregnated or coated with the nutrient. Riboflavin may colour the food. Nicotinamide is usually preferred to nicotinic acid.
Vitamin A or beta-carotene	Dry cereal products, flour, bread, pasta, milk products, margarine, vegetable oils, sugar, tea, chocolate, monosodium glutamate	Vitamin A must be protected from air and or added in water-miscible form to non-fatty products. (It may be added as gelatin-based beadlets together with stabilizer as a coating on the food product or mixed into a simulated kernel such as rice.) Carotene may colour the products. Losses due to heat may be great in cooking oils.
Vitamin D	Milk products, margarine, dry cereal products, vegetable oils, fruit drinks	See comments for vitamin A. Multiple sources of this vitamin may be undesirable.
Calcium	Cereal products, bread	The quantity to be added usually limits the range of vehicles that can be used.
Iron	Cereal products, bread, canned and dried milk	Availability varies with the form in which the iron is added. Iron may cause colour or flavour changes in the food.
Iodine	Salt	Iodide is usually used. Iodate is more stable in crude salt.
Protein	Cereal products, bread, cassava flour	Protein concentrates of various types are used. The amount to be added usually limits the range of vehicles that can be employed.
Amino acids	Cereals, bread, meat substitutes	Other vehicles have been proposed. The use of lysine, cysteine or methionine is authorized in some areas. Interest in amino acid fortification has diminished from the early 1970s.

[a] In addition, a wide range of nutrients have been added to infant foods and formulations.

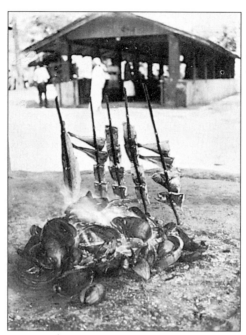

PHOTO 67
Traditional way of smoking fish using coconut shells for fuel

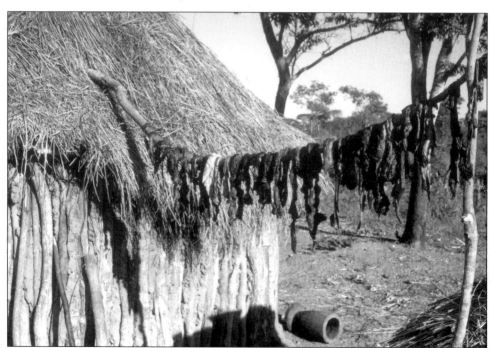

PHOTO 68
Meat drying in Angola

Part V
Nutrition policies and programmes

Chapter 33
Assessment, analysis and surveillance of nutrition

Nutritional problems are complex in their aetiology, and there are many different nutritional deficiency diseases. Knowing how they occur is one vital part of solving and, better still, preventing nutritional problems. The ability to predict their occurrence makes prevention a more realistic prospect.

A great variety of data can throw light on the risks of malnutrition in a community or a nation. Between 1946 and 1975 large national nutrition surveys were conducted in many countries. They often included the collection of a broad range of dietary, clinical, biochemical, anthropometric and socio-economic data. The surveys were often designed to detect evidence of a range of vitamin and mineral deficiencies as well as protein-energy malnutrition (PEM). The surveys were expensive to conduct; they required well-equipped laboratories and numerous personnel. Many of the earlier surveys in over 20 countries were supported and largely conducted by the United States Inter-departmental Committee for Nutrition for National Defense. Subsequently, international agencies such as FAO helped countries conduct large national nutrition surveys. In the United States, major nutrition surveys were conducted in ten states between 1968 and 1971.

All of these surveys provide a wealth of data on nutritional status, usually for a representative sample of the population. Unfortunately, in most cases the data collection did not seem to result in a broad set of actions to deal with the nutritional problems found in the surveys.

By about 1975 it was generally agreed that such detailed surveys were not necessary and that, because PEM in young children was thought to be the most important problem, simplified surveys, using mainly anthropometry and selected dietary and socio-economic indicators, would be more appropriate. Nutritional assessments were increasingly based on measurements of weight and height. There also was a move away from national surveys to more local surveys and in some countries, such as Kenya, to regular data collection to assess trends. Anthropometric surveys were to some extent replaced in the 1980s by rapid appraisal methods which involved the collection of a broader range of data but used new methodologies. At about the same time there was a move to collect qualitative as well as quantitative data and to conduct surveys related to a single micronutrient deficiency, such as iodine deficiency disorders (IDD).

In working to assess the nutritional status of a community, it is important to decide on the objectives of the assessment, how the analyses will be done and what actions are feasible. It is important to draw from experience and to design the most appropriate data collection exercise. For example, in an assessment in a large, newly established refugee camp, it might be advisable to collect more than just anthro-pometric data; in the past, when nutritional status in refugee camps was judged only on anthropometry, deficiency diseases such as scurvy and pellagra were missed. Social scientists might be consulted to help decide what qualitative data would be most useful and how these might be gathered and analysed.

Large and expensive surveys, in which a wide variety of nutrition-related data are collected, are seldom justified and should never be done unless there is reasonable assurance that the data will be used for an action programme and that adequate resources and funds are available. In many countries expensive surveys have been carried out and little action has followed. It has been suggested that ten times the amount spent on a survey should be available for programmes aimed at overcoming the deficiencies identified by it. It is therefore important that the information collected be kept to the minimum required to assess or monitor the situation, and that surveys be simplified as much as possible. Some information used for the assessment of the nutritional status of a community can also be used for evaluation of programmes and for nutritional surveillance.

TYPES OF DATA FOR ASSESSING AND ANALYSING NUTRITIONAL STATUS

Today the main interest in a survey might be to determine nutritional status at the household and local level, rather than at the national level. The following ten types of information can be useful in assessing the nutritional status of a community:

- clinical examination data;
- anthropometric data;
- laboratory tests of nutritional status;
- dietary surveys;
- vital statistics;
- additional health statistics and medical information;
- food availability and market surveys, including agricultural data relevant to food production and food balance sheets;
- economic data related to purchasing power, food prices, food distribution, etc.;

- socio-cultural data, including food consumption patterns and food practices and beliefs;
- food science information such as the nutrient content of foods, the biological value of diets, the effects on nutrients of common food processing practices and the presence of toxic or harmful factors such as aflatoxins and goitrogens.

Only the first five are discussed here since a nutrition survey comprehensive enough to collect all these types of information would very seldom be undertaken.

Clinical examination

Clinical examinations are often given low priority as a means of assessing the nutritional status of a community. Moreover, most countries in Africa, Asia and Latin America suffer a lack of vital statistics, accurate figures for agricultural production and laboratories where biochemical tests can be performed. Records of local food habits and practices are difficult to obtain. Under these conditions clinical and anthropometric examinations are the most simple, most practical and without doubt the most sound means of ascertaining the nutritional status of any particular group of individuals.

The nutritional status of a community is the sum of the nutritional status of the individuals who form that community. However, in any survey only a representative group of persons needs to be examined. To give a true picture, these people should normally be chosen completely at random, not taken from any particular age group, sex, religion, social class or area within the community. Stratified sampling is valid under certain circumstances. For example, if a survey is being carried out to determine the importance and prevalence of PEM among the young in a given area, it would be sound to restrict examinations to children up to five years of age. If the exact date of birth of the child is unknown, the age should be estimated using local historical, agricultural or social events as time indexes.

The clinical nutrition examination should be carried out by a person with medical training. Although it may be possible to train non-medical personnel to recognize such conditions as angular stomatitis, mottled teeth and even oedema, collection of clinical data by people with inadequate medical knowledge could lead to incomplete survey results. For example, a person looking for the dermatoses of kwashiorkor or the skin changes of pellagra should also be able to recognize scabies and eczema. However, non-medical persons can be entrusted to collect anthropometric data (physical measurements).

In order to avoid overlooking important details, the clinical examination should be systematic. The examiner should look for specific signs, and their presence or absence should be recorded on a standardized form. A modified sample of a form that has been found useful in East Africa is presented on the following page.

Using this form, examinations should start at the head (i.e. hair, eyes, mouth), move down the body and end at the feet. Central nervous system (CNS) signs may in some instances be omitted; they are relatively rare and the tests may be difficult and time consuming to perform.

Anthropometric data

Anthropometric data can be collected by medical or non-medical personnel. In the former case, they can be included as part of the clinical nutritional examination. However, it is often simpler and faster if a reliable person other than the medical examiner records the height and weight during a survey.

Weight. The weight of a person is the most important single anthropometric measurement that can be taken. In children its interpretation is dependent on knowing the age of the child with some degree of accuracy. Weight should be measured with the subject nude or wearing the minimum of clothing (shorts only for males, light dress for females). Footwear should be removed.

Spring scales are less reliable than balance scales. In many countries, balance scales have been supplied to clinics and health centres by the United Nations Children's Fund (UNICEF). At boarding schools a good scale is often available in the kitchen, where it is used for weighing sacks of food. Similarly, in a village the local market master or the owner of a small shop will usually have a produce scale that can be borrowed. Special baby-weighing scales are necessary for accurate weight measurement of children under two years of age.

Height. Height is also a very important measurement in the assessment of nutritional status. As with weight, its interpretation in children is dependent on knowing the age of the child. Height should be measured with the subject barefoot. Though many different types of equipment are available, height can be fairly accurately measured with a tape-measure or a ruler. The following method may be used.

Locate a vertical wall rising from a truly horizontal floor. Make a horizontal pencil line about 2 cm in length at a height of 1 m from the floor (60 cm for children). Then, using sticking plaster, sticky tape or a drawing-pin, secure the bottom of a 1-m length of tape-measure to correspond with the line. Similarly fasten the top, which will now be 2 m from the floor. The person being measured stands against the wall facing outward (Figure 17). The height of the individual is ascertained using a block of wood having a true right angle. A rectangular block with the dimensions 30 × 10 × 20 cm is adequate, although a

Clinical nutrition examination (for use of medical personnel)

Name ....   Date ....

Sex ....   Age ....

Pregnant? ....   Lactating? ....

Height ....   Weight ....

Haemoglobin ....   Upper-arm circumference ....

Haematocrit ....   Triceps skin thickness ....

Hair

1. Lack of lustre? ....
2. Depigmentation (colour change)? ....
3. Texture change (thinness ....
   or sparseness)? ....
4. Easily pickable? ....
   ....

Face

1. Moonface? ....
2. Pallor? ....
   ....

Eyes

1. Xerosis conjunctivae ....
   or xerophthalmia? ....
2. Keratomalacia? ....
3. Conjunctival thickening ....
   or wrinkling? ....
4. Bitot's spots? ....
5. Conjunctival injection or ....
   vascularization? ....
6. Corneal scars? ....

Mouth

1. Angular stomatitis? ....
2. Cheilosis of lips? ....
3. Angular scars? ....
4. Spongy or bleeding gums? ....
5. Mottled teeth? ....
6. No. teeth decayed (D) ....
7. No. teeth missing (M) ....
8. No. teeth filled (F) ....
9. Total DMF teeth ....

Glands

Thyroid ....

Goitre ....

Grade (0, 1, 2, 3) ....

Parotid enlarged? ....

Skin

1. Xerosis (dry scaly)? ....
2. Follicular hyperkeratosis? ....
3. Mosaic (crazy pavement)? ....
4. Pellagrous dermatosis? ....
5. Skin haemorrhages (petechiae or
   ecchymoses)? ....
6. Flaky-paint dermatosis? ....
7. Scrotal or vulval dermatosis?
8. Oedema? ....
9. Ulcers? ....

Muscles

1. Wasting? ....

Skeleton

1. Epiphyseal enlargement? ....
2. Beading of ribs (rickety rosary)? ....
3. Skeletal deformities? ....
4. Subperiosteal haematomas? ....

Central nervous system (CNS)

1. Psychomotor change (apathy,
   misery, etc.)? ....
2. Sensory loss? ....
3. Calf tenderness? ....
4. Loss of ankle or knee jerks? ....
5. Motor weakness? ....

Internal system

1. Hepatomegaly? ....
2. Splenomegaly? ....

Remarks (include other abnormalities)

....

....

....

....

triangular block of the same dimensions, as shown in Figure 17, is easier to handle.

The measurement of the length of young children presents more difficulty. A suitable apparatus consists of a flat board of dimensions 120 × 40 × 2 cm with a head-board 30 cm high fixed at a right angle to one end. The triangle used for height measurements can be used as a sliding foot-piece. A metal tape-measure is nailed to the board for readings in centimetres.

A less satisfactory alternative is to push a flat wooden bench, available in most dispensaries and schools, up against a wall in the corner of the room and measure it off in centimetres, starting about 50 cm from the wall and going up to 150 cm. The triangle is again used as a foot-piece.

When the length of an infant or toddler is being measured, the child must lie flat and straightened out to full length (see Figure 17). For research purposes or where

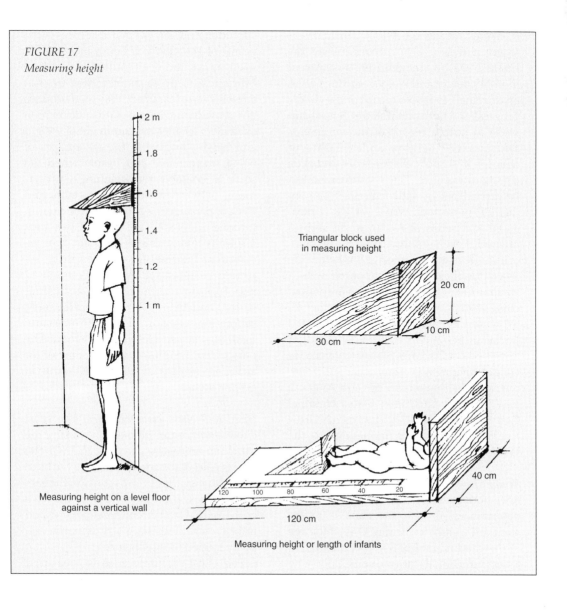

FIGURE 17
Measuring height

Triangular block used in measuring height

20 cm

10 cm

30 cm

2 m

1.8

1.6

1.4

1.2

1 m

Measuring height on a level floor
against a vertical wall

40 cm

120   100   80   60   40   20

120 cm

Measuring height or length of infants

adequate funds are available, commercially made length boards can be used.

Series readings. A series of readings of weight and/or height of an individual taken at, for example, monthly intervals gives valuable information. In an adult, weight loss indicates that energy intake is below energy output. Gain in weight indicates a more than sufficient energy supply. In adults a series of weight readings might be used, for example, during a famine to ascertain whether relief measures are adequate, or in a normal year to see if weight drop occurs during the hungry season. In children a series of monthly height and weight readings gives an extremely valuable record of the child's progress and nutritional status. It is worthwhile to keep a record of measurements taken of the heights and weights of children in schools, dispensaries and even community centres. The measurements can be carried out by either medical or non-medical personnel. When weight is measured in a series of readings, the figures are useful even without those for height.

If single readings of weight or height are available, they can be compared with a standard weight or height. The individual child's actual weight or height can then be expressed as a percentage of that expected for his or her age or in terms of standard deviations or Z scores. Standard tables for weight, height and certain other anthropometric measurements are given in Annex 2, based mainly on United States National Center for Health Statistics (NCHS) reference values as recommended by the World Health Organization (WHO).

Weight for height. When weight and height have both been measured, it is possible to determine how near the child is to the standard weight for height. Even if the age of the child is not known, it is possible to assess nutritional status to some degree by expressing the weight as a percentage of that expected for the child's height or length or in terms of standard deviations or Z scores. This figure gives a relative measure of how thin the child is. Another commonly used method is to calculate the body mass index (BMI) (see Chapter 23 for details).

Mid-upper-arm circumference (MUAC). The measurement of the circumference of the left upper arm midway between the acromion process (the bony tip) of the shoulder and the olecranon process (the point) of the elbow is being increasingly used as an index of nutritional status. Fibreglass tape-measures that do not stretch should be used. This method does not provide nutritional status information as reliably as does measurement of weight and height, but it has the advantages of being inexpensive and usable where no scale is available for weighing. Furthermore, between about eight months and five years of age the standard arm circumference increases very little. An arm circumference above 13.5 cm can be considered normal for children from one to five years of age. MUAC between 12 and 13.5 cm indicates moderate malnutrition, and below 12 cm indicates more serious malnutrition. The MUAC measurement may be especially suitable for use by persons with a minimum of training or for gross assessment of nutritional status in famine areas.

Head and chest circumference. The head circumference can be measured using the same tape-measure used for MUAC. The tape is placed horizontally around the head at a level just above the eyebrows, the ears and the most prominent bulge at the back of the head. Head circumference is related to brain size, but brain size is not necessarily related to intelligence.

The chest circumference is measured

horizontally at the nipple line. Up to six months of age the head circumference is usually larger than the chest circumference. Children over 12 months of age having a head circumference larger than the chest circumference are abnormal; this is evidence of poor growth of the chest.

Skinfold thickness. The skinfold thickness can only be measured if a pair of skinfold callipers is available (Photo 69). This instrument is designed to measure the thickness of the skin and subcutaneous fat using constant pressure applied over a known area. The two most common sites for measurement are over the triceps and in the subscapular region. The measurement is of considerable value in assessing the amount of fat and therefore the reserve of energy in the body. Unfortunately this instrument is rarely available in small hospitals, let alone health centres and dispensaries. This situation could easily be rectified, since the instrument is not expensive. The two most common skin callipers used are the Harpenden, made in the United Kingdom, and the Lange calliper, made in the United States.

Laboratory tests

Many laboratory tests have great value in determining nutritional status, but few of them can at present be performed outside large hospitals. Only those tests that are widely available are discussed here.

Haemoglobin. An accurate assessment of haemoglobin level is by far the most important laboratory information that can be obtained in any nutrition survey. Accurate haemoglobinometers are rarely available in district hospitals, health centres and dispensaries. However, some cheap and simple-to-use haemoglobinometers which are reasonably accurate are now available.

In hospitals and for field research the cyanmethaemoglobin method is recommended. Blood is collected from a finger, ear lobe or heel prick. Two measured samples of 0.02 ml of blood are added to Drabkin's solution (a cyanide-ferricyanide solution). The specimen should be stored cool and protected from sunlight. The haemoglobin is determined later the same day using a spectrophotometer or other apparatus.

Haematocrit or packed cell volume (PCV). This determination is also important in the diagnosis of anaemia. A capillary tube is filled with blood from either a vein or finger prick. The sample is spun in a standard electric or hand centrifuge, which separates the red cells from the plasma. The haematocrit or PCV is the percentage of the blood volume composed of red cells.

Red cell counts and blood films. Red cell counts are not easy to do and add little information to the above tests. However, it is easy to prepare a thin blood film on a glass slide. Such slides are useful, since they enable the size and uniformity of the red blood cells to be seen. Use of such slides may facilitate the diagnosis of malaria and the haemoglobinopathies that may also cause anaemia.

Serum protein. Determination of total serum protein and especially of the serum albumin and globulin levels can only be undertaken in a well-equipped laboratory. These data are useful in cases of kwashiorkor, but they have not been found helpful in the diagnosis of mild or moderate PEM.

Examination of stools, urine and blood for parasites. After haemoglobin estimation, the next most important laboratory tests in a nutrition survey are strictly non-nutritional. There is little doubt that parasitic infestation and malnutrition are closely linked. The medical nutritionist must examine the individual and the community on all aspects related to public health. Laboratory examination should therefore be made of stools for the ova of hookworm, roundworm, *Trichuris* species, *Schistosoma mansoni* and other parasites; of urine for albumin, casts and *Schistosoma haematobium*; and of blood for malaria parasites. These tests are all easily performed in most dispensaries. They require only a microscope, a hand centrifuge, some laboratory glassware and a few simple reagents. Precautions should be taken in collection and disposal of specimens. Quantitative tests to assess the parasite load should be performed if possible.

During a nutrition survey it may be preferable to do these examinations on a separate day or during the afternoon following clinical examinations in the morning. In a large community it is advantageous to restrict these examinations to one particular group, such as all the children at the local school. The results will give a reasonable picture of the prevalence of diseases such as malaria and hookworm in the community. It is easier and more hygienic (especially with regard to stool examinations) to deal with a selected group than to collect specimens from people scattered over wide areas who have assembled in large numbers at a centre for clinical examination.

Biochemical tests. Certain biochemical tests (see Chapters 13 to 20) are useful for assessing deficiencies of almost all the minerals and vitamins. Even though in many developing countries vitamin A deficiency and IDD are important public health problems, very few local hospitals have laboratories that can conduct tests to assess these deficiencies. Similarly, in countries where pellagra, ariboflavinosis and rickets occur there are very few laboratories that can assess these deficiencies.

Table 37 lists the important nutrient deficiencies and indicates laboratory tests used for their assessment.

Dietary surveys

Accurate assessment of the dietary intake of a community takes much longer than getting a picture of the community's nutritional status by clinical or anthropometric examination. There are two main types of dietary survey. One relies on direct observation of a sample of the population, with their food measured and weighed over a given period of time. The other relies on inquiry, with a larger group of people questioned about their diet. Each type has a disadvantage: the former is very time consuming, and the latter depends on the memory, integrity and intelligence of the subjects questioned. Neither method takes account of past consumption or of uncertainties of food composition. Such involved methods are rarely justified or practical. It is often better to use cruder, simpler methods that provide data that reveal the causes of malnutrition and suggest corrective measures. The various methods of dietary survey are discussed below.

Observation. The only way to assess the diet accurately is to weigh and measure all the food that individuals eat over a representative period of time. A survey team goes to households and weighs and measures all food that is prepared, cooked and eaten, as well as that which is wasted or discarded.

If possible, the proportion of the total quantity of food prepared that is eaten by each individual should be weighed. (This is difficult in countries where household members often feed from one large communal dish or pot.) When the food eaten by each person on an average day has been ascertained, it is necessary to calculate the amount of each nutrient eaten by each subject or each family, using quantitative tables of dietary constituents.

A dietary survey of this kind requires a survey team of at least two persons that can cover two to four families at one time and perhaps 20 families in a month. It is essential to obtain truly representative households as samples and to cover a small, statistically acceptable sample of the population properly, rather than to try to cover more families in a less thorough manner.

Inquiry or recall. Direct inquiry cannot give very accurate information on amounts of energy or nutrients consumed. However, it can give an indication of the frequency of meals and the methods of food preparation and cooking, as well as providing details of the foods commonly consumed.

In developing countries it is most usual for a survey worker to go to a household and ask questions of the wife of the head of household. The answers are recorded on a form. This kind of inquiry depends heavily on the memory of those giving information and also on their attitude towards the person inquiring. False answers are often given unconsciously, or the subject may have some concealed reason for misleading the inquirer. For example, if the subjects believe that the inquiries are being made to ascertain whether famine relief food should be issued or increased, then quite naturally they will indicate that they are eating a small quantity and variety of food. If, however, they believe that the questioner is attempting to assess their standard of living or their degree of development, local pride may influence them to overstate the quantity and variety of food that they eat.

The most common method is to ask the subject to recall what was consumed during the previous 24-hour period. This is termed the 24-hour recall method. It is useful to have available local measures (bowls, cups, spoons) so that the respondent can indicate the approximate amount eaten.

Another survey method is to have literate people fill in a questionnaire. For example, schoolchildren may be given a questionnaire on which they are asked to record each morning for a week what they ate during the previous 24 hours. The process should be repeated at different seasons of the year. Such an inquiry gives no indication of quantities consumed, but it may provide useful information about meal patterns, the staple foods of each household, the frequency of consumption of certain foods such as meat, fish, eggs, fruit or vegetables, seasonal variations in diets, etc. Food frequency surveys of this kind can be performed on other groups of people. They provide qualitative, not quantitative, information.

Combined observation and inquiry. In a combination method, the observer goes to previously selected households and asks the wife of the head of household to show what food she intends to cook for the family that day. This food is then accurately weighed. The worker also records the number, sex and age of the people in the household. He or she then moves on to the next household. Clearly much more ground can be covered per day using this method than with a full-scale dietary survey as described above.

However, the respondent may have no idea of how much food she is going to use that day, or she may exaggerate the amount. This type of survey takes no account of food loss or wastage and gives no indication of what individual members of the family consume. The medical nutritionist is often very keen to know what the toddler or the pregnant woman actually eats, not what is prepared for the whole family.

One survey using this method, carried out in East Africa under the direction of statisticians, reported that the people surveyed consumed over 5 000 kcal per

TABLE 37

Manifestations of important nutrient deficiency diseases

Disease	Nutrient	Prevalence	Clinical manifestations	Laboratory tests
Protein-energy malnutrition: kwashiorkor, nutritional marasmus	Protein and energy	Very high	Growth retardation and wasting; in kwashiorkor: oedema, flaky-paint dermatosis, hepatomegaly, hair changes, mental signs; in marasmus: loss of subcutaneous fat, extreme wasting	In kwashiorkor: low total serum protein and very low serum albumin levels; low levels of digestive enzymes; in marasmus: low urinary hydroxyproline
Xerophthalmia	Vitamin A	High	Night blindness; conjunctival xerosis; Bitot's spots; corneal xerosis and ulceration; keratomalacia, corneal scarring	Low serum vitamin A levels; altered relative dose response; changed cytology of conjunctival cells
Beriberi, Wernicke's encephalopathy	Thiamine (vitamin B_1)	Moderate/low	Weakness; peripheral neuropathy; loss of reflexes; ataxia; weight loss; oedema; dyspnea; heart failure; in infants: tachycardia, aphonia, heart failure; in Wernicke's syndrome: ataxia, ocular signs, psychosis	Low whole blood or erythrocyte transketolase activity; low urinary thiamine in 24-hour urine collections or per gram of creatinine; low thiamine in whole blood
Ariboflavinosis	Riboflavin	High	Cheilosis of the lips; angular stomatitis; glossitis; seborrhoeic dermatitis, often of genitalia	Raised levels of erythrocyte glutathione reductase; low urinary riboflavin levels in 24-hour urine collections or per gram of creatinine
Pellagra	Niacin	Moderate/low	Photosensitive dermatitis on light-exposed areas; diarrhoea; stomatitis; mental confusion, depression and psychosis	Low levels of urinary N-methyl-nicotinamide in 24-hour urine collections or per gram of creatinine; low niacin in whole blood
Scurvy	Ascorbic acid (vitamin C)	Low	Swollen fragile papillae between teeth; bleeding gums; petechial and other skin haemorrhages; depression; weakness; in infants: tender swellings of bones; frog-leg position	Low leucocyte vitamin C; low serum ascorbate levels
Megaloblastic anaemia	Folate, vitamin B_{12}	Medium	Anorexia; tiredness; dyspnea; ankle oedema; cheilitis	Low haemoglobin; hypersegmentation of polymorphonuclear leucocytes; megaloblastic red blood cells; macrocytic red blood cells; low levels of serum folate

TABLE 37 (*continued*)

Disease	Nutrient	Prevalence	Clinical manifestations	Laboratory tests
Rickets, osteomalacia	Vitamin D	Moderate low	In rickets: craniotabes, bony deformities, rickety rosary because of enlargement of costochondral junctions, bow-legs, kyphosis, bossing of skull; in osteomalacia: bone tenderness and pain; kyphosis and bony deformities, waddling gait, tetany	Low plasma 25-hydroxycho ecalciferol levels; increased plasma alkaline phosphatase
Microcytic anaemia	Iron	Very high	Tiredness, weakness, dyspnea, pallor of tongue, nailbeds and conjunctiva; occasionally pica	Low haemoglobin; low serum ferritin; low transferrin saturation; ra sed free erythrocyte protoporphyrin; hypochromic macrocytic red blood cells
Iodine deficiency disorders, goitre, cretinism	Iodine	Very high	Enlargement of thyroid gland; in children born of iodine-deficient mothers: cretinism, mental retardation, deaf-mutism; strabismus	Low urinary iodine levels
Zinc deficiency	Zinc	Low	Acrodermatitis enteropathica with bullous dermatitis; dwarfing; hypogonadisim	Decreased plasma zinc levels
Dental caries	Fluoride (plus other causes)	Very high	Tooth cavities; tooth decay; loss of teeth. Excess fluoride causes dental fluorosis	

head per day. Malnutrition and under-nutrition were known to exist in this area, and the likely intake of those questioned was 2 200 kcal. Clearly the average householders in this survey area had tried to impress the observer with how well they were living.

Reducing random and systematic errors.
In almost all methods of obtaining dietary information there are common errors which make the data unreliable or even lead to wrong conclusions. These errors can be random or systematic. Various precautions including quality control can be taken to reduce some errors. No dietary assessment measurements are completely precise.

Random errors are related to the precision of the dietary method used. If the number of observations made is increased, the influence of the random errors on conclusions reached will be reduced. Many such errors cancel each other out, and they are therefore of less concern than systematic errors.

Systematic errors cannot be reduced by increasing the numbers of observations, and they do not usually cancel each other out. They are often cumulative and may be increased when more observations are taken. They therefore constitute a more worrying problem than random errors.

Systematic errors may result from several kinds of bias. Possible biases on the part of the interviewer include improper writing down of answers; neglecting to ask certain questions; and failure to ensure that the subject understands the questions. Those on the part of the subject include provision of information that is not true but is believed to be the "desired" answer (perhaps to try to create an appearance of being either better off or worse off); underreporting or overreporting of the consumption of certain foods; and lack of understanding of certain questions.

Other major sources of error in dietary surveys include difficulties in estimating the size of food helpings or the size of an item eaten; poor memory of what foods were eaten; and failure to remember or to mention foods eaten between meals. Errors may also arise in translating the results recorded on the survey form into amounts of food in grams and millilitres and into nutrients consumed. There may also be coding errors.

Methods that should be used to try to minimize errors include quality control; training, retraining and checking of interviewers, coders and data analysts; use of standard questioning methods and good data collection forms; consistent use of good and appropriate food models of different sizes and commonly used house-hold measures and utensils; and finally instilling into survey workers and study subjects the vital importance of accurate information. Interviewers should understand that it is much better to admit errors rather than to hide them or falsify data. Respondents should be convinced that it is preferable to admit not knowing or not remembering rather than to provide an untrue answer.

Vital statistics
Vital statistics are those related to births and deaths in the community. Complete and accurate vital statistics are not maintained in all countries, nor are they likely to be in the near future. However, vital statistics are so important as an index of nutritional status and for other public health reasons that they serve a useful purpose even if collected in small areas only. Infant mortality rate (death during the first year of life) gives a good indication of the state of nutrition and the health of the community. The neonatal mortality rate (death during the first month of life) and stillbirth rate are also useful.

In developing countries, figures for the

toddler mortality rate (TMR) (deaths between the first and fifth birthdays) are far more useful to the nutritionist than the other rates. TMR values often give a good indication of the prevalence of PEM, although they do not necessarily illustrate the nutritional status of the whole community.

TMR often provides a clear indication of the comparative state of development of a country. For example, in Scandinavia, the former Soviet Union, North America and the United Kingdom, TMR is below 1 per 1 000, while in much of Asia and Africa it is at least 35 times as much. The infant mortality rate is around 7 per 1 000 in Sweden and from 35 to 150 per 1 000 in most African countries.

Although it is normally impossible for an individual worker or a survey team to collect accurate vital statistics, some information of value regarding birth rate and death rate is usually available. For example, during a survey, one can easily ask all married women of child-bearing age two simple questions:

• To how many live children have you given birth?
• How many are still alive today?

From these figures a percentage of children that have died and also some indication of the fertility rate can be obtained. Careful questioning might also elicit the approximate ages of the living children and a rough estimate of the age at which the others died. Questioning as to the cause of death, if carefully done, may produce useful information.

It must be emphasized that information gathered in this way provides only rough estimates of the true figures, but these are nevertheless useful and will have to suffice until such time as proper vital statistics are maintained.

Other useful data

As indicated above, many other types of information are helpful in assessing nutritional status. These include other health statistics and medical information. Diarrhoea rates, measles incidence and other disease data have implications for nutritional status. (See Chapter 3 for the relationship of nutrition to infection, health and disease.)

Since food security (see Chapters 2 and 35) is partly dependent on food production, agricultural data are useful in judging the likelihood of food security and its relationship to nutrition. Economic data provide information for judging the nutritional climate in a community or a country. Figures on incomes, purchasing power, food prices and food distribution are useful. Data normally obtained by food scientists are helpful in judging nutritional status, food quality and food safety.

Participatory and rapid appraisal techniques

In the field of nutrition, as in social, agricultural and other fields, it has been increasingly realized that participatory methods of collecting information have many advantages. Involving members of the community, the potential beneficiaries, at the stage of data collection can prove extremely valuable. The active participation of the community in assessment and analysis, rather than only in the action stage of a project or activity, is likely to be very helpful. It assists in educating the public, in mobilizing local resources, in empowering people and in sustaining the success of actions taken. The community members, whether villagers or urban dwellers, come to understand their health and nutrition situation and the underlying causes of various problems. They offer alternative options for change and play the central part in implementing actions. This kind of participatory development, which is now suggested for nutrition, was well described 30 years ago by Paulo Freire working in Brazil. He termed it "conscientization" of the community, or helping community members become more aware of the causes and consequences of nutritional problems and, more important, how they can work together to prevent and overcome such problems.

A new series of techniques have emerged in the last decade as tools for participatory appraisal exercises. Semi-structured interviews, with either selected individuals or focus groups, are combined with observation (e.g. transect walks) and visualization techniques (such as mapping, seasonal calendars, ranking exercises, time charts and Venn diagrams). These techniques are particularly useful to gain an understanding of people's food habits and related beliefs, food entitlements and existing constraints and the role of the different family members in relation to nutrition (household food security, health and care). The choice of the techniques and their combination will be determined by the information needs and time constraints of community members. It is essential to cross-check the information gathered through different techniques. The information must be analysed on a regular basis to identify inconsistencies and remaining gaps, to be addressed in the next stage of the appraisal.

Participatory appraisal can best be carried out jointly by the community and local development staff, as it is a continuous process and should be an integral part of development activities at community level (for identification and selection of activities to promote household food security and nutrition, monitoring and evaluation, and reformulation).

Another major change in data gathering for assessing the nutrition situation of communities is the acceptance of rapid appraisal methods. Rapid appraisal exercises can help develop a first understanding of the situation and identify issues on which further information is needed. They can

then be complemented by formal surveys or routine data collection. The rapid methods borrow from anthropology and the other social sciences to obtain both quantitative and qualitative data. They offer promise because if properly used, they can provide useful information without the need for more complex survey methods or very large sample sizes. Even though rapid appraisal is usually carried out by international or national experts, it should involve local development staff who will be in a position to ensure follow-up of the process within their regular activities.

NUTRITIONAL SURVEILLANCE

Nutritional surveillance is a set of activities to assemble information to assist in policy and programme decisions to influence the nutritional status of a population. It usually includes the regular and timely collection, analysis and reporting of nutrition-relevant data. Surveillance differs from surveys in that it involves the periodic or continuous collection of data.

For many years various kinds of nutritional information have been collected, often for decision-making, but nutritional surveillance did not become a central activity in national nutrition planning until after 1976, following the report of a Joint FAO/UNICEF/WHO Expert Committee entitled *Methodology of nutritional surveillance* (WHO, 1976).

Because nutritional status is influenced by many different factors, nutrition monitoring and nutrition indicators may come from many different disciplines and may be of many different kinds, ranging from meteorological data, to food production, to nutritional status of people and so on.

Because nutrition is an outcome of social, economic, health, agricultural and other conditions, the nutritional status of a population can be used as an indicator of the overall development of a society. Specific nutritional status indicators are often better indicators of equitable development than are traditional economic indicators such as gross national product.

Information for decision-making

Nutritional surveillance, like nutrition surveys, is not useful if the data collected are not used to improve the nutritional status of the population. The weakest part of many nutrition surveillance programmes has been that the data collected have not been used to solve nutrition problems. For various reasons decision-makers have not used the information to take action. Why? It may be that lack of information was not the problem, that the kind of information needed is not being provided, or that there is a lack of commitment and resources to solve the nutritional problems. In general, it is agreed that the information needs to be provided in an easily understood form and in a timely manner.

In the past, nutritionists, health workers and others collected data and passed them to decision-makers in the expectation that action would follow. Some rethinking is strongly recommended. It is suggested that the first step after identifying the important nutritional issues should be to discuss and review possible policies and programmes and to identify how decisions will be made to influence these policies and programmes. This exercise would influence decision-makers to identify for themselves the information that they need in order to make decisions. If this approach were taken, the data collected would be what the decision-makers needed and would be likely to be used by them. The data would be analysed and would be discussed with the decision-makers, and decisions could be made to take appropriate actions. Later the impact of the actions would be determined.

Before surveillance is initiated, there should be an assurance first that there will be good communication between the people and institutions collecting the data and second that the data will reach the people and institutions that have the power to make decisions.

Assessing and monitoring nutritional problems

There are a huge number of possible indicators of nutritional status. The following are some typical indicators of different kinds that have been used in nutrition monitoring (FAO/WHO, 1992b).

- food crises:
  - production patterns,
  - market prices,
  - food stocks,
  - fall in body weights;
- protein-energy malnutrition:
  - children's anthropometry (weight for height, weight for age, height for weight),
  - children's growth,
  - infectious disease rates,
  - food intake relative to need,
  - body mass index;
- household food security:
  - employment levels,
  - market prices,
  - changes in real income and purchasing power,
  - dietary energy supply;
- caring capacity:
  - maternal education,
  - literacy rates,
  - maternal employment,
  - public expenditure,
  - breastfeeding (duration and percentage);
- malnutrition-infection complex:
  - incidence of diarrhoea,
  - immunization coverage,
  - availability of clean water,
  - children's weight for age;
- micronutrient deficiencies:
  - iron deficiency: rates of anaemia,

- vitamin A deficiency: night blindness/ xerophthalmia in children,
- iodine deficiency: goitre, cretinism;
• non-communicable chronic diseases:
- cardiovascular disease, diabetes, obesity, some cancers: rates of morbidity and mortality, comparison with some infectious disease rates,
- age distribution of population,
- age-specific mortality,
- changing dietary and lifestyle patterns.

Local decisions need to be made on which indicators to use. It is best if only a few indicators are chosen and if these are suitable for relatively easy regular collection. In developing countries the most widely reported indicator of malnutrition is low weight for age. However, data used are often not representative of the population and have been gathered from hospitals or growth monitoring clinics. For nutritional surveillance the data should be representative of the targeted population (for example, children six to 36 months of age of a particular district) and should be collected periodically. The use of well-chosen sentinel sites where data are regularly collected is a means of obtaining such data. However, although weight-for-age data provide a picture of the nutritional status and, if collected regularly, give important information on trends, they do not reveal the causes of the malnutrition identified. These underlying determinants can be grouped into those related to food security, health factors and child care (see Chapter 1). Data are often collected routinely on some of these causes.

In food crises early warning indicators may allow action before overt starvation. Indicators may be based on forecasts of food availability and food prices in the market. In countries where droughts are common, data on rainfall provide an early warning; these data are followed by food crop status and harvest yield estimates plus monitoring of food stocks, reserves,

marketing and prices. Sentinel households can provide useful information, some quantitative (e.g. crop yields and food stores) and some more qualitative (e.g. subjective views about family food security and reporting when they have to sell their personal possessions to purchase food).

In relating health factors to nutrition the focus is usually on infections and on monitoring infectious diseases such as measles, whooping cough, diarrhoea, respiratory infections, intestinal worm infections and malaria. Important health interventions also deserve monitoring; these include immunizations, oral rehydration for diarrhoea, attendance at clinics and preventive measures such as health and nutrition education, sanitation and improvement of water supplies.

To monitor caring practices and their impact on nutrition, data could be collected on breastfeeding and weaning, time available to the mother for child care and competing activities, differential treatment of girls and boys, family responses to poor appetite or poor health in their children, etc.

Many of the indicators discussed above are rather directly related to PEM, but many are also associated with micronutrient deficiencies. Lack of food security, high rates of disease and deficient caring practices have a negative impact on vitamin A and iron nutritional status as well as on PEM. Specific micronutrient deficiencies may also be monitored, for example by monitoring night blindness rates for vitamin A deficiency or haemoglobin levels for iron deficiency. Objective data might be collected from sentinel households. Data on food consumption also provide useful information.

The use of rapid appraisal methods is potentially valuable in monitoring nutrition. Some of the data collected in this way might be qualitative, including some that provides information on the functioning of relevant programmes.

TABLE 38
The four types of nutritional surveillance

Objective	Type
Io prevent short-term critical reductions in food consumption	Timely warning and intervention
To enhance the nutritional effects of development policies as expressed through programmes, to assess policies and programmes	Policy and programme planning
To rationalize and maximize effectiveness of health and nutrition programmes	Management and evaluation
To assess and/or monitor indicators related to nutritional status as a basis for directing funds towards particular nutritional problems	Advocacy

Nutritional surveillance systems

There are four types of nutritional surveillance, distinguished by their different objectives (Table 38). A number of countries have only one type of surveillance system, while others have several or even all four. Where several types are used, they may be coordinated in an organized way and may use some common data.

Timely warning and intervention. Nutritional surveillance was first established to warn governments of poor nations of imminent nutritional crises. It was in part modelled on health surveillance for important infectious diseases. Certain infectious diseases such as plague and cholera are notifiable to WHO; countries require that each district or province notify the national ministry of health on a weekly basis of the number of cases of notifiable diseases. In famines or severe crises, data on famine deaths or serious famine-related malnutrition can be collected and reported. Unlike outbreaks of serious infectious diseases, famine brings with it many cases of serious malnutrition.

Nutritional surveillance reports on indicators that would warn a government of an approaching nutrition disaster. As listed above, production patterns, market prices, food stocks and fall in body weights are possible indicators of food crises.

The types of data needed for an early warning system must be decided in the individual country or the affected region of the country. They cannot just be prescribed. It is important that the indicator system be sensitive and that it be able to predict food crises, even if warning is sometimes given of a crisis that does not then occur.

The first indicator may be rainfall below a certain level over a period of two or three agriculturally critical months. The next set of indicators might relate to the important crops in the field prior to harvest. These may be followed by estimates of food production and indications of food consumption. Finally, actual indicators of nutritional status such as the weight of adults and children in poor families may be monitored.

In some countries indirect indicators have proved useful, such as the pawning of household items, the movement from the consumption of a preferred food such as rice to a less desirable food such as cassava or the actual measure of food stores of sentinel households.

In Indonesia a timely warning intervention was introduced at the district level in drought-prone districts. Data collected at the district level could be provided quickly to the district official, who was given authority to take immediate action. A district-level food security system was established so that surveillance data indicating a shortfall in the food supply would result in delivery of a supply of rice to the local markets to prevent price rises and unavailability of rice. If the data had had to go to the capital city for review before decisions were taken, as is the case in many countries, long delays would have occurred. This example illustrates the need for data to be provided rapidly to officials authorized to take action speedily. Unfortunately the need is not often satisfied; data often end up as reports considered by people far from the scene, on which little action is taken.

Nutrition surveillance for policy and programme planning. Many kinds of indicators, including those listed above, can be used by governments or local authorities for surveillance to influence policy and programme planning. The data may be on nutritional status or on a variety of factors that influence nutrition. For example, anthropometric data may be collected on a regular basis to describe PEM trends over time. The data may be analysed to discern groups of the population most severely affected. They might be used to show which five provinces in a country have the worst malnutrition; which social groups are worst off; or what health factors are related to the most serious PEM. The next step might be to decide on direct interventions (perhaps supplementary feeding or nutrition education) for the most seriously affected groups and to suggest ways in which

existing policies (for example, regarding credit for small farmers to improve agricultural productivity or subsidies for staple foods for the poor in urban areas) might be modified or strengthened to influence nutritional status.

Costa Rica has had a national nutritional surveillance and information system since 1978. The system is designed to target activities to the poorest parts of the population and the poorest areas of the country. The anthropometric data used include child height, collected when children enter primary school, and the weight of younger children, collected by home visiting. A goal of the surveillance has been to use existing programmes more effectively by targeting activities to the poorest families who have the most PEM.

In these types of programmes interventions may be clearly nutritional (supplementary feeding; iron supplements) or non-nutritional but expected to have an impact on nutritional status (measles immunization; improved sanitation and water supplies; actions to reduce women's work load).

Nutritional surveillance for management and evaluation. Surveillance can be used to evaluate programmes aimed at improving nutrition and to assist in their management. For example, data from growth monitoring over a period of five years might be used to evaluate whether an agricultural credit scheme has improved the nutritional status of children; or night blindness data might be used over time to evaluate whether horticultural activities are influencing vitamin A nutritional status.

Data collected might be used as an internal management tool to judge the efficiency with which programmes in different parts of a country reach their objectives, or to compare the effectiveness of two alternative interventions aimed at solving the same nutritional problem.

Nutritional surveillance for advocacy. Scientists are often reluctant to be advocates, believing falsely that advocacy is unscientific. It is highly desirable, however, that most of those involved in nutrition be advocates for action. If serious problems of malnutrition are found in areas where food and health services are available the situation is unacceptable, and it is right to advocate interventions to reduce malnutrition.

Conducting surveillance for advocacy mainly involves collecting data on the prevalence of PEM or micronutrient deficiencies or on related indicators and using these data to get support for action. Support can be solicited in different ways including making the government aware of the problems found or embarrassing the government into taking action by publicizing a serious nutrition problem in the news media. The objective is to influence policy-makers to allocate resources and to provide the needed assistance to allow interventions or programmes to be imple-mented to improve the nutritional status of the communities affected. For example, in Chile it appeared that a reduction in supplementary foods provided to poor families was adversely influencing nutritional status. Advocates used anthropometric data from the health monitoring system which showed a recent rise in the rates of malnutrition in children. When the government was presented with these findings, it reinstituted the supplemental food benefits.

Nutritional surveillance cycle
Table 39 illustrates ten basic steps in nutritional surveillance or in nutrition monitoring. These steps form a cycle; when Step 10 is reached, the cycle needs to continue. The first five steps involve assessment, data collection and analysis, while Steps 6 to 10 move to decision-making and the enactment of interventions based on the decisions.

Nutritional surveillance is part of a data or information management system. It is designed very concretely to provide the data and the information that will help decision-makers ensure that actions and

TABLE 39
Basic steps in carrying out nutritional surveillance

Scope	Assessment	Implementation
Impact	1. Problem identification, including desired impact of action taken	10. Actual impact
Intervention	2. Proposed policies and intervention strategies	9. Intervention enacted based on decision
Decision	3. Potential decisions regarding policies and interventions	8. Decision(s) made based on information
Information	4. Information needed to aid in decision-making	7. Data analysis: the transformation into information
Data	5. Data needed to generate information	6. Data collection action

interventions are implemented based on good information. It is hoped that nutritional surveillance properly used will help ensure good decisions aimed at improving nutrition, and that the decisions will be made by senior officials who have the authority, the ability and the resources to ensure proper action.

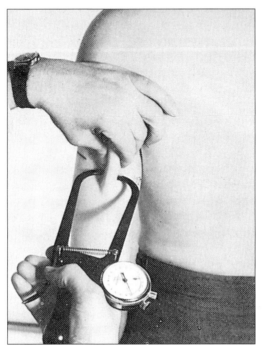

PHOTO 69
*The skinfold calliper is used to measure
the thickness of the triceps skinfold*

Chapter 34
Improving food quality and safety

Food production and food demand receive a great deal of attention in agriculture and nutrition. Clearly for people to have a healthy diet enough food has to be produced and families have to have access to sufficient food which then is consumed in adequate amounts by each family member. These issues are discussed elsewhere in this book. What receives less attention in writing, in training and in action is the fact that the food and water that people consume need not only to be adequate in amount, but also to be safe and of good quality.

Most industrialized countries have well-developed systems to ensure a reasonable level of safety and quality of foods consumed. Most developing countries have rudimentary systems that need strengthening. For a food system to work effectively, all those involved in it – from production, through processing, to marketing and eventual consumption – must be educated about food safety and quality and must implement actions to ensure them. Consumer education is a part of this effort.

Consumers, the food industry, government ministries and international agencies all have important, interrelated roles in ensuring food quality and safety. Food control measures can help reduce food losses and food spoilage, promote appropriate food processing and help ensure food safety and quality for the local consumer, for local markets and for export.

These lofty goals require appropriate legislation, regulations and food standards. These in turn demand a means to ensure compliance, which entails surveillance or monitoring, usually carried out through food inspection and in many cases laboratory analyses. Poor countries may not have the trained staff or the facilities to do a very good job in this respect, so they often decide to limit their activities in the area of food safety by trying to avoid serious outbreaks of food-borne illnesses and serious food contamination. Without much laboratory backup, public health inspectors and related staff may visually inspect meat at abattoirs or in meat markets; visit shops to find spoiled food; and inspect restaurants, hotels and stalls that sell food. They can insist that reasonable standards of hygiene are observed.

Appropriate national authorities should at the very least take steps to educate the public about food safety and quality so that consumers can insist on safer, better foods. These practices may begin with the education of the farmers who grow the foods and continue with education at various stages along the food path, up to the family kitchens in rural and urban areas. Education and assistance to food processors and manufacturers are also important. All should be made aware of standards, food laws and existing regulations and how to adhere to them.

In many rapidly urbanizing poor nations, more and more food is sold, processed, cooked and even served by small-scale entrepreneurs such as market or street-corner vendors. At street-side stalls or tables food safety and quality practices are not infrequently ignored. As many students are frequent street-stall users, food safety and food quality should be included in nutrition education activities and in the curriculum in schools to empower students to recognize food that is of doubtful quality or safety.

ENSURING FOOD QUALITY IN POOR NATIONS

Poor countries often do not have the institutions or the personnel to ensure food safety and control, although most do have some legislation, standards and regulations on the books. Governments would be wise to seek help internationally to improve their capacity in this regard. Small, poor countries can sometimes, with international assistance, share food microbiology and toxicology laboratories. The larger, emerging developing countries, sometimes called middle-income countries, should devote much more effort than they do now to ensuring food safety, and many can afford to do so. These countries are becoming highly urbanized and commercialized. The centres of the cities often appear modern and Western, with high-rise buildings, paved streets and running water in every household. However, nearby are often slums and squatter settlements which do not have safe water or satisfactory sanitation. In these areas the food that is sold is very likely to be contaminated and unsafe.

The food industry has an important part to play in food quality and safety at every stage of the food path from agricultural production onwards. For example, in the fields where crops are grown chemical fertilizers and pesticides need to be properly used; appropriate methods of preservation and storage need to be adhered to; and good technologies must be adopted to ensure food products at low cost but of high quality and safety.

International organizations can provide expert technical assistance and advice on various aspects of food quality and food safety, including the use and control of food additives; cut-off points for acceptability of food contaminants; and monitoring of simple hygienic practices in particular industries.

FAO and other organizations have a very important role internationally in advising member countries about appropriate legislation and regulations, which may include specific standards and guidelines related to quality, safety and labelling of foods put up for sale. Many of the standards and guidelines have been developed by the Codex Alimentarius Commission, a joint body of FAO and the World Health Organization (WHO) that provides international standards designed mainly to protect the health and welfare of the public while ensuring fair trade practices. These food standards help in international trade of food products. FAO, almost since its inception 50 years ago, has helped member countries improve the quality and safety of foods available for consumption by their people, through its staff expertise, meetings and expert consultations, numerous publications, assistance in standards development and numerous other activities. But for the countries themselves, adhering to standards and codes that help ensure the safety of foods must surely be considered a part of national or local food security.

An epidemic of a serious food-borne disease can have a significant negative impact on food trade within a country or internationally. A good recent example is the cholera epidemic which was first reported in Peru in 1991 and then spread first to other Andean countries and then to a wide group of Latin American and Caribbean countries. Peru is a major exporter of seafood, and very soon its trade was greatly affected, areas were quarantined and internal trade was limited. The result was a major negative impact on many poor people involved in the trade of seafood and later of other foods as regulations became extended. The epidemic led Peru to pay much greater attention to urban water supplies, sanitation, food handling and sale of street foods.

Food or water introduces health risks if it is contaminated with pathogenic organisms, toxins, pesticides or poisons. Any of these can lead to illness, sometimes in a few hours and sometimes a long time after their consumption. Perhaps the most common symptom or sign of illness resulting from consumption of contaminated food is diarrhoea. Diarrhoea can be caused by viruses, bacteria, parasites, toxins or poisons. An example of disease occurring a long time after the consumption of contaminated food or water is the development of certain cancers because of carcinogenic toxins.

Contaminated foods eaten at home or in public eating places may appear to be safe or may have evidence of contamination. If food, beverages, dishes or utensils are obviously unclean, if the food looks or smells bad, if a food that is meant to be eaten hot is served cool or lukewarm, if the environment where the food is served has flies, cockroaches or evidence of rodents or if food servers have dirty hands and clothes, then it is likely that the food being served is contaminated.

Sometimes it is difficult for people to refuse to eat food that they suspect may be contaminated. However, there are some steps that consumers can take, for example, at a stall selling street foods.

• Choose a food that is served at a very high temperature. If it is cold, ask the vendor to heat it more. Heat kills many organisms.
• Of uncooked foods, choose only those that are eaten peeled. Choose a banana rather than a slice of watermelon, for example. Even if both are crawling with flies, the banana can be peeled and then kept free of flies.
• Ask for a drink that comes in a bottle or can that can be opened by the consumer, or order tea or coffee that is served very hot.

Remember the old saying, "If you can't boil it, bake it or peel it, then forget it!" This saying makes a lot of sense.

SIMPLE STEPS TO IMPROVE FOOD SAFETY

In every household, but especially in those with less than ideal sanitation, some knowledge about food-borne disease is very important. It should be imparted in every school and should be an element of health education at every level. Many people in developing countries have very little understanding of the germ concept of disease, i.e. that serious illness can be caused by unseen organisms. An important challenge for health educators is to ensure that people understand that microorganisms cause disease.

Diarrhoea is commonly caused by a variety of microorganisms which are in human faeces and get into food and water. The following simple preventive steps can be taken.

Latrine and faeces disposal

The first sanitary essential in the household is a latrine and a well-organized system of safe disposal of human excreta. Measures are needed to prevent human faeces from contaminating the household and its environs. Very young children may not be able to use a pit latrine, but their faeces can spread disease and therefore need to be disposed of safely. Animal faeces are not nearly as dangerous as human faeces, but they can spread disease.

Personal hygiene

All members of the household should understand the basic rules and practices of good personal hygiene and practise them. Hands should be washed after use of the latrine and before each meal, and by people preparing food. All aspects of personal hygiene, however, including a clean body and clean clothes, also have a role. Personal hygiene is much easier if adequate water is available.

Household hygiene

A third form of protection is to ensure a good level of household hygiene, which is especially important in the kitchen and wherever food is stored, prepared and eaten. These places need to be kept clean and as free as possible of vermin such as flies, cockroaches and rodents. A clean house is a protection against food contamination and resulting disease.

Food preparation and storage

Various aspects of food preparation and storage have been described in Chapter 32. In the home, irrespective of its circumstances, the best possible efforts should be made to store, prepare and serve food in a way that minimizes the dangers of contamination and to make the meals as nutritious and as appealing as possible. This is relatively easy for an affluent household that has a refrigerator, a gas stove, running hot and cold water in the kitchen and a flush toilet. For a poorer household where there is no refrigerator, where food is cooked outside over a wood fire, where water is carried for two hours from a contaminated stream and where there is a pit latrine, food hygiene is a struggle.

FOOD PREPARATION TO ENSURE FOOD SAFETY

Bacteria that cause disease multiply rapidly in many foods, but more rapidly in foods of animal origin that are warm and wet. Small amounts of sugar enhance bacterial breeding, while larger amounts reduce it. If foods are not stored at low temperatures millions of bacteria will breed in them. Meat stew will deteriorate very quickly, stiff maize porridge moderately quickly and bread less quickly.

Uncooked dry rice granules will not deteriorate quickly. It should be understood that parasitic eggs (such as those of roundworm) or parasitic cysts do not multiply in food, but they do cause disease.

Four steps to improve food hygiene

Cleanliness along the food chain is the major preventive measure to avoid disease from contaminated food. People should be advised to observe the following household tips.

- Buy fresh food that looks clean and uncontaminated and has a good appearance. It should not have a bad smell, mould or discoloration. If the food is canned, the can should not be bulging, dented or discoloured.
- Store the food in a safe cool place. Many foods are best stored in a refrigerator. Dry foods such as cereal grains and flours or legume seeds should be left in a cool dry place in containers that prevent rodents and other pests from gaining access to them.
- Prepare the food for eating in a clean environment, with clean hands and clean utensils, and cook foods such as meat thoroughly to kill all organisms. Uncooked foods are safe to eat if peeled; if they are not peeled, then washing thoroughly, perhaps in a chlorine solution, will increase their safety. Tomatoes can be dipped in boiling water for two minutes or soaked in a chlorine solution. Lettuce is very difficult to clean thoroughly and presents a danger. Bananas are peeled and are safe.
- After the meal, leftover food should be stored safely, and some foods that cannot be stored may be fed to domestic animals. Food areas should be cleaned, utensils well washed and garbage buried or burned some distance from the house.

These tips apply almost equally to the small vendor or to those who prepare and sell street foods, although they are not easy to enforce.

Although many cooked foods in a poor household without a refrigerator should not be stored for very long, it is helpful to cover food, perhaps with gauze, to let in air but not flies. Alternatively, food can be kept in a simple "meat safe" which can be a simple wooden box on legs with metal or plastic screening on the sides or across the front. Each leg of the meat safe can be stood in a bowl or can of water to prevent ants and cockroaches from entering the safe.

BIOLOGICAL CONTAMINATION OF FOOD

Organisms are much more common contaminants of food and causes of disease than toxins or chemical poisons. More than 25 organisms, including bacteria, viruses and parasites, infect humans and cause specific disease after being consumed in contaminated foods. Microorganisms are ubiquitous, but only some of them are pathogenic (disease-causing) in humans.

Many of the pathogenic microorganisms are passed out of the body in faeces; they infect another human being when they reach the mouth, taken there perhaps by unwashed hands, utensils or flies. This type of transmission is termed faecal-oral transfer.

Gastro-enteritis or diarrhoea resulting from toxins produced by microorganisms can be distinguished from diseases caused by microorganisms invading the lining cells of the gastro-intestinal tract. The spread of both types is similar. The most important types of microorganisms are listed below.

Viruses

It is now clear that many outbreaks of diarrhoea, particularly in children, are caused by virus infections, mainly rotavirus or Norwalk virus. These viruses do not multiply in food, but they do in the intestine. The measles virus can also cause diarrhoea.

Bacteria

Many different bacteria are food borne and cause gastro-enteritis and other diseases.

Many different types of salmonella have been identified and found to be pathogenic. In some countries salmonella is the main cause of food poisoning. It may be transmitted through consumption of raw or undercooked eggs or through contamination of foods with salmonella by food handlers. Usually symptoms begin less than 48 hours after the food has been consumed. The disease is self-limiting, usually ending within six days. *Salmonella typhi* leads to the serious disease called typhoid fever, which is also spread by faecal-oral transmission. It is characterized by intermittent fever, a rash, abdominal pain and great, sometimes lengthy, debilitation.

Some staphylococci, such as *Staphylococcus aureus*, a widespread organism, can lead to diarrhoea and vomiting. Clostridium (*Clostridium perfringens* or *Clostridium welchii*) is a common cause of food poisoning. These bacteria are anaerobic and produce spores which can be widespread. *Clostridium botulinum* causes a very virulent form of food poisoning. It is usually food borne, but it can also infect wounds. If consumed its toxin produces serious neurological and muscular signs and symptoms, and the disease is often fatal. In food-borne infections, the contaminated food, often a preserved meat, becomes the site for toxin production by the clostridia. The spores are resistant to heat, but the toxins are destroyed by thorough cooking.

The disease that used to be called bacillary dysentery is caused by four *Shigella* species that infect foods: *S. sonnei*, *S. flexneri*, *S. dysenteriae* and *S. boydii*. These bacteria lead to marked diarrhoea, sometimes accompanied by vomiting and blood in the stools.

A very serious bacterial infection is

cholera, caused by the organism *Vibrio cholerae*. The infection involves much of the small intestine. Cholera is an acute infection leading to profuse and frequent watery stools, vomiting and abdominal pain. The patient may soon become severely dehydrated and may die rapidly. Oral rehydration can be life saving.

Other food-borne bacteria incriminated in diarrhoea or other diseases include certain serotypes of *Escherichia coli* (although many forms of *E. coli* are non-pathogenic); *Campylobacter* species; *Bacillus aureus*; and other vibrios such as *Vibrio parahaemolyticus*.

Parasites

Parasitic infections can be transmitted in food and water. The most prevalent intestinal worm infection is *Ascaris lumbricoides* (roundworm), which infects about 1 200 million people worldwide. Female worms in the intestine of an infected person produce millions of eggs which pass out in the faeces. If faeces are not properly disposed of, the eggs can get in the household environment or in dust being blown around, can get into food and can infect new subjects. Whipworm (*Trichuris trichiura*) and the protozoan infection *Giardia lamblia* are spread in the same manner and can cause serious disease.

Other parasites are transmitted through consumption of raw or undercooked food. Pork or beef that is not thoroughly cooked may be infected with *Taenia solium* (pork tapeworm) or *Taenia saginata* (beef tapeworm) which if eaten will infect the consumer. Pork tapeworm is a particular danger, because it can cause cysticercosis with serious complications. Undercooked or raw freshwater fish may be infected with a tapeworm called *Diphyllobothrium latum*. The tapeworm in the human gut competes with the host for vitamin B_{12}, so the infection may lead to macrocytic anaemia.

NON-INFECTIVE FOOD TOXICITY

Non-infective toxins or toxic substances in foods for human consumption can be "natural" in that they occur in nature. In certain fungi, lathyrus, cassava and fish, for example, these are the most common toxins. Less common but of great importance are toxins that are artificially added to food, such as various chemicals used to assist in food production, including fertilizers, weed killers, insecticides and fungicides. Other toxins that cause problems for humans include metals such as mercury or lead, which may get into the food supply or be consumed inadvertently.

Below is a summary of some of the more important non-infective substances that have resulted in ill health when consumed in food.

Aflatoxins

A toxin produced by a mould called *Aspergillus flavus* was found in 1960 to kill poultry fed groundnuts contaminated by this mould. A flurry of research followed, and it became clear that aspergillus grows on many foods, including cereal grains, when stored damp in tropical countries. In animals aflatoxin produces liver damage and carcinoma. It is not yet clear if aflatoxins are a determinant in primary carcinoma of the liver in humans; it now seems more likely that the high rates of primary liver cancer in Africa are a result of hepatitis earlier in life. Aflatoxin does cause disease, however. Some countries attempt to monitor the aflatoxin content of foods. Other hepatotoxins are found in food but they are not as important as aflatoxin.

Lathyrus

Lathyrus sativus is a vetch that grows wild, but it is also cultivated, particularly in India, where it may be planted in wheat fields. A neurotoxin in the plant, when consumed in large amounts, causes a neurological disease which can first result in weakness or spasticity in the legs and eventually lead to crippling and paralysis. The disease, lathyrism or neurolathyrism, has been widely discussed in Indian medical literature.

Fungal toxins

Some forms of fungi such as mushrooms are delicious foods and perfectly safe to eat. Other fungi, some of them resembling mushrooms, are highly toxic and lead to gastro-intestinal symptoms and perhaps kidney damage. Consumption of food contaminated with the fungus *Claviceps purpura* leads to the disease ergotism, with nausea and vomiting, and also to more serious neurological and vascular problems.

Antivitamins

Certain substances in food can act as antivitamins, inactivating vitamins or limiting their absorption in the human gut. The best described is thiaminase, present in certain fish. It has been shown that animals fed raw fish containing thiaminase can become thiamine deficient. It has not been clearly demonstrated that anti-vitamins are a major problem in humans. Haemorrhages have been observed in cattle that consumed feed containing dicoumarol, a substance that can have a negative impact on vitamin K and lead to bleeding.

Cassava toxicity

Cassava is not indigenous to Africa, but it is widely used as a food in both East and West Africa, as well as in Asia and Latin America. It is usually eaten without any toxic effects, either because of the varieties used or because of local preparation measures that remove the toxin. Some types of cassava contain a cyanogenic glucoside which can result in acute toxicity with serious symptoms and death. It may

cause nerve damage leading to paralysis, or it may behave as a goitrogen, aggravating iodine deficiency disorders (IDD) and causing goitres. In many African societies people know how to remove the toxin, mainly by soaking and sometimes also by grating and drying the cassava. Peeling cassava also helps remove the toxin. Toxicity occurs less frequently in Asia and the Americas.

Goitrogens

Some foods other than cassava contain substances that have been termed goitrogens, which appear to make those consuming them more likely to get goitre or IDD. The main goitrogens are thiocyanide, which reduces the levels of iodine in the thyroid gland, and thiouracil, which reduces the secretion of thyroid hormone. These goitrogens are most common in vegetables of the genus *Brassica* such as cabbage, cauliflower, mustard and rape (see Chapter 14).

Allergens in food

Many people are allergic to one or more foods. Allergens vary in composition and in the foods in which they are found. Shellfish and other seafoods are especially common causes of allergic reactions.

Metals in food

Industrialization, urbanization and the improper disposal of waste from factories and other businesses have caused metals which may be toxic to enter the food supply. A classic example is mercury in fish. In the early 1970s in the United States, various kinds of fish, such as swordfish, could not be sold because they had more than the permissible level of mercury, 0.5 parts per million (ppm). Mercury poisoning has also been a problem in fish in Japan.

Of much greater prevalence worldwide, especially in poor urban areas, is the problem of lead poisoning. Some of the lead consumed comes from foods, particularly animal foods such as meat and milk from animals that have consumed lead. Lead is also inhaled, for example from lead-containing fuels, and it can be ingested from water which has flowed through lead pipes and from the lead-based paints used in old houses. Lead poisoning causes long-term neurological problems, reduced psychological development in children and bone changes.

Other metals that have occasionally caused problems are cadmium, arsenic and selenium. The topic of fluoride excess causing dental or skeletal fluorosis is described in Chapter 21.

Agricultural chemicals

The green revolution, which has led to higher yields of cereals and other agricultural advances, has enhanced farmers' ability to produce food in adequate amounts to feed the rapidly increasing population in the world. Some of the advances are dependent on the use of chemical pesticides, which are used to control weeds and a variety of pests, from marauding animals such as rodents, monkeys and elephants to disease-causing organisms such as parasites, moulds, fungi, bacteria and viruses. Farmers also use externally applied medications such as insecticides and oral or injectable medicines such as anthelmintics to rid their domestic animals of, for example, ticks on the skin and worms in the intestinal tract. These chemicals, their residues or metabolites may end up in the food that humans consume; some of them present health hazards. Textbooks of toxicology cover these in detail, and only a few are mentioned here.

The Joint FAO/WHO Expert Committee on Food Additives (JECFA) is responsible for reviewing the safety of residues of veterinary drugs in foods for human

consumption and from time to time recommends safe limits. The Codex Alimentarius Commission can then adopt these limits as recommended international standards.

Under optimal agricultural and animal husbandry practices the residues of chemicals used would not present a risk either to agricultural workers or to consumers. Most countries have regulations regarding the permissible use of these chemicals. Some have monitoring systems. The efforts of the Joint FAO/WHO Meeting on Pesticide Residues (JMPR) have resulted in authoritative reviews of the safety of agricultural pesticides. JMPR has assessed the potential health problems from these chemicals based on the current literature and has recommended maximum residue limits both for adoption by the Codex Alimentarius Commission and for broad dissemination to member countries. In poor countries the regulations are often not adhered to and monitoring fails to detect many potential or actual problems.

In the use of farm pesticides, the first risk is to the agricultural workers who use them. They need to have clear instructions for the use of the chemicals. They need to know how to protect themselves, and they must have protective clothing and facilities to clean their bodies and clothes after working with pesticides.

Pesticides may also contaminate food. They are used in food storage to prevent spoilage or loss of food, and in this way too may present a danger to the consumer.

Most countries have regulations for pesticide residues in foods, and these need to be monitored and enforced. For example, the United States Environmental Protection Agency lists maximal residue levels of some 90 pesticides in foods sold for human consumption. DDT (dichloro-diphenyltrichloroethane), which was used both for agriculture and also to kill mosquitoes in anti-malaria programmes, has been banned by many countries (and by all countries for use in agriculture), but others have felt that the risk from malaria was greater than the risk of toxicity from DDT. Now there is greater concern for other insecticides. Of particular concern now are polychlorinated biphenyls (PCBs); the organophosphorus pesticides such as malathion and parathion, widely used in agriculture; dieldrin; and the herbicide chlorophenoxy acid. In most countries the Acceptable Daily Intake (ADI), set by FAO and WHO (via JMPR), is the standard for monitoring.

Although there have been a few industrial accidents involving workers accidentally being sprayed with pesticides and an occasional poisoning of a child who drank a pesticide solution, both are rare. Extremely few cases of pesticide poisoning from eating food have come to the attention of JMPR.

Food additives
Chemical or other substances are added to foods for human consumption for many different reasons. The most important perhaps is to preserve the food, but additives may also be used to change the colour, the taste or some other quality of the food. Some countries have very strict regulations governing the approval of a new food additive for use by the food industry. For those additives that are approved, the regulations usually state the maximum level that is permitted. Again it is JECFA that has established the safe levels which then have been used by the Codex Alimentarius Commission. Concerns regarding food additives are that they might be carcinogenic (stimulate cancer) or have a negative impact, including genetic or teratogenic effects, on the foetus if consumed by pregnant women. In the United States food additives approved for use by industry are listed as "Generally

recognized as safe" or GRAS. The GRAS list includes many additives in use before 1958 which evidence suggested were safe, and new items introduced since 1958 which are rigorously tested to show among other things that even rather large amounts are not carcinogenic in laboratory animals. JECFA has prepared specifications for food additives which guide Member Governments to establish the identity and quality of additives being used. These specifications are also used by industry.

Radioactive contamination of foods
Happily, the contamination of foods with radioactive fallout, either from explosions of atomic bombs or from accidents at nuclear power plants, is rare. The accident at Chernobyl in the former Soviet Union in 1986 was the worst well-described accident of this kind. When radioactive dust is liberated into the atmosphere, it is blown by the wind and falls to earth where it may contaminate food crops such as cereals, fruits and vegetables, but also grass which is then eaten by cattle and other livestock. As a result the milk and the meat of these domestic animals may contain unacceptable levels of radioactive materials. Following the Chernobyl accident, elevated levels of diseases such as thyroid cancer (presumably because of fallout of radioactive iodine, ^{131}I), particularly in children, and other malignancies have been reported.

Very soon after the Chernobyl accident FAO convened an expert consultation which recommended action levels for radionuclide contamination of food in international trade. No guidelines existed previously, so this rapid action was important. In the event of a nuclear disaster, people living in the area of the fallout should avoid eating foods that were growing in the affected area. They should also avoid consuming milk and meat produced in the area and foods that might have been exposed to dust fallout. Foods stored in sealed containers, including tins, are safe. The authorities should bring food into the area from unaffected areas as soon as possible. People all over the world should be made aware that a nuclear accident has occurred and that it could make their usual food dangerous.

CONSUMER PROTECTION

Many of the actions discussed earlier in this chapter will help protect the consumer and ensure a safe diet of good quality. Some other specific activities might further help the consumer. In many countries greater attention is now being given to food labelling, which may be controlled by regulations. FAO has had a leading role.

Recommended nutrient reference values for labelling purposes were established at an FAO consultation in 1988. Food packaging that provides useful information for the consumer can be helpful. It should, if possible, express in simple terms the amount of nutrients in the food, perhaps as percentages of the requirements or allowances of each important nutrient per serving of the food. The energy, protein, carbohydrate and fat content of one serving should also be included. In countries where there is concern about arteriosclerotic heart disease, this information might be broken down further to indicate the amounts of different kinds of fat, cholesterol and fibre. Food labelling might also include the amount of additives in the food.

Food advertising should use only truthful information and should not make claims for the food that are not true. Foods that can be harmful should perhaps not be advertised.

In 1981 at the World Health Assembly in Geneva, 118 nations voted in favour of adoption of the International Code of Marketing of Breast-milk Substitutes, which calls for the cessation of all promotional advertising of breastmilk substitutes to the public. (Only one country, the United States, voted against the code.) Many countries have introduced legislation to limit the promotion of infant formula, because it is generally agreed that breast-feeding is very important for good health and good nutrition and that promotion of infant formula has greatly eroded and undermined breastfeeding (see Chapter 7). The multinational corporations that manufacture infant formula continue strenuously to promote infant formula in other ways than advertising to the public, for example by offering free samples and by providing literature to the medical profession.

IMPROVING FOOD QUALITY AND SAFETY IN DEVELOPING COUNTRIES

Most countries have legislation to help ensure the safety, and sometimes the quality, of foods from production to retail sale. Farmers, food processors and the public, however, are not always conversant with the regulations. Moreover, dishonest traders may seek to ignore the regulations. As a result, unsafe foods that are contaminated or spoiled or have dangerous levels of chemicals are reaching consumers, sometimes widely, putting the public at risk of illness.

Most countries have established institutions or branches of ministries (such as a bureau of standards or a branch of the ministry of agriculture) designated to ensure food quality and safety. These mechanisms often need strengthening, and there are often too few well-trained people or well-equipped laboratories to monitor the situation. In some countries an interdisciplinary, interministerial committee could be established to examine all areas related to food safety, to ensure that the most important aspects get covered and perhaps to suggest the most important and most feasible priority areas. Such a committee could have many functions, but the main ones might be to promulgate and implement food safety standards; to establish means of monitoring, including inspection, sampling and testing; to recommend a programme for educating both food industry personnel and the public on food safety; and to find ways to involve and obtain assistance from international agencies such as FAO and WHO (with the Codex Alimentarius Commission) and other foreign institutions.

The following actions might be given priority for immediate strengthening because they would cost little and seem feasible and important:

- greater attention to food hygiene practices at all places where cooked food is sold to the public (restaurants, stalls, street carts);
- education of employers and employees in the food processing industry and monitoring of their food safety practices nationwide;
- ensuring improved meat inspection at all abattoirs;
- collaboration with the ministry of education to produce a syllabus and perhaps a booklet on food hygiene for primary and secondary schools;
- seeking fellowships to send university graduates overseas for high-level training in food science with emphasis on food safety;
- teaching specific steps to improve the quality and especially the hygiene of street foods.

Steps to improve the quality and safety of food are important if people are to have good health and nutrition in developing countries. Such steps will also benefit food trade because contaminated or unsafe food should not be traded either in internal markets or for export. The FAO/WHO Codex Alimentarius Commission can assist non-industrialized countries in implementing standards and codes with the objective of protecting consumers and promoting food trade. FAO can assist governments in modernizing their food regulations, in designing compliance systems, in training food inspectors and related personnel, in improving food analysis laboratories and training their staff and in actions to ensure better quality control by food producers, manufacturers and processors. Food quality needs to be protected from the farm to the consumer. FAO, with WHO, can also help with the scientific evaluation of food additives, various contaminants and medicinal products. In the years ahead countries will need to give consideration to the agreements of the General Agreement on Tariffs and Trade (GATT) regarding sanitary, technical and other regulations which may be barriers to food trade.

In conclusion, consumers have a right to expect that their food is safe and of good quality, and both the food industry and governments have a responsibility to honour that right. To do so will require knowledge on food safety on the part of farmers, food processors and the public plus effective food safety control activities by the food industry and government. Control of food safety requires that there be in place laws, regulations and standards related to food quality and safety plus a system for food inspection and for monitoring to ensure compliance. Some inspection and monitoring can be achieved without extensive facilities, but there will be a need for laboratories to undertake the important analyses recommended. International agencies such as FAO may be called upon for technical and other assistance. FAO's very important efforts in helping to establish and strengthen food control systems internationally and particularly in member countries must be recognized. The Organization's work and actions over many years have contributed substantially to significant improvements in the overall quality and safety of the food consumed in many countries, especially in developing countries worldwide.

Chapter 35
Improving household food security

Food security is frequently defined as access by all people at all times to the food they need for an active and healthy life. Household food security, in turn, means adequate access by the household to amounts of food of the right quality to satisfy the dietary needs of all of its members throughout the year. A family can secure food in two main ways: food production and food purchase. Both require adequate resources or income. Other less important, less common ways of obtaining food are through food gifts or charitable or government food allocations, in free school meals or with food stamps.

In Chapter 2 lack of food production and lack of food security were discussed as underlying causes of malnutrition. The importance of agricultural food production to underpin national and local food security was outlined. Food security was shown to be important at all levels, but particularly at the household level.

This chapter outlines some ways of improving household food security to improve nutritional status or to prevent malnutrition. As discussed in Chapter 1, food security for the individual child (or for the family) is one of the three essential ingredients (along with adequate health and adequate care) in preventing malnutrition. Individual food security is essential for good nutrition, but it does not ensure good nutritional status, because other factors such as disease, infrequent feeding, lack of care and poor appetite may adversely influence nutrition.

The achievement of food security requires:

• a sufficient supply of food;

• stability in the supply of food, both throughout the year and from year to year;

• access, both physical and economic, to food, which requires the ability and wherewithal to produce or procure all the food needed by the household and each of its members.

The main underlying determinant of household food insecurity is poverty. In Asia, Africa and Latin America a large proportion of the population in both urban and rural areas is affected. It has been stated that not all poor people are undernourished, but most undernourished people are poor.

Household food security in each country, even if the country is food secure, depends partly on the extent to which the country pushes for greater equity in incomes, in land distribution and in access to services. National policies may not only help farmers achieve increased food production, but may also help people satisfy their food demands. Although household food security is most influenced by actions at the household level, factors and actions at the local, national and international levels also have effects.

FORMS OF FOOD INSECURITY
Household food insecurity takes different forms which require different responses or actions. The approaches may be different depending on whether food insecurity is chronic (with households almost always short of food) or transitory (resulting from temporary adverse circumstances). Food insecurity may be seasonal; a family may have insufficient food

perhaps each year or most years, but only in certain seasons.

The consequences of household food insecurity are as different as the causes. Which members of the household are most affected will vary, sometimes as a result of intrahousehold food distribution. Thus two families each with a mother, a father and two young children, with similar moderate but not severe insecurity, may respond in different ways, with different outcomes. The first family may believe in "children first" and despite food shortages may make certain that the two children receive all the food necessary for good growth and health; the adults then may develop signs of undernutrition or more likely will reduce their energy expenditure by reducing their activities and productivity. In the second family, the father may always satisfy his desires for food first, leaving the remaining food for the mother and, last, the two children, who get less food than required. In this family the children would show evidence of malnutrition. Sometimes, however, ensuring the energy and nutritive intake of the food producer and wage earner may be necessary for the family to get the food it needs for survival.

WHO IS AT RISK?

Households most likely to be food insecure, or at high risk of food insecurity, are the poorest. In rural areas these may be landless households; those with such small plots of land (sometimes marginal land) in relation to family size as to make adequate agricultural production impossible; sharecroppers or tenant farmers who get relatively little of the crop produced; pastoralists, fishermen, forestry workers and others who earn too little money or produce too little food for the needs of their families; female-headed households where the mother has many responsibilities for child care as well as farming;

and poor households with a high dependency ratio or that have no or few active adults because of age, disease, disabilities or other reasons.

In urban areas also the most food insecure are the very poor, including households where there is unemployment or underemployment; single female-headed households with dependent children; elderly people living alone; destitute and homeless individuals; and those with chronic debilitating disease or serious disabilities.

Increasingly the acquired immunodeficiency syndrome (AIDS) epidemic is contributing to food insecurity, sometimes because adults who were breadwinners have become seriously ill or because orphaned children as young as 12 years of age have become household heads caring for younger children. In addition, where human immunodeficiency virus (HIV) infection is prevalent, the disease is having a major negative impact on agricultural production, on economics and on health services.

VARIABLES AND ISSUES IN HOUSEHOLD FOOD SECURITY

Many variables influence household food security, and all of them can be manipulated to some degree to improve it. However, there are few easy answers or prescriptions for alleviating food insecurity. Recommendations often depend on local circumstances. Solutions will almost always involve participation at the local and household level.

Among the issues that influence household food security are adequacy of local food supplies; potential for cash crops and home gardens; urban versus rural food supplies; producer and consumer prices; available means of improving food production; food storage and stabilization of food supplies; employment questions; and labour-intensive versus labour-saving work. Agricultural and planning ministries and other organizations need to address some of these issues at the national level.

Other issues of great importance to food security involve gender. What roles do males and females have in the society? To what extent are females discriminated against? Do women have an unfair labour burden? Who controls household finances?

People have different ways of dealing with food insecurity depending on their systems of earning a livelihood or procuring needed food. There are major differences between subsistence farmers and pastoralists; between sharecroppers and urban workers; and between welfare recipients and those working in the informal economy. Clearly urbanization and migration from rural areas have a role in food security.

Evidence about household food insecurity and its causes strongly suggests that in many instances attempts to improve food security should start not at the national level alone – the classical approach – but at the household level, or preferably at both. Emphasis must be on local-level planning of community interventions and on using a participatory approach.

The three important requisites of household food security – an adequate local supply of food, stability in the food available and accessibility of food – are discussed below. For nutritional security there must also be adequate health and adequate care, and the food must provide all the nutrients needed for good nutrition.

Food supply

If there is an insufficient quantity of food to meet the food needs of a population, then some persons or some households will be food insecure. Various steps along the food chain need to be considered in relation to supply.

To improve household food security,

various methods of increasing sustainable agricultural production of food (or other methods of food acquisition) need to be promoted. It is also necessary to ensure good harvesting and storage of food with the smallest possible losses; an effective and efficient marketing system; and good food processing and preparation. All these topics are discussed in detail in many publications, of which some are listed in the Bibliography.

At the national level food supply also depends in part on government and private-sector decisions and actions concerning what and how much food to import and export, when to do so and how to allocate resources. These decisions in turn depend on whether domestic food

---

Policy measures related to food supply

Some policy measures related to food supply include:

- national macroeconomic policies and overall development strategies that ensure adequate public- and private-sector investment in agriculture and food production, including the much-discussed structural adjustment policies and greater consideration of equity issues, which is necessary if household food security for the poor is an objective;

- appropriate agricultural and trade policies to enable expansion and diversification of food and agricultural production and availability, a proper balance between food and cash crops, an adequate and stable food supply, sustainability in light of environmental issues, adequate employment for the rural poor and improved market efficiency and opportunities;

- policies that improve access to land and to other resources important for increased production, including credit, fertilizers and other agricultural inputs.

production is able to meet local needs. If imports are necessary, the amounts and types of food imported will depend on many factors including political considerations, availability of funds and foreign exchange, trade policies, world food prices and perhaps availability of food aid.

Often government economists and planners, considering the supply side of food security, address only the need for adequate energy for the population in terms of cereal grains and perhaps legumes. For good nutritional status, however, the production, supply and availability of other foods, including fruits and vegetables, need consideration.

Stability of food supplies

A reasonable degree of stability in the supply of food during the year and in all years is a necessary ingredient of food security. This stability can be ensured in various ways, including:

- adequate stockholding by ensuring strategic food reserves;
- a good food marketing system at all levels, including the village level, throughout the year;
- protecting or introducing a variety of cropping strategies such as mixed cropping, proper rotation and use of appropriate agricultural inputs;
- promoting good post-harvest food handling, transportation, distribution, preservation, storage and safety;
- assisting where appropriate with increased production of fish and animal products for human consumption (which includes attention to animal health);
- promoting household, school and community gardens, especially stressing production of fruits and vegetables;
- ensuring the sustainability of food supplies using agricultural, industrial and marketing strategies and relying on renewable resources with proper concern for the environment.

Access to food

Household food security depends on access by all household members to food that satisfies their nutritional needs at all times. Each household needs to have the resources, the ability and the knowledge to produce or to procure the foods that it needs to provide for the energy needs and the nutrient requirements of every member. It is important that households be able to acquire adequate quantities of food all year and in all years. The food must be culturally acceptable.

The acquisition of adequate food depends on how much a person, family or household:

- owns (land, resources, etc.);
- produces;
- receives (gifts, government aid, charities, etc.);
- trades, barters or exchanges;
- inherits.

There are obvious differences in how urban dwellers and rural farmers usually obtain access to sufficient food for themselves and their families. Most urban households usually need to obtain sufficient money to purchase enough food to satisfy the nutritional requirements of all their household members. By contrast, the rural landowner or farmer must have enough land, resources and labour to produce sufficient food to feed all household members or to sell for cash with which to buy the ingredients of an adequate diet for all. The rural family that has neither land nor labour usually needs to obtain enough money to purchase food, much as urban households do. Many farming households are also dependent on off-farm income-earning opportunities.

Where household insecurity is prevalent among both urban and rural people, attention has to be given to ensuring that farmers are paid remunerative prices for their produce; that processing and distribution systems are expanded and efficient;

that minimum wages are adequate; that prices of staple and perhaps other important foods are reasonable, or even subsidized; and that other essentials (such as housing, health care, education and transport) are affordable for those receiving the minimum wage. Programmes that provide social security, welfare and unemployment payments or that provide free or subsidized food (through food stamps or school feeding, for example) will help the poor and disadvantaged obtain access to food.

Rural farming households can take measures, and authorities can help them, to optimize production from their land and to get the most food and money from farm production. In some parts of the world implementing land reform policies to allocate adequate land to poor rural families and ending sharecropping might help families become food secure. In many areas livestock are integral components of farming systems and may provide insurance against bad agricultural years, as a form of asset that can be exchanged for money to purchase food. Rural families may also be assisted with credit, subsidized foods, food stamps or charitable help, especially in bad agricultural years.

It has been observed that where there is food shortage and famine, families with money and resources do not suffer from starvation. Very poor families have the fewest assets and thus are usually the most food insecure and the most vulnerable to serious food crisis.

RESPONSIBILITIES FOR THE RIGHT TO FOOD
Sustained improvements of household food security are likely to depend on actions at the local and household level and on the participation of the poor in bettering their own lives. However, this idea should not allow those who are better off to forget that adequate nutrition is a basic human right and that the occurrence

of malnutrition among so many people in the world is an indictment of all who permit it. The world is divided into nation States, each of which has a major influence on its own inhabitants. Each State has the responsibility to respect, protect and fulfil human rights, including the right to adequate food and nutrition. Respecting means that the State does not take actions or have policies that make it more difficult to procure food for the needs of its people, even in times of crisis or conflict. Two examples of protection would be preventing individuals from being deprived of their abilities to produce food or to earn money to purchase food; and establishing and enforcing regulations to ensure consumers a safe food supply. Fulfilment of the right to food and adequate nutrition includes the State's obligation to provide assistance to the vulnerable to meet their food needs even at times of shock or crisis.

MEETING DESIRABLE ALLOWANCES FOR ENERGY
It cannot be stressed enough that humans have a right to sufficient food and good nutritional status. "Sufficient" food, moreover, must provide not only for basic energy requirements, but also for the energy requirements of an active and healthy life.

Dietary needs have been discussed elsewhere in this book but deserve mention in regard to policies and programmes to improve food security. For good health and optimum nutritional status a person must consume food to satisfy all essential nutrient requirements or nutrient needs. In terms of energy, however, food has to be sufficient to satisfy not just the basic needs, but also the individual's wants for energy, provided that this does not lead to overconsumption and obesity. These energy wants, i.e. energy intakes sufficient both for basic requirements and also for the desired activities of each person, are now widely termed "desirable allowances".

The concept of desirable allowances has important implications for improving food security. If only energy requirements or needs are considered, a person in energy balance who is not clinically undernourished or does not have low body mass index (BMI) or low weight for height might be considered food secure. However, such a person may be foregoing desired activities to conserve energy. That person has unfulfilled energy wants, does not have enough energy to satisfy desirable allowances and is food insecure.

Energy balance is not an indicator of adequate energy intake. A person may be in energy balance, with energy intake equalling energy expenditure, but may in fact be greatly reducing his or her activity levels to remain in balance. Consciously or unconsciously he or she may choose to do less work on the farm, to reduce household chores, to play less with the children, to refrain from participating in sports and to curtail social and community activities, and instead may rest more and sleep more. This individual, though in energy balance, is nonetheless in a state of energy deprivation and is therefore not food secure; yet a physical examination may indicate no physical evidence of malnutrition or undernutrition.

There is a difference between affluent and poor people who are in energy balance over time. Generally, affluent people adjust energy and food intake to meet energy expenditures, while very poor people with food shortages adjust their activity to their energy intake (foregoing activities to conserve energy). Where food is plentiful, people may forego food or increase exercise to maintain balance (the jogger's syndrome); where food supply is deficient, they may forego activities to maintain balance.

Very little research has been conducted to determine what activities are foregone, and to what extent, in order to maintain energy balance when too little food is available. Policies and programmes are needed to ensure that energy wants as well as energy requirements are satisfied. Providing women with the opportunity and freedom to control their own fertility is also important. These issues are all highly relevant to any consideration of food security.

INDICATORS OF HOUSEHOLD FOOD SECURITY
As stated, adequate supply, stable availability and proper access to food are essential requirements of household food security. Indicators of household food security are then those related to food production and supply on the one hand, and food demand and access on the other. Manuals and books have been written on agricultural production, nutrition surveys, food balance sheets, household economics and other topics related to specific indicators of food security. Here a few key indicators are briefly mentioned.

Indicators related to food supply include:
• measurements of agricultural production (similar to those collected for food balance sheets);
• inputs that influence agricultural production in the area or country (such as credit, irrigation, fertilizers and pesticides);
• climatic data (especially the amount of rainfall compared with that usually expected and the timing of the rainfall, but also temperature and other meteorological data);
• market factors, including food sales and prices;
• security (whether there are areas of conflict or parts of the country where movement of people and food is restricted or limited);
• data on crop diseases and agricultural pests.

Indicators related mainly to household access to food include:

- food consumption data;
- clinical assessment related to signs of nutrient deficiencies;
- anthropometric data such as BMI;
- assessment of food stores;
- selling of assets (or loans obtained for assets) including livestock and household goods;
- greater consumption of low-status foods (a move from rice to cassava consumption, for example);
- increases in food foraging and gathering of wild foods;
- migration from rural to urban areas;
- data suggesting frequent perception of food insecurity or food crisis by household members.

In many countries with diverse topography, agricultural conditions and peoples, indicators may need to be rather specific for particular areas of a country or particular groups of the population.

Nutritional surveillance may be established as a system for regular monitoring of the food situation, the functioning of the food system and also some aspects of the nutritional status of the population (see Chapter 33). This system will then, depending on the data being collected, provide indicators of household food security. Sometimes nutritional surveillance is established as an early warning system to help predict serious food shortages and to trigger action. Some countries have established nutritional surveillance as a means of providing data to influence government policies.

COPING AT THE HOUSEHOLD LEVEL

Often poor households have amazing resilience and an impressive ability to cope with short-term crises and to survive on low incomes and what appear to be relatively low availabilities of food.

Transitory or short-term food insecurity is often the result of a shock that has struck a blow to the household. The coping mechanisms adopted depend partly on the nature of the shock and partly on the household's circumstances. Different members of the household may respond to a shock in different ways. It has been suggested that there are four main types of shocks (Maxwell and Frankenberger, 1992):

- work shocks, when there is a sudden fall in the availability or the amount of work on which a family is dependent for income, or a fall in the wage rate;
- output shocks, when the production output of different family members or the money received for a given output from work declines suddenly and significantly;
- food shocks, when food in the marketplace is less available and/or when food prices rise, either of which results in less food in the household;
- asset shocks, when the assets of the household are reduced in quantity or value because of fire, theft, the death of livestock or small animals owned by the family, inflation or sale of assets to raise money.

Where shocks cause transitory food insecurity, and also when families face chronic food insecurity, families take actions to ensure adequate food. Examples of such actions include:

- using labour differently, perhaps having one or more family members move from the rural area to town to earn money;
- using money differently, perhaps by purchasing cheaper foods (such as yams in place of bread or cassava in place of rice) and foregoing non-food purchases (e.g. not buying school uniforms or not paying school fees);
- purchasing less kerosene (for lighting or other uses);
- selling or pawning household assets

(farm animals, bicycles or luxury items such as watches and radios);
- securing credit or loans, which for the poor is often very difficult;
- entering the informal economy, either legally (having older children shine shoes or clean automobiles) or illegally (through prostitution or thieving);
- seeking assistance from government or non-government programmes (e.g. feeding programmes, food subsidies or food-for-work programmes).

Imaginative programmes to assist poor families to overcome the results of shocks will help reduce food insecurity.

GOVERNMENT ACTIONS TO IMPROVE HOUSEHOLD FOOD SECURITY

Food security may be influenced by anything that governments do to improve income and reduce poverty; to increase agricultural production, especially by poor rural families; to ensure prices that are fair to producers and consumers; and to make services available to people.

Some examples of more specific government actions include:
- increasing agricultural food production, preferably using sustainable methods (see Chapter 2), in such a way that poor subsistence farmers who are most vulnerable to food insecurity derive benefit;
- taking steps, if necessary, to import more food and to limit the export of food where this will improve food security;
- promoting improved marketing of food and better food distribution in a manner that addresses problems of food insecurity;
- in times of modest food crises when shortages of food are predicted, releasing or moving foods into the crisis area to prevent price rises and profiteering and to stabilize supplies so that market mechanisms protect the poorer people from a food shock;
- if the preceding strategy is not working or is deemed impossible, effecting food price controls, subsidization or rationing, but only if doing so is unlikely to be a disincentive to food production;
- improving equity by ensuring that all people pay a fair share of taxes and perhaps by increasing minimum wages and offering subsidized or free services to poorer people;
- streamlining the purchase of cash crops produced by small farmers so that most of what is paid goes into their pockets rather than lining the pockets of intermediaries or being spent on bureaucratic marketing practices.

Besides these specific measures, governments need to have a sound overall development strategy which creates conditions for economic growth with equity. Poverty alleviation programmes need to be sustainable. This book is not the appropriate place to discuss how the poor countries of the South strike a balance between macroeconomic policy objectives and food security needs. Clearly the rate of exchange of currency in a country, the nation's export and import policies, the rate of inflation, the budget deficit and debt repayment obligations can all influence prices, unemployment rates and incomes of the poor. Much recent discussion has focused on structural adjustment programmes, sometimes mandated for poor countries to promote economic growth. These programmes have caused major problems for the poor, often through reductions in producer and sometimes consumer subsidies. Of great concern also has been the reduction in social services: previously, many countries in the South had free primary and secondary education and free health services, including both out-patient care and hospitalization, but by 1992, with implementation of structural adjustment and sometimes for other reasons, school fees and charges for health services had become common or even the norm. These changes have had a marked impact on the poor, in some cases worsening the problem of food insecurity.

In some countries, particularly in Asia and Latin America, economic development has progressed and the creation of wealth has resulted in a reduction of malnutrition and a lowering of infant mortality rates. However, in other countries, particularly in Africa, economic policies, in concert with very adverse socio-economic and ecological conditions, appear to have sometimes aggravated malnutrition. When this outcome can be predicted, governments need to consider taking early measures to compensate for likely adverse effects, to lessen the hardships for the poor.

Promoting rural development with a special focus on sustained reduction of poverty among the rural poor can improve food security. Appropriate technologies and sometimes producer incentives to increase both production and employment in rural areas can help to reduce food insecurity and poverty. These strategies need to be imaginative and innovative, but there have been successes which give grounds for optimism. For example, credit is often a serious problem for the rural poor, but the Grameen Bank in Bangladesh has made thousands of loans to poor people, many of them female-headed households. The bank has achieved a good record of repayment and has helped lift many people out of poverty. Agricultural extension aimed at poorer farmers has moved research results from universities and research institutions into the fields of poor farmers. Attitudes in many countries have changed, so that strengthening local leadership and empowering women are on the agenda of many countries. Participation and community involvement are increasing rapidly. Non-governmental organizations (NGOs) which work well with people at the local level are absorbing external funds that previously were poorly utilized by major government or international agencies. Some of these organizations are promoting participatory projects and attempting to empower women. Successes in any of these areas can improve household food security.

Agrarian reform remains a problem, particularly in certain Latin American and Asian countries. In several countries, lack of tenancy reform, continuing bias against females and social discrimination, including caste differentials, still contribute very significantly to food insecurity. Redistribution of land is still much needed. Lower-caste families need to have full access to all services. In certain countries, such as Indonesia, the strategy of resettlement on new lands, often on less-populated islands, can reduce food insecurity.

Government and the private sector can reduce poverty by increasing employment opportunities in both rural and urban areas. They should aim to improve both the incomes of the poor and also where possible their capacity to earn income. Some governments can invest in public works, particularly labour-intensive ones, and in programmes focused on parts of the country that have high rates of poverty.

At the local level community mobilization is probably the best approach to improving household food security and nutrition. Chapter 41 includes a detailed discussion on social mobilization to improve nutrition and gives a good example, that of a project in the United Republic of Tanzania aimed to improve nutrition by improving food security (particularly for children), care, health and health services.

Chapter 36
Care and nutrition

Very young children depend for their nutrition on good care. Of course, everyone benefits from care: health, nutrition, and general well-being blossom in a caring environment. Clearly very young children, certain older people, some sick people and some physically or mentally ill people are especially dependent on care. For young children the relationship between care and nutrition is especially strong. In this chapter special attention is given to the young child and how care may influence his or her nutrition.

Infants and young children up to age three years are almost totally dependent on others for food and therefore for good nutrition. Children three to five years of age have some ability to gather food, to select a diet and to feed themselves, but in most societies children up to the age of about six years, or school age, would also be considered in need of feeding care. Thereafter, care is highly desirable but not essential for survival. However, good care will always positively influence nutritional status and well-being.

Of the three underlying causes of malnutrition, namely food, health and care (see Chapter 1), the one with the least investigated and the least understood role is care. Food security (see Chapter 2) and health (see Chapter 3) have long been known to have an important relation to nutrition, and a huge literature and extensive range of interventions focus on them. Few programmes designed to improve nutrition include a set of actions to address problems related to care.

The English word "care" is both a verb and a noun. In *The Oxford English dictionary* definitions of the verb include to feel concern or interest, to provide food, attendance, etc. for (children, invalids, etc.), to look after and to provide for, and meanings for the noun include solicitude, anxiety, serious attention, heed, caution, charge and protection. Engle (1992) provided a working definition referring to the care of young children: "Care refers to caregiving behaviours such as breast-feeding, diagnosing illnesses, determining when a child is ready for supplementary feeding, stimulating language and other cognitive capacities and providing emotional support".

In most developing countries the mother is usually the main care-giver for the infant and the very young child, but in the common extended family grandmothers, siblings, the father, other family members and people outside the family often contribute to child care. As the child gets older care may be increasingly provided outside the home, for example, in day care facilities.

Adequate care is important not only for the child's survival but also for optimal physical and mental development and good health. Care also contributes to the child's general well-being and happiness, otherwise termed a good quality of life. Care influences the child and the child influences the care.

The inadequate food, health and care which lead to malnutrition can be factors at the international, national, local and family level. Child care may be influenced by international factors such as war, blockade or global determinants that keep nations in poverty; national factors such as equity issues and availability of good health services and education; local factors such as land distribution, climate, water supplies and primary health care; and family factors such as the presence of other family members, type of housing, availability of water, household hygiene and mother's knowledge.

PROTECTION, SUPPORT AND PROMOTION OF GOOD CARING PRACTICES

Care-giving behaviours that contribute to the good nutrition, health and well-being of the child vary enormously from society to society and from culture to culture. A first assumption can be made that almost all societies value children and wish to see them grow to be healthy, intelligent and productive adults. A second assumption, which is more debatable, is that societies in general have traditional or culturally determined caring practices of which most are good and contribute well to child development, including good nutritional status.

Besides these two assumptions, it is submitted that in Africa as well as in most of Asia and Latin America, problems with good child care in the 1990s may be related more to an erosion of traditional caring practices than to the fact that important caring practices in the society were, or are, wrong or inappropriate, or important contributors to malnutrition. (There are exceptions; for example, a traditional caring practice that has been an important contributor to malnutrition is the favouring, in terms of diet, health and care, of male over female children in some areas of South Asia.) Traditional caring practices in their broadest terms have been altered, often for the worse, as a result of modernization, westernization and increasing urbanization (see Chapter 5). A good example, and the one most written about (see Chapter 7), is the decline of breast-feeding, which was a good traditional

practice almost everywhere. Its decline has in large part been influenced by modernization, including promotion by infant formula manufacturers and the medical practices of Western-oriented health professionals.

Protection of good practices

Protecting is an essential part of any strategy for optimal care to ensure good nutritional status. Good practices need to be protected from erosion by many different factors. For example, in a society where most mothers breastfeed their babies for 18 months or longer (Photo 70), with no or few other foods introduced until the child is four to six months of age, protection should take priority over support and promotion of breastfeeding. Similarly, protection is warranted if a society traditionally provides a lot of stimulation for children; if the infant is seldom left alone but is carried on the mother's back (Photo 71); if fathers, grandmothers, older siblings and other relatives frequently help in child care (Photo 72); and if traditional weaning foods of groundnuts, green leafy vegetables and legumes with a local cereal gruel are the norm. These practices may be threatened by modern or Western influences. A new television set in the family may result in adults neglecting to stimulate their children; advertising and promotion of expensive manufactured weaning foods may lead families to poorer diets at higher cost; or work away from home may cause long separations of the mother and her infant.

Support

Support is particularly appropriate when mothers' or families' good traditional caring practices are threatened or being eroded because of changes in society, which may result from modernization, westernization or urbanization. Support includes activities, both formal and informal, that may help women in changing circumstances to follow those good caring practices that were once considered normal and are now threatened. Support may involve restoring confidence in mothers, strengthening their belief that traditional good caring practices may be better than new practices that may seem modern and up to date but are in fact inferior. For example, westernization and modernization may suggest that a modern woman does not breastfeed her baby in a public place; that canned baby foods are superior to home-prepared foods; that salt and sugar comprise a better treatment for mild diarrhoea than family soups and breast-feeding; that it is better for a child to stay at home and watch television than to go with the mother to the village market; and that eating with a fork is preferable to eating by hand after traditional hand-washing. In fact none of these "modern" practices is better for the child than the traditional alternatives.

In many developing countries paid employment for women away from home is an important factor in the erosion of traditional good caring practices. It has certainly made breastfeeding more difficult (see Chapter 7). Three months of maternity leave would help support mothers in providing initial infant care. Then, during the eight hours mothers are away from home, a crèche or day care centre at the place of work would be supportive. Support for good traditional care may include mothers' support groups or arrangements for adequate child care while the mother is away from home. Staggered working hours for different family members and a greater role for the father in child care could also help.

Promotion

Promotion is particularly important when some, many or most good traditional caring practices have been abandoned or lost. Promotion involves motivation or re-education of mothers, other family members or whole communities. It is the most difficult and the most expensive of the three strategies.

It may be important to start by identifying the most important factors that led to the decline or disappearance of good caring practices. There must be evidence that the new caring practice is less desirable and less beneficial. A lack of such knowledge will almost certainly lead to failure of a promotional campaign. Properly applied social marketing methods and techniques may be useful. Political commitment and will may be necessary. The promotion of good caring practices will often involve public education and mass media efforts.

Some of the best examples of promotion of a good traditional caring practice that had been seriously eroded concern breast-feeding where it had markedly declined and been replaced with infant formula and bottle-feeding. Promotional campaigns in Brazil in the 1970s and in Honduras in the 1980s proved successful. Other practices for which promotion might be attempted include traditional breastfeeding and family feeding for children with diarrhoea; the carrying of children on the back of the mother where this has been replaced by leaving the child at home; and the use of good home-prepared weaning foods in place of expensive, less-nutritious manufactured foods.

IDENTIFYING GOOD CARING PRACTICES

Mothers, fathers, families and communities (as well as governments and international institutions) take actions all the time that influence nutrition. These actions are in the area of food, health or care. They are based on, or arise from, everyday decisions. They may have a positive or negative influence, or they may be neutral.

The first step in making decisions that

will lead to actions to protect, support and promote good child care is to assess current caring practices that may influence nutrition. For many countries where there is fairly good knowledge about the food situation and about health status and health care, there may be very few published findings on child care, especially as it relates to nutrition. There will often be some information on breastfeeding and weaning practices, but there are usually very few data or even descriptions concerning caring practices that influence psycho-social and motor development, maternal factors such as mothers' self-esteem and mothers' beliefs and attitudes regarding child care, or household and community factors that greatly influence child care. There may be ways of obtaining such information rather quickly; this may be the first activity, and it is an important one.

A useful approach for identifying child-caring practices that seem to be desirable may be an investigation of "positive deviants" in a community. Positive deviants are young children who have good nutritional status even though they come from very poor households, have uneducated mothers, have limited access to food and health services and live in a community where most children have malnutrition. If it can be found that the mothers and families of positive deviants have a set of caring practices not usually used by other families, then it can be assumed that all or some of these caring practices are good and deserve protection, support and promotion. A comparison of negative deviants and positive deviants may also be useful.

ACTIONS IN FAVOUR OF GOOD CARE TO ENSURE GOOD NUTRITION

Actions in favour of good care can be divided into three groups: delivery of services, capacity-building and empower-ment. All three can operate at different levels in society (from national to family), and each contributes to the others.

Delivery of services in support of child care may address the most immediate causes and may sometimes be curative rather than preventive; examples include oral rehydration for diarrhoea, deworming and child feeding targeted at malnourished children. In other cases delivery of services may address problems from the top down and may be preventive to some degree; examples include immunization and organized day care centres. It should be accepted that delivery of services may not be sustainable or if sustainable may have to remain in place for a long period unless other changes prevent or permanently cure the problem in society, not just in the individual child. Oral rehydration prevents death in a child and treats dehydration, but it does not reduce prevalence or incidence of diarrhoea in society. Acknowledging the limitations of an action is just as important for its effectiveness as recognizing its successes.

The next level of action, capacity-building, is aimed to deal not with the immediate causes but more with the underlying causes of malnutrition. Consequently actions at this level are often preventive rather than curative and are likely to be more sustainable. These actions are also likely to be most successful if they work mainly from the bottom up, not from the top down. Capacity-building is seen as of very great importance for improved care in relation to nutrition and may involve protection, support and promotion. Examples include infant feeding practices that permit a smooth transition from exclusive breastfeeding to mixed feeding to exclusive feeding of home foods; child care practices that are stimulating and influence good psycho-social development; health education to provide knowledge about protection against disease; and home hygiene and sanitation to prevent diarrhoea and intestinal parasitic infections.

The third level, empowerment, crosses the boundaries of service delivery and especially of capacity-building. In general, however, actions that are empowering for mothers often address the more basic causes of child malnutrition. Empowerment for women involves ensuring that they have rights that women in many societies lack. Every woman everywhere should have the right to earn income; not to be overburdened with work; to breast-feed freely and easily; and to have reasonable access to services and resources and to capacity-building activities. Possible actions at the level of empowerment include those that improve mothers' income or control of family income; providing good access to health care for women and their children; managing water supplies to lessen the burden on women; and also many activities that reduce poverty and increase equity (including some trade and price policies). Some actions that are empowering are top-down and others are bottom-up activities.

Investigations on current good caring practices, on how they might be threatened by new influences and on how they might be protected in changing, modernizing, urbanizing societies deserve a very high priority. Support for good caring practices is undoubtedly also an important action, but it is perhaps not such a high priority for research, although some investigations will be needed.

Relatively little is known about which good caring practices that are not now the norm for particular families should be promoted or how to promote them. Where caring practices are inadequate and are causes of malnutrition, studies are needed on appropriate alternatives, how they might be promoted and their potential impact on child nutrition.

Some research has been published on intrafamily food distribution, meal frequency, energy density of foods and some other practical topics; but very little is known about some other important subjects that are related to care and that may influence nutrition. The following are some of the unanswered questions.

- How do maternal psychological characteristics and mental health influence child feeding?
- How do modernization, westernization, urbanization and mothers working away from home influence child care and nutrition?
- What is the impact of poor maternal nutrition and health on the development of the child?
- What is the importance of mothers' and other family members' strategies for allocating time for child care versus competing needs?
- What impact do factors related to exclusive or prolonged breastfeeding have on the health and nutrition of the baby?
- Which maternal and family practices help protect children from illness?
- What are the extent and causes of child anorexia, and how do mothers respond to poor appetite in different cultures?

The world's children, born and as yet unborn, depend on the finding of answers to these questions.

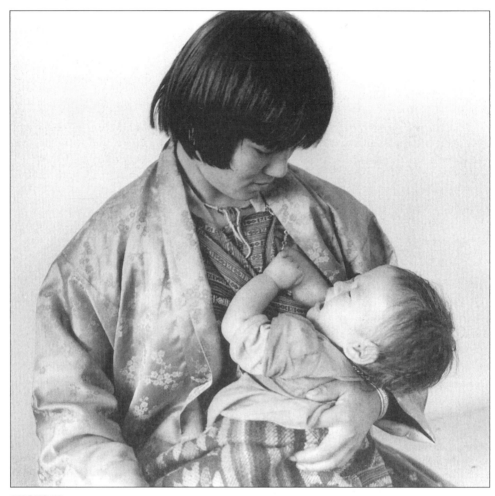

PHOTO 70
Mother breastfeeding her child in Bhutan

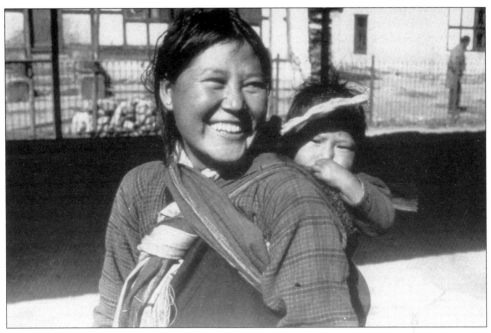

PHOTO 71
Mother in Bhutan carrying her child on the way to market

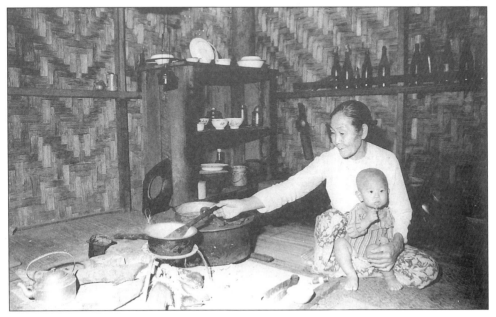

PHOTO 72
Burmese grandmother cooking while caring for her grandchild

Chapter 37
Protection and promotion of good health

The conceptual framework discussed in Chapter 1 suggests that adequate food, adequate care and adequate health are all essential to good nutritional status. The important ways in which the protection and promotion of good health can contribute to optimum child growth and development and to good nutritional status of all humans are the focus of this chapter.

Chapters 3, 12 to 24 and 34 have dealt with particular health and nutrition problems and how they may be prevented or treated as part of primary health care or in other ways. Other chapters examine food-based approaches for improving nutrition and health. Those discussions are not repeated here. Rather, this chapter highlights certain appropriate health strategies to promote good health with special reference to good nutrition. Topics include current thinking on primary health care, hospital treatment of malnutrition, nutrition rehabilitation centres, growth monitoring and promotion, immunization, oral rehydration, control of parasitic infections and acquired immunodeficiency syndrome (AIDS).

In developing countries the prevention of infections is a priority area for health workers and is very important also for nutrition. Actions to control infections include health education, hygiene, safe water, sanitation, immunizations and appropriate curative services. Disease transmission can often be reduced by behaviour change, so health education aimed at informing the public about the cause of disease and preventive measures is vital. Some of the messages may be directly related to nutrition, for example encouraging breastfeeding as a means of preventing diarrhoea, and others are directly related to food, including those regarding the many food-borne diseases which can be reduced by improved food hygiene. Food-safety programmes can help control faecal-oral disease transmission.

Although public health measures to prevent infections and other diseases deserve the highest priority, treatment needs to be easily accessible and adequate. Essential drugs, including some nutrient supplements such as ferrous sulphate and vitamin A, need to be available at health facilities.

PRIMARY HEALTH CARE
Alma-Ata – a watershed
In 1978, at Almaty, Kazakstan (then Alma-Ata, Soviet Union) the World Health Organization (WHO) and the United Nations Children's Fund (UNICEF) held the International Conference on Primary Health Care. The conference helped define primary health care (PHC), placed it firmly on the world agenda and recommended it as a central strategy for the ministries of health of most developing countries. Nutrition is recognized as a vital part of PHC.

The overall goal of PHC is the attainment of the highest possible level of health by all people. Health is defined as a state of complete physical, mental and social well-being rather than just the absence of illness or disease. PHC, which deals with the primary causes of ill health, is the first interface between people and the health care system. Programme planners stress the need for preventive measures, local initiatives and intersectoral approaches to address the social and economic factors that contribute to ill health. Participants at the Alma-Ata conference concluded that PHC should include assurance of an adequate food supply and proper nutrition for all citizens; provision of safe water supplies and training in sanitary education; support of maternal and child health programmes, including family planning and immunizations; introduction of health education; appropriate care of disease and injury; and prevention and control of endemic disease, as well as the provision of essential drugs.

Past experiences

Primary health care was widely practised in many forms throughout the world prior to the Alma-Ata conference. However, no one had named the set of practices that make up PHC, nor did world health leaders collectively recognize the importance of PHC programmes to world health and well-being. Following the colonial period, some countries were left with more effective health care systems than others. Attempts were made to institute programmes that stressed preventive care and community health workers. These programmes were similar to PHC programmes today.

A small number of African nations, notably the United Republic of Tanzania, had some success in the 1960s in diminishing the urban bias by restructuring their health services. They also stressed preventive over curative services and the use of village-based health workers in place of doctors and hospital-based medicine. Programme planners concentrated on nutrition, maternal and child health and the control of infectious diseases, all of which are now considered part of PHC. This approach to health care was described in various publications.

The Alma-Ata conference was organized

for a number of important reasons. First, during the 1960s and early 1970s, hope in the development strategies espoused by leading economists was dashed. These strategies stressed industrial development including the construction of expensive, capital-intensive infrastructure such as large factories, huge dams, electric power stations and superhighways linking the capitals to other major cities. Development based on the economists' blueprints failed more often than it succeeded, and those most in need of aid were overlooked. Huge amounts of resources were squandered on national stadiums, international airports and plush conference centres that did little to improve the quality of life of the majority of the people. Meanwhile, health, social services and agriculture-related activities languished. Health expenditures were concentrated on capital-intensive urban hospitals or "disease palaces" providing curative services, often serving mainly affluent and urban people. This model of development made the rich richer and the poor poorer. Now, however, the poor in many countries are increasingly better organized and are beginning to demand larger, more equitable shares of health and other resources. Interest in PHC has increased because it aids those most in need.

Second, many came to feel that modern technology alone was not the solution to major health problems in the developing world. At the same time, the Western medical model, the appropriateness of Western medical training for the conditions in developing countries and the ethics and intentions of some pharmaceutical companies were questioned. Gradually, people realized that social conditions were closely linked with the incidence of disease and that improvements in social and economic conditions bettered health. Improvements in agriculture and rural development began to receive more attention. China's successes in raising the health status of its population illustrated the role that socio-economic change (in this case, increased access to land and employment opportunities for the poor) could have in improving health and in allowing local communities to generate the resources needed to provide health services. Increased agricultural production was seen to be at the heart of most rural development. Health professionals began to recognize that auxiliaries and traditional medical practitioners have a critical role in maintaining health, particularly in remote rural areas. (WHO began to use the term "traditional healer" rather than "witch doctor".) Scientists learned that both traditional and modern medical practices contribute less importantly than socio-economic improvement to the prevention or cure of disease and malnutrition. PHC, with its emphasis on prevention rather than treatment coupled with the extensive use of auxiliary or paraprofessional health workers, clearly can help to implement needed changes in the medical establishment.

A third factor that led to the organization of the conference and its endorsement of PHC was an increased recognition of the importance of self-reliance at the community and family levels. For example, in Tanzania the Ujamaa approach, in which the process of empowerment of people and communities is key, became a national effort to promote self-help. The concept involves people learning about, and gaining control over, the factors that create and maintain conditions responsible for malnutrition and ill health. The "barefoot" doctors in China appeared to be a good example of a successful system of local involvement. With only limited technical training, local inhabitants improved the health of rural populations and returned control over health care to the local level.

These changes in attitudes, beliefs and health practices sprang up in socialist and capitalist countries alike, both developing and industrialized. [The WHO publication *Health by the people* (WHO, 1975b) highlights several encouraging examples of health programmes based on community participation and self-reliance.] However, more assistance from international organizations was clearly needed to spread the message around the world, to provide assistance to initiate programmes and to coordinate programme efforts among countries.

Alma-Ata declaration on primary health care

On 12 September 1978 the Declaration of Alma-Ata, the credo of primary health care, was adopted by delegates representing more than 100 countries with the objective of improving health worldwide. The declaration, setting out an ideal vision of PHC, contained a broad but rather vague array of objectives for attaining "Health for All". These objectives can be divided into two main categories: those designed to aid in restructuring health systems to promote effectiveness and equity (medical impact); and those designed to build local self-reliance through the promotion of community participation and control over health care and resources.

Objectives in the first category were mainly concerned with improving the health status of populations in as short a time as possible. Based on definable criteria, such as infant mortality rates and disease prevalence, these objectives allowed for the quantitative assessment of PHC programmes and could be used to encourage communities, health workers and political decision-makers to address health. Increased coverage of services, appropriate health technologies and new approaches towards making health systems more efficient and equitable were stressed.

The objectives concerned with self-reliance emphasize local participation by encouraging the development of human resources (social empowerment), not just technical infrastructure. Decentralization of health planning and decision-making and the growth of local institutions to provide community input are also included in these objectives.

Seven essential features of primary health care

- Perhaps most important is universal availability; this implies the redistribution of health resources from more affluent urban centres, where they are now concentrated, to the rural and urban poor. Clearly, attention to concerns of equity is essential because a reduction in poverty and the provision of basic needs often improve nutritional status and general health. In addition, special efforts must be made to reach those who are usually overlooked, such as slum dwellers, inhabitants of remote rural areas and people without transport.
- Local people should participate in the planning and implementation of any programme that directly affects them. Involvement of the entire community is likely to ensure the continuation of programme activities.
- Prevention rather than cure should be stressed. Essential to any prevention programme are nutrition education and an adequate diet. Immunizations, maternal and child health services, provision of sanitation and ensuring safe water supplies are all examples of preventive programmes.
- Coordination with programmes in other sectors, such as agriculture, economics and social services, should be an important part of any PHC agenda. Nowhere is this more important than in the area of nutrition. Although nutritional problems are health related, to prevent malnutrition it is essential to give attention to agriculture, economics, education and social services and to confront political issues such as land tenure and access to economic resources.
- The use of simple low-cost but appropriate technologies needs to be stressed. For example, simple equipment can be locally repaired and is not as expensive to maintain; generic medicines are cheaper and often preferable to brand-name products; the breast is superior to a feeding bottle; the baby is often better off in a bed than in a bassinet; and oral rehydration at home is preferable to intravenous fluids in the hospital.
- Applied research and investigation, including evaluation, monitoring and surveillance, can contribute to primary health care. Health workers can participate in much-needed research activities such as the development of growth charts for children; maintenance of disease prevalence and incidence statistics (used to pinpoint important health problems); the upkeep of immunization records (to chart successes and failures); and surveillance of disease and nutrition. All of these activities contribute to modifications and changes in the PHC system based on new knowledge or demonstrated alterations in the health or nutritional status of the population.
- If reliance on cure-oriented medical professionals is to be reduced, an essential component of any primary health care programme will be training programmes for health auxiliaries. Personnel can thus be used more efficiently, and local people will have the opportunity to participate directly in community health care.

Implementation – rhetoric versus reality

Endorsement of the PHC concept has had major implications for participating governments, committing them to:

- reallocation of health resources away from the traditional beneficiaries – the urban élite – towards a health system that benefits the majority;
- instigation of political action to address the causes of ill health outside the health sector;
- decentralization of decision-making power in health away from central authorities and the medical establishment towards communities and local health workers.

Experiences in implementing primary health care over the last 15 years showed that many governments, while adopting the rhetoric, made only slow progress in institutionalizing its concepts in practice. There is a large and growing gap between the intentions that governments express and the health care policies that they are actually willing or able to implement. Although the Declaration of Alma-Ata clearly defined PHC, its objectives, components and overall concept, in practice the principles have been applied in many different ways.

While many government officials have orally supported the concept, their implicit objectives are often in sharp conflict with those of primary health care. For those controlling many political systems, the maintenance of stability, the preservation of existing social and economic structures and relations and the monopolization of political powers are all high priorities. When primary health priorities are added they often create major contradictions, inhibiting the development of health care along the lines envisioned at Alma-Ata.

In the 18 years following the Alma-Ata conference, tremendous progress has been made in recognizing the importance of primary health care as an essential part of promoting food, nutrition and health care strategies that benefit those left out of previous development efforts. It has been very difficult, however, to institutionalize the concept of primary health care. When PHC is practised in line with the principles implicit in the Alma-Ata declaration, it is perceived as a threat by established interests such as the traditional medical profession and the urban élite.

Even countries with a substantial governmental commitment to health care, such as Thailand, find the implications of resource reallocation, community control and concern with the broad structural reasons for ill health too threatening to be accepted or tolerated. In Viet Nam, which radically restructured its health and economic systems, it has proved very difficult to overcome the urban bias, to change the attitudes of medical professionals and to sustain earlier health and nutritional improvements. Both cases demonstrate that strong political will is necessary to ensure the success of PHC, and both highlight some of the many obstacles in the way.

The numerous goals and objectives that are part of PHC often conflict, creating contradictions between programme rhetoric and programme reality, between self-reliance and equity and between the delivery of health care services and allowance for meaningful community participation. Overcoming these problems requires a balanced approach applied over a prolonged period and a recognition that different situations require different strategies and approaches.

In recent years there have been new international influences which have led to a move away from free health services in developing countries, including the structural adjustment programmes of the International Monetary Fund, UNICEF's Bamako Initiative and a move in many countries to capitalist, free-market economic systems. Hospital fees and payment for medicines are now common. However, by contrast, health is now regarded less as a welfare service and more as a development priority. The World Bank has now indicated a very significant attempt to increase assistance to countries for improvement of health services and public health. The next decade could see preventive medicine, with nutrition at its heart, move forward both as part of PHC but also in new programmes designed to deal with specific health and nutritional problems. Health for the poor will benefit if PHC programmes strongly directed from the centre (usually the ministry of health in the capital) are devolved to the local level. Then the local health establishment needs to involve communities in planning and implementing their own health actions.

MEDICAL TREATMENT OF MALNUTRITION

The ultimate objective of most comprehensive nutrition programmes should be to reach a stage where no children require treatment for malnutrition in hospitals, in other centres or as out-patients. No country has reached that goal, so treatment must remain a part of control. Treatment of malnutrition can be viewed as taking place at three levels: first, hospital treatment for severe and life-threatening malnutrition; second, nutritional rehabilitation or similar treatment for moderate malnutrition or after severe cases are discharged from hospital; and third, preventive care and treatment of mild malnutrition in maternal and child health and nutrition clinics or growth monitoring centres. At each level, prevention should be a component of the services offered. Not all countries have an organized system for providing all three levels of treatment.

Hospital treatment

It is generally agreed that admission to hospital is necessary for cases such as: a severely ill child whose life is in danger because of kwashiorkor or marasmus; a pyrexial toddler with a cornea near to perforation as a result of xerophthalmia; or an infant almost moribund from dehydration.

Some nutritionists have painted a bleak picture of hospitalization and its results. They suggest that hospitals may contribute more to mortality than to cure of malnutrition. In many countries high case fatality rates occur in children hospitalized for severe protein-energy malnutrition (PEM). The length of the hospital stay is often long, and discharged patients frequently die at home in the weeks following discharge or return with a relapse of their condition. Data do show that these problems are real. There has been no controlled study in which cases of severe malnutrition were randomly assigned to hospital or out-patient treatment. Nevertheless, poor results should not lead to a universal condemnation of hospital treatment for the very sick child. Rather, the criticisms should be used by paediatricians, doctors and nurses to determine what can be done to improve conditions and to reduce case fatality rates. There are too many paediatric wards where existing conditions offer little hope for the severely malnourished child. Rare is the hospital that provides the ideal treatment and environment for care and future prevention.

Case fatality rates for malnutrition vary greatly from hospital to hospital. The rates reflect not only the quality of the health care but also the severity of the cases admitted. Some parents only bring their children to hospital when they are almost moribund. Sometimes there is so much demand for hospital beds and such a heavy out-patient load that only extreme cases can be admitted to the wards. Hospitals with equally good staff and treatment regimes can have different fatality rates if one of them admits moderate cases of PEM and the other admits only very severe cases.

Many hospitals report case fatality rates from severe PEM of around 25 percent, although rates are sometimes as high as 40 percent and sometimes as low as 10 percent. In most hospitals, the majority of deaths from PEM occur within 48 or 72 hours of admission. Attention needs to be given to controlling hypothermia, recognizing hypoglycaemia and treating infections (see Chapter 12). Staff at all levels need to be well trained in the practical management of cases. Good nursing care is essential, but a large part of this, especially feeding, can be provided by well-trained auxiliaries.

During the recovery phase the treatment of the child needs to include an educational component. The mother, or a responsible guardian, should be admitted to hospital with the child and participate in the treatment, especially regarding the dietary measures. As recovery progresses the child is fed solid or semi-solid foods; these should be locally available, cheap and acceptable. Few paediatric wards have the design, staff or policy to provide nutrition and health education for patients or parents, yet it is an integral part of therapy which may prevent relapse in PEM, xerophthalmia, nutritional anaemias and many other forms of malnutrition. Where possible, learning by doing should be a part of the instruction.

Every attempt should be made to minimize the length of the child's stay in hospital. A shorter stay will reduce the cost of treatment that has to be borne by the State or the family and the time that the mother, entering hospital with the child, has to spend away from home, where other child health problems may exist or may be aggravated by her absence. Many hospitals keep malnourished children for months rather than weeks, increasing the risk of cross-infection. It is appreciated that recovery from marasmus is often very slow, usually much slower than recovery from kwashiorkor. Even so, it is seldom essential for children to stay in hospital longer than a few weeks.

Perhaps the main reason for the slow recovery of hospitalized children is a failure to provide an adequate total intake of energy. Children can benefit from very high intakes of energy and to a lesser extent protein until they reach near-normal weight for length. A reliable staff is essential to ensure that feeding is properly carried out at regular intervals.

Many relapses will be prevented and physicians will be more willing to consider early discharge if good follow-up services are available. Hospital staff should try to provide clinics at the hospital or in the community where food supplements are supplied free (or highly subsidized) for the child and sometimes for the whole family, and a system of home-visiting using auxiliary workers with suitable training.

Nutrition rehabilitation centres

In the 1960s and 1970s nutrition rehabilitation centres (NRCs) were widely promoted as a major answer to the problem of PEM in developing countries. This approach was unrealistic. Now such centres exist in many countries, but they play a rather small part in overall nutrition services worldwide. Each country needs to decide if such centres are of value or if some alternative measures can be used to rehabilitate moderately malnourished children before hospitalization is necessary and after serious cases are discharged from hospital.

NRCs when first established were described as centres organized either to have sleeping accommodation where children could be kept overnight or to resemble day nurseries or kindergartens where malnourished children could attend for a few hours each day, with the objective of educating the mothers through the nutritional rehabilitation of their children. The centres, established mainly in the 1970s in countries in Asia, Africa and Latin America and the Caribbean, differ quite markedly in their manner of functioning, but most of them have a common thread of objectives.

An NRC differs from a day care centre in several important respects:

- the selection of children attending the centre is based mainly on nutritional criteria, whereas children are selected for day care centres based on social, educational, economic or other criteria;
- the duration of attendance is usually based on the time necessary to rehabilitate the child and is therefore limited;
- nutrition education of the mother is an important feature of the centre.

The NRC provides the second level of treatment: the most severely malnourished are at first admitted to hospital, and the less malnourished attend health clinics. The NRC takes severely malnourished children after discharge from hospital during the important period of recuperation; moderately malnourished cases from the community; and less severely malnourished cases that are failing to make adequate progress following treatment as out-patients or at clinics. In this graded system of treatment, children discharged from an NRC continue to attend an out-patient facility or clinic. In certain cases such a service is provided at the NRC.

The NRC has always been envisaged as providing important nutrition education. It should also be economical to run and should provide services at a fraction of the cost of hospitalization. It is suggested that a centre should be an ordinary village or urban house, staffed with one or two village women who have received some practical training in nutrition and child

feeding. A typical centre can accommodate about 30 children, who receive three or more good meals a day and attend five or six days a week for eight to ten hours a day for three to five months. Mothers of children attending the centre may be required to provide one day a week of work to assist with the running of the centre. The participation of the mothers not only can reduce the number of staff needed but can also provide them with an active learning experience. The opportunity can be used to teach improved child feeding practices using local foods and other aspects of health and hygiene.

An NRC can play an important part in improving nutrition. However, the average centre taking 30 children for three months will provide services for only about 120 children per year. Very few countries can provide enough centres for all children with moderate malnutrition. If NRCs are to have a real impact on nutritional problems in a country, they must offer effective nutrition education and function also as demonstration and teaching centres.

Child health clinics

Child health clinics have been in existence in various countries for many years, and some have had an important role in reducing the incidence of certain deficiency diseases. In industrialized countries rickets was highly prevalent and was a major cause of child mortality a few decades ago. The establishment of clinics where cod-liver oil was dispensed and where attention to child health was provided was one of several factors responsible for its control.

Healthy children, whether from wealthy or poor families, benefit from regular visits to child health clinics. In many industrialized countries well-baby clinics provide this valuable service. For poor families and in developing countries generally, there may be no great advantage in separating attendance of well babies from that of sick babies.

Health clinics are meant to draw together the curative and preventive components of child health care. However, they also have the advantage of separating these important activities from the often over-loaded out-patient services of many hospitals.

There is no universal rule to indicate what services a clinic should provide, but if at all possible, it should be linked with some more sophisticated health unit, often a hospital. The relationship might be close, as for example when a clinic is run as part of a general or children's hospital; or it may be remote, involving simply occasional supervision from a hospital in the region or district. If the link is remote, a well-organized referral system and a means of transporting patients to hospital should be features of the clinic. The professional staff in charge of child health clinics ranges from well-trained paediatricians to auxiliaries with some special training in child health and nutrition.

Much has been written about the means of communicating nutrition and health facts to those with little education. Important aspects of nutrition teaching by clinic staff would be to stress the value of breastfeeding, to emphasize the control of family size and spacing of children, and to pay attention to nutritional and health problems specific to the particular area. In areas where childhood diarrhoea is an important cause of morbidity, attention needs to be given both to preventive measures and to simple treatment with home fluids or oral rehydration therapy.

Child health clinics, often called "under-five clinics" in developing countries, should provide curative services at least for minor illnesses. Preventive medicine provided at the clinics should include at least two major components: immunizations and nutrition services.

Immunizations should be available, preferably free, and parents should be encouraged to use this service for their children. In most countries the young child would receive triple antigen against diphtheria, pertussis (whooping cough) and tetanus (DPT vaccine), BCG vaccine against tuberculosis, oral vaccine against poliomyelitis and live attenuated virus vaccine against measles. In certain areas vaccination against other diseases such as cholera may be warranted. (Vaccination against smallpox is not now necessary, because smallpox has been totally eradicated worldwide.) Some clinics may provide prophylaxis against malaria.

Nutrition services are basically of two kinds: making available nutritional supplements for malnourished children, and providing attention to growth and development of the child.

Supplements are designed to complement and add to the foods available at home for young malnourished children from poor families. The most widely used supplements have been protein-rich foods. It has been realized that growth deficits in children do not often result purely from protein deficiency and that mild or moderate malnutrition is almost always caused by poor total food intake and energy deficiency. Therefore, a supplement that provides a concentrated source of energy balanced with other nutrients including protein is most frequently needed.

In addition to food supplements, clinics may make available certain nutrient supplements. In areas of the world where xerophthalmia is endemic, children may be given a dose of vitamin A every four months. The vitamin A is usually provided in capsules each containing 200 000 IU (60 000 RE) of retinyl palmitate with 20 IU vitamin E added. If the child is unable to swallow the capsule, the end may be snipped off with scissors and the tasteless contents squeezed on to the tongue. In some areas specific vitamins or minerals may be given, such as iodine to prevent iodine deficiency disorders or iron to prevent iron deficiency anaemia.

The second and perhaps more important nutrition activity of health clinics is specific attention to good growth and healthy development. The promotion of good physical growth and optimum psychological development is of the greatest importance and should not be confined to clinics. It is mainly the responsibility of parents, families and communities.

GROWTH MONITORING AND PROMOTION

Many different strategies, programmes and actions are undertaken by international agencies, national governments, individual families and others to promote good growth and development. However, there is one strategy above others that both in name and in stated objectives focuses specifically on the growth of children. This is growth monitoring and promotion (GMP).

In the 1980s, the use of the Morley growth chart (see below), used mainly at under-five clinics, began to be promoted in many developing countries as growth monitoring (GM). GM was the first of UNICEF's GOBI (growth monitoring, oral rehydration, breastfeeding and immunization) strategy to improve child health worldwide. Because growth monitoring itself does not improve growth, GM is now usually referred to as growth monitoring and promotion.

GMP should, where possible, be closely integrated into primary health care activities; it should not usually be a separate programme. It should focus on maintaining good growth in infants and children and not, as is often the case, be used mainly for rehabilitating children whose growth is poor. If growth monitoring of all children is to be the aim, it is essential that

infants enter the programme soon after birth, because infants up to five months of age who are breastfed generally have satisfactory growth.

The GMP strategy has become controversial, with strong proponents and opponents. The many other actions taken to support or promote growth and development, although very widely practised, are not as visibly advocated as strategies for growth monitoring. Because of this, growth monitoring is deserving of attention, but not at the expense of limiting consideration of other actions that foster good child growth and development. It is also necessary to recognize that good growth is often related to other aspects of good child development and that those situations, environments and actions that promote good child development usually also help promote optimum physical growth. The two are intertwined. However, because physical growth is relatively easy to measure, much more reliance is placed on physical growth than on other aspects of child development as a gauge of childhood well-being.

Growth charts

In the 1960s under-five clinics became widely used around the world to promote good growth, nutrition and health in children. The growth chart became the centre-piece of these activities. In the 1980s this concept was further developed, and UNICEF and many countries promoted growth monitoring using growth charts. This was seen as a major action to reduce malnutrition and also to rehabilitate malnourished children.

On each visit to a GMP centre, every child should be weighed and measured. Accurate balance scales and good simple equipment for measuring length or height are essential. Recording the weight (and height) of children may serve three important purposes. It may help to detect children at high risk of developing PEM; it may be an important tool in assessing the effects of treatment; and most importantly, it can be used to follow the growth of the individual child.

Maintaining an adequate rate of growth has replaced prevention of malnutrition as the goal towards which clinics should direct their work. Experience has shown that the clinical syndromes of kwashiorkor and marasmus are usually preceded by months, and sometimes years, of failure to gain weight. The common exception is when a child develops kwashiorkor suddenly after an illness such as measles, whooping cough or diarrhoea. It is also now known that children with mild or moderate PEM have much higher mortality rates than do well-grown children.

Maintaining an adequate rate of growth has become a positive objective for both the clinic staff and the mothers who attend. A child who has failed to gain weight for several months is given special attention. In clinics the mother may be provided with a temporary supply of a food supplement and with instruction on improving the child's diet. The nurse or assistant uses the trend in the weight curve to assess the effectiveness of food supplements and of education in nutrition. When failure to gain weight is persistent, the child is referred to a physician or to the next level of health care.

Many countries use the growth chart developed by Morley in Nigeria (Figure 18). It has several unusual features in its design and use which help to make it more acceptable than previous charts. These include a calendar to record the child's age and a graphic and easily understood record of the child's recent and past medical history and state of nutrition and of the inoculations received. The fact that the mother, rather than the clinic, keeps the chart and that home visits are made to evaluate the work of the clinic stimulates interest. The appearance on the chart of certain factors that indicate whether the child is in a high-risk category and the indication of channels of growth that are based on weight standards are extremely useful.

The advantages of the calendar over many other methods of age charting are several. Formerly the most common charts in use around the world recorded the age of the child in months. After one year of age this becomes increasingly difficult; the necessity of a calculation at each visit led to errors and was a deterrent to graphing weight, especially in a busy clinic. On Morley's chart a simple calendar is constructed when the child is first seen. Against the growth curve, entries are made of important incidents such as cessation of breastfeeding, birth of a sibling or major diseases. With this chart, the worker can absorb the important facts of a child's medical history in a matter of seconds.

The chart should be colourful and durable and supplied to the mother in a tough open-ended plastic envelope. It is considered to be her property and not that of the clinic. Experience in several centres has shown that few charts get lost, probably fewer than the number of records mislaid in the average small hospital's card filing system.

The chart has an upper line representing a satisfactory weight for a healthy, well-fed child at each age. A lower line indicates the tenth centile or some other arbitrary standard which the child's growth should exceed. The standard is probably relatively unimportant. Of more significance than the position of the child's weight curve in relation to the standards is the relation of each weighing to the previous weighings of that particular child. The important point for the health worker to watch is whether the weight of the child is following a path that goes approximately parallel to the channel and steadily upward.

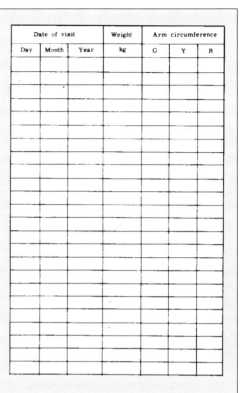

Date of visit			Weight	Arm circumference		
Day	Month	Year	kg	G	Y	R

FIGURE 18
A simple growth chart

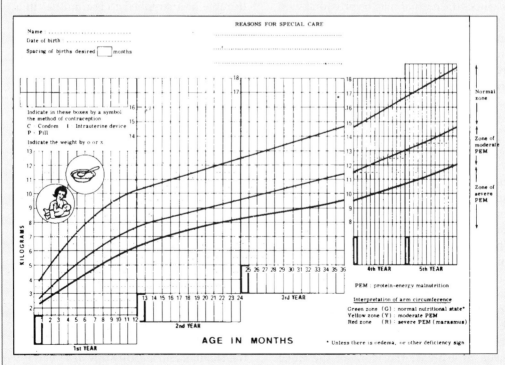

Name : ....

Date of birth : ....

Spacing of births desired ☐ months

REASONS FOR SPECIAL CARE

Indicate in these boxes by a symbol
the method of contraception
C · Condom   I · Intrauterine device
P · Pill

Indicate the weight by o or x

AGE IN MONTHS

1st YEAR   2nd YEAR   3rd YEAR   4th YEAR   5th YEAR

Normal zone
Zone of moderate PEM
Zone of severe PEM

PEM : protein-energy malnutrition

Interpretation of arm circumference

Green zone (G) : normal nutritional state*
Yellow zone (Y) : moderate PEM
Red zone (R) : severe PEM (marasmus)

* Unless there is oedema, or other deficiency sign

A positive approach

GMP is viewed as a strategy to empower mothers to maintain good nutritional status in their children and to prevent growth retardation. It is a preventive, not a curative, strategy; it is designed mainly to promote good growth and health, not to deal with malnutrition and ill health. Workers should obtain information on how mothers and families are managing to achieve good growth rather than mainly finding the reasons for growth failure. Praise and reinforcement should be an important feature of the programme.

Although the major emphasis is on maintenance of good growth, which can be viewed as a pre-emptive strategy, the programme should include a strategy for dealing with those few cases where the programme has failed and where children are not doing well and need special attention. This will usually involve some special advice from health workers regarding behavioural change aimed to achieve rehabilitation, and in some cases treatment or referral will be necessary. In some programmes the strategy may include dietary supplements.

In GMP programmes, much of the action should consist of positive reinforcement rather than corrective action. As a diagnostic exercise, GMP should serve as much to find out what mothers are doing right as what is going wrong. It is also used to detect early growth faltering, to find the likely reasons for it and to suggest to mothers corrective actions that are realistic and that they might try. GMP is likely to be relatively unsuccessful if used mainly to try to correct the growth of older children who are moderately or severely stunted, especially if these children are not wasted.

In all cases, meaningful involvement of mothers and families should be the heart of a GMP programme. It is a participatory exercise. It involves dialogue and discussion, not lecturing and scolding, and mothers should help in decision-making, for example, about the location, hours and organization of growth monitoring sessions. Mothers also need to be consulted about such matters as the need for privacy and confidentiality and whether it is appropriate in their culture to weigh children nude or clothed.

This is a view of the concepts of what good GMP should be, rather than what it usually is in practice in countries in Africa, Asia and Latin America. Growth monitoring continues to be practised in ways that ignore these principles. Too often growth monitoring is used mainly as a weighing and charting exercise and advice is given only to mothers whose children are doing badly. Often the mothers are scolded publicly, and advice is frequently impractical and does not recognize what would be useful to them. Inadequate time is devoted to dialogue, advice and education. In some parts of the world, GMP is regarded by health workers mainly as a tool for diagnosis of malnutrition. In other places, it is used to select children to receive free or subsidized weaning foods. Feeding can be a component of a GMP programme, but the full potential benefits will not be realized without the level of communication, dialogue and empowerment of mothers and communities described above.

At worst, growth monitoring consists of the routine exercise of weighing and charting with no advice given and with no use made of the chart, often because of lack of time or because of lack of training or knowledge regarding the proper use of other needed interventions. Where this is the case GMP is useless and wasteful of resources, including the mothers' time. In some societies, cultural prejudices against weighing of young children may be a reason for not introducing GMP or at least for sensitive efforts to overcome this difficulty.

Improving GMP

In a properly run GMP programme, most infants should be enrolled as soon after birth as possible. Children seen for the first time in their second or third year of life often will already have evidence of growth failure, and at this stage GMP can do relatively little to improve the situation, especially in stunted older children. When breastmilk is adequate and breastfeeding is the normal feeding practice, infants under four months of age usually show good growth. The first four months are therefore the most valuable period to establish dialogue and to provide positive reinforcement. This becomes most useful in the months ahead, during the nutritional danger period, which is usually between four and 18 months of age. The mother should be encouraged to tell the health

worker about how long she expects to breastfeed, when she intends to introduce other foods, whether she wants to get the infant immunized and how she will deal with illnesses such as diarrhoea and respiratory infections. The worker at the GMP session should then cautiously advise the mother and discuss with her a strategy for maintaining good growth and health in her infant during the danger period, rather than concentrating on the rehabilitation or cure of malnutrition.

If dialogue is to be the heart of the programme, it is important that the health worker have a good understanding of existing child raising practices and the cultural, social and dietary environment of the community. Otherwise the messages may not be relevant, practical or feasible to implement and may not even be credible to the mothers. The health worker must also have a minimum of knowledge about the factors most likely to lead to growth faltering. For example, he or she should understand that after about six months of age breastfeeding alone often provides inadequate nutrition and needs to be supplemented; that too much supplementation may reduce suckling and lead to insufficient milk; that certain foods are bulky and have low energy density, but that there are ways to increase energy density; that as breastfeeding becomes less important, frequent feeding with other foods is important while breastfeeding should continue as long as possible; that infections in themselves may lead to growth faltering, but that starvation as a treatment for diarrhoea and other infections contribute to this; and that breastmilk and other foods should be provided during most illnesses.

To discuss these issues properly, the health worker needs to have enough time with each mother, adequate training and understanding of health and nutrition beyond charting. The right temperament and attitude are perhaps the most important qualities.

An operational rule might be that health workers must be given at least five to 15 minutes to talk to each mother and must be equipped with certain basic knowledge and reasonable communication skills. It is important that they know how to listen to the mother and how to elicit information from her, as well as how to provide positive feedback, encouragement and appropriate advice. Many of the skills can be imparted in training, but obviously some individuals are better listeners and communicators than others.

Another operational rule that follows is that GMP be integrated into PHC. Many of the messages and advice suggested are an integral part of PHC. In general, mothers should not have to attend separate sessions on different days for treatment of common infections, to have their children immunized, to receive vitamin A or anthelmintics, to get advice about oral rehydration, to have a prenatal examination or to obtain family planning advice. In fact, it should be the duty of the GMP staff to ensure that all children attending have been immunized against the six diseases covered in the WHO Expanded Programme on Immunization (see below), that mothers know how to prevent dehydration caused by diarrhoea, etc. GMP can be a part of PHC or it can encompass PHC activities. GMP can serve as an activity that brings the child into contact with the health services at frequent intervals. GMP can act as a catalyst in the strengthening of PHC activities. It is also much easier to carry out GMP as part of a well-functioning PHC system. Therefore, efforts to strengthen and improve PHC will also improve the feasibility of well-run GMP.

A good principle is that advice, nutrition and health education should be rather specific and aimed at the particular circumstances of each mother and child.

The dialogue should give the mother the feeling that she herself is developing a realistic, achievable strategy to maintain the good growth and health of her child, and in this way she will see the benefits of the time that she has invested in the exercise. The content of the messages should be simple and must take account of the child in a family situation.

Finally, GMP should be conducted as near as possible to people's homes; at a time convenient to parents; in small enough groups to allow adequate individualized dialogue and short waiting periods; and in a way designed mainly to suit parents, not health workers. For example, in an urban setting where mothers work away from home, the sessions could be on a Sunday and the health workers could have Monday off. Unless some means are provided for combining GMP with simple therapy and other preventive services (for example, deworming, administration of vitamin A, provision of antimalarial drugs and possibly also simple treatment of common illnesses), attendance may be poor. In all cases, rural GMP activities based in a small village must be linked with and have backup from a health centre, dispensary or clinic.

Some physicians have stated that food supplements should not be provided at GMP sessions even for a child who is faltering, because supplements may have negative consequences for the programme. This view is not shared by all those involved in GMP. In the much-heralded Tamil Nadu Integrated Nutrition Project funded by the World Bank in India, free food supplements are provided to the most needy children, with the targeting based largely on the weight charts.

Under some circumstances GMP may be conducted not at a health centre, but by visits to people's homes. Home-based GMP is often popular with mothers, and it results in wider coverage, especially of the most neglected families; however, it is usually more expensive, because field workers can cover fewer children per day.

Although growth monitoring is simple in concept and is a relatively low-cost technology for helping to reduce the extent of malnutrition, it is very seldom done well. It requires good organization, adequate resources, an appropriate existing infrastructure and careful training and proper supervision of workers. In some locations cultural barriers may have to be overcome.

The success or failure of GMP depends on how the information and the chart are used. The weighing and plotting have to result in action, generally on the part of the child's mother (or parents or guardian) or the health worker, if there is to be a benefit. GMP is one among several means of attempting to achieve the desired goal of healthy growth. Are there other easier, cheaper and more feasible ways to promote good health and development in poor societies? This question should only be answered at the local level or by national ministries of health.

IMMUNIZATION

Immunization is not a direct nutrition intervention; therefore it is not discussed in detail here, nor are recommendations given for how immunizations should be provided. However, because childhood infectious diseases contribute importantly to malnutrition, immunization needs to go hand in hand with more direct nutrition interventions. In fact it would be negligent for a nutritionist or for any organizer of a set of nutrition interventions to fail to make certain that children have been immunized.

Measles, tetanus and whooping cough (diseases for which vaccines have existed for many years) kill close to 3 million children worldwide each year and result

in compromised nutritional status for many of those who survive. Despite these figures, it is encouraging that many countries, some of them very poor, have immunized as many as 80 percent of their children.

Measles remains the biggest killer among the diseases that can be prevented by immunization, and it is also the most closely related to malnutrition. Measles is particularly lethal for children who have vitamin A deficiency and serious PEM. It is also clear that provision of medicinal vitamin A to malnourished children with measles will lower case fatality rates.

In developing countries the main immunizations recommended and given are those to prevent diphtheria, pertussis (whooping cough) and tetanus (DPT),

---

Immunization timetable of the WHO Expanded Programme on Immunization

For immunizations in maternal and child health clinics the EPI schedule is as follows:
- BCG: as soon after birth as possible, up to 12 years;
- DPT and oral polio vaccine: at two, three and four months (with the possibility of starting at one month if one of the diseases, e.g. whooping cough, is highly endemic);
- measles: at six to nine months of age;
- tetanus toxoid: two doses one month apart in the last trimester of pregnancy, and one booster dose in subsequent pregnancies.

In mass campaigns, and to all children presenting after six months of age, immunizations should be given as follows:
- first contact: measles, DPT, polio;
- second contact, one month later: DPT, polio;
- third contact, one month later: DPT, polio, BCG;
- tetanus toxoid to pregnant women during the last trimester of pregnancy.

measles, poliomyelitis and tuberculosis (BCG). The immunization schedule recommended by the WHO Expanded Programme on Immunization (EPI) is provided in the accompanying box.

There are, of course, many other diseases for which there are immunizations. These are discussed in textbooks dealing with infectious diseases.

ORAL FLUIDS FOR DIARRHOEA

Diarrhoea, which can have many causes (viruses, bacteria, parasites, toxins and others), is a major public health problem in almost all developing countries (see Chapter 3). It usually contributes very substantially both to morbidity and mortality. The control of diarrhoea deserves high priority (Photos 73 and 74). The interaction between diarrhoea and malnutrition is well known.

Oral rehydration therapy (ORT) has for 20 years been strongly advocated and promoted by WHO and UNICEF and has also been a strategy at the national level. Diarrhoeal disease causes death, particularly in children, because of dehydration (Photo 75). Frequent liquid stools, sometimes combined with vomiting, lead to severe loss of water and electrolytes.

Until 20 years ago, the main life-saving medical measure in the treatment of severe dehydration was to provide intravenous (IV) fluids, often containing electrolytes, and glucose to provide energy. It was then found in studies, particularly in cholera patients with very profuse watery diarrhoea, that providing a glucose electrolyte solution by mouth will often rehydrate the patient just as well as IV fluids. In 1978 an editorial in the prestigious medical journal *Lancet* stated that "the discovery that sodium transport and glucose transport are coupled in the small intestine, so that glucose accelerates absorption of solutes and water, was potentially the most important medical advance in this century".

Oral rehydration packets are now widely available and extensively used. WHO recommends that these contain:
- 3.5 g sodium chloride,
- 2.5 g sodium bicarbonate,
- 1.5 g potassium chloride,
- 20 g glucose.

A packet should be added to one litre of boiled water.

There is no doubt that in hospitals the use of ORT in place of intravenous treatment for the dehydrated patient has been a major scientific and medical advance. Under medical supervision it can also work well in an out-patient setting for the dehydrated child or adult, provided good instructions are given and followed.

In recent years it has been shown that infants and young children with diarrhoea should continue to be breastfed as much and as frequently as possible. Thinking has also changed in terms of feeding during diarrhoea. Doctors often used to advocate "resting the intestine" during diarrhoea. Now experts agree that this is wrong and that both food and drinks should be provided. More recent research has shown that ordinary sugar (sucrose) and starch, which is the carbohydrate in cereal grains and root crops, also enhance fluid and solute absorption. For this reason cereal-based solutions and traditional rehydration mixtures are gaining acceptance.

It is now evident, however, that in many societies ordinary food and fluid are provided to children and others with diarrhoea. This should be encouraged, not discouraged. In such situations there is no need to promote the use of ORS packets for the home management of diarrhoea.

The aggressive promotion of ORS in packets as a treatment for diarrhoea needs re-evaluation. ORS was developed for treatment of dehydration in the hospital, and it works well there; but it is being promoted for the treatment of diarrhoea in the home, where it may be unnecessary and where alternatives are often available (see Figure 19). Breastfeeding, home fluids and local foods if given early in diarrhoea may prevent dehydration.

It should also be remembered that ORT does nothing to prevent diarrhoea. It is curative medicine to prevent diarrhoea deaths. To reduce diarrhoea requires improved sanitation; safe water supplies; good personal, environmental and food hygiene; health education; and improved standards of living for the poor.

DEWORMING AND CONTROL OF INTESTINAL PARASITIC INFECTIONS

At this moment over 2 000 million persons worldwide carry a burden of worms. High prevalence of infection occurs mainly in the non-industrialized countries, particularly in the tropics and subtropics. *Ascaris lumbricoides*, the large roundworm, is the most prevalent and is estimated to infect 1 200 million individuals – about one-fifth of the world's population. The two main forms of human hookworm, *Necator americanus* and *Ancylostoma duodenale*, infect approximately 800 million people. Ascariasis and hookworm disease have received much less attention than they deserve from doctors, public health officials and international agencies. These parasites and others such as the whipworm (*Trichuris trichiura*) and flukes of the genus *Schistosoma* have a negative impact on nutritional status and on child development. The control or alleviation of these and other common helminthic infections deserves a high priority because it would benefit millions of people and it is feasible and relatively cheap. Programmes to reduce the prevalence and especially the intensity of infections would be economical and would positively influence development.

There is now very strong evidence to show that ascariasis, especially when

FIGURE 19
Home management of diarrhoea

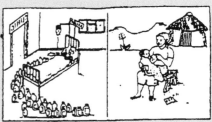

ORT was developed as an alternative to IV fluids in clinical settings for treatment of dehydration.

It was then presumed to be equally effective in community settings for treatment and prevention of dehydration.

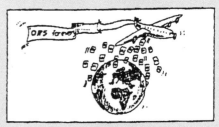

Ideally every household would have a few packets of glucose electrolyte powder.

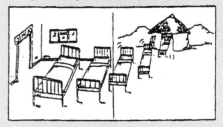

However, the community is not an extension of the clinic.

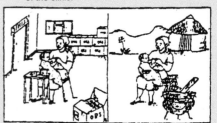

In clinical settings, ORS is as effective as IV fluids for treatment of dehydration.

In community settings, home-based fluids and foods are probably more effective than ORS for prevention of dehydration.

worm burdens are high, retards the normal growth of children and contributes to malnutrition. Several well-conducted studies have shown that children treated for *Ascaris lumbricoides* infections grow better after deworming than do untreated children. There is some evidence also that ascariasis is associated with poorer fat and lactose digestion and with reduced absorption of vitamin A and some other micronutrients. Heavy burdens of worms contribute to PEM and other deficiency diseases (Photos 76 and 77).

Hookworm constitutes the most important of the human helminthic infections mainly because the parasite is an important cause of iron deficiency anaemia, a condition that has a high prevalence worldwide. It is extremely prevalent and often results in marked debilitation of the host. Iron deficiency anaemia is one of the world's leading nutritional deficiency diseases.

Both roundworm and hookworm may contribute to poor appetite, decreased food intake, intestinal abnormalities and poor absorption or increased loss of nutrients, which may result in PEM, anaemia or other deficiency states. Trichuriasis infections can cause diarrhoea and debilitation. These conditions may in turn lead to decreased energy, low physical fitness and decreased work output in adults and poor school performance in children. The decreased productivity may in turn lead to a reduced ability to grow or procure food. Infections aggravate poverty and malnutrition, and poverty and malnutrition worsen infections. This vicious cycle may adversely affect the development of whole communities (Figure 20). There is now more appreciation of the economic costs of these infections.

Control programmes that involve either reducing the prevalence of parasitic infection or deworming those infected will have an impact on the nutrition of whole communities where prevalence rates are high and large worm burdens are common.

In many parts of the world people often harbour several intestinal parasites at the same time. Polyparasitism is very common. In over 1 000 primary school children examined in seven schools in Kenya, 96 percent had hookworm, 95 percent had *T. trichiura* and 50 percent had *Ascaris lumbricoides* eggs in stool specimens examined. Half of these children had mild or moderate PEM, and about 40 percent had anaemia with a haemoglobin level below 120 g per litre.

In the long term, control of ascariasis, trichuriasis, schistosomiasis and hookworm disease will require measures to reduce simultaneously other infections spread by faecal contamination. Improvements in sanitation, water supplies, housing, personal and environmental hygiene and levels of living are needed, together with improvements in people's knowledge of disease transmission and prevention. Latrine construction has been on the agenda of health ministries in Africa, Asia and Latin America for over 50 years. However, in many countries the prevalence (and sometimes also the intensity) of helminthic infections remains as high as ever. With huge continuing population increases, the numbers of persons infected rise.

In the past 50 years there have also been major advances in the drug treatment of these conditions. Whereas in the 1950s it was necessary to use toxic medicines such as tetrachloroethylene for hookworm and antimony for schistosomiasis, there are now safe oral drugs such as albendazole and praziquantel. For intestinal helminthic infections, the new drugs mean that regular treatment is now feasible, safe and often highly effective. Large-scale deworming is a strategy whose time has come. It is not only a treatment measure benefiting

FIGURE 20
Worm infection, malnutrition and lack of development

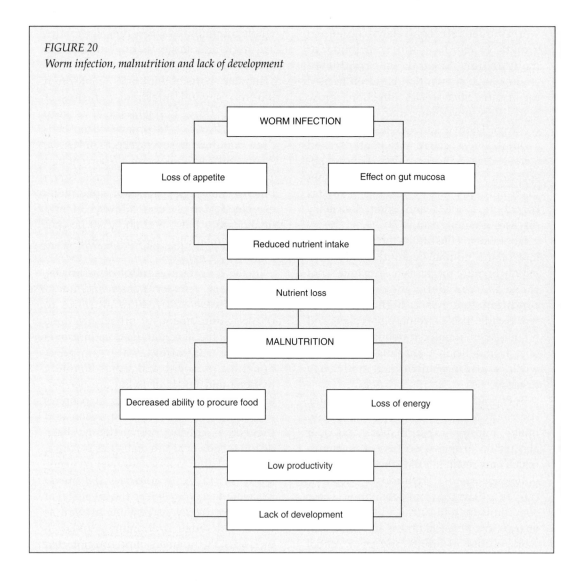

individuals, but also a public health measure. If large numbers of people, particularly children, are regularly dewormed in a community, then there will be reduced contamination of the environment. It is true that reinfections will occur, but it often takes time to build up the heavy parasite burdens that are most harmful. Over time infections will be reduced in terms of both prevalence and intensity.

In the last 15 years whenever and wherever large numbers of children have been dewormed, the intervention has been very popular and the demand for deworming from neighbouring communities has been intense. Most mothers want their children to be rid of worms. Teachers report that treated children do better in school.

Deworming may be a useful entry point for primary health care. In 12 villages in Tamil Nadu, India, women were found to be much more willing to have their children weighed and to participate in growth monitoring after their children had received albendazole treatment.

Many anthelmintic drugs are now available. Piperazine salts, effective mainly against *Ascaris lumbricoides*, and bephenium against hookworm (though less effective against *Necator* infections than against *Ancylostoma duodenale*) are giving way to newer drugs. Levamisole, given in a single dose, is effective in ascariasis but much less so for hookworm. Pyrantel in a single dose is effective for ascariasis and relatively useful against *Ancylostoma duodenale* but less so against *N. americanus*. Mebendazole is highly effective against ascariasis and both forms of hookworm; it is usually given in doses of 100 mg twice a day for three days. Albendazole is equally effective and is given as a single dose of 400 mg.

A parasitic infection that is even more important than these worm infections is malaria. It kills millions of people each year, causes severe illness in many others and is very difficult to control. Its relationship to nutrition is less clear than that of worm infections. However, malaria is known to cause a haemolytic (not an iron deficiency) anaemia, which may be particularly important in women of child-bearing age and in children. The control of malaria requires a partnership of persons in the community and in health ministries, plus those involved in environmental issues, in education and in other fields. Work is progressing on a vaccine. Treatment is becoming more difficult because of drug resistance. Impregnated mosquito-nets over the bed to protect people from the insects at night are useful. Attacks on mosquitoes and mosquito breeding sites are important.

HIV AND AIDS

The AIDS pandemic is a world problem. It is a health problem, a social problem and an economic problem for many developing countries. It has some nutritional implications. The human immunodeficiency virus (HIV) destroys the immune system and in adults results in overt signs of the disease AIDS often five to ten years after infection. As the disease progresses it causes anorexia; infections in the mouth make eating difficult; and wasting becomes a disease sign. In Uganda, AIDS is called "slim disease" because AIDS sufferers are usually very thin. It is said that male customers now favour plump prostitutes rather than thin ones, because they are thought to be safer.

One way in which HIV is transmitted is from mother to infant. It can be transmitted *in utero* or at the time of birth, but the HIV virus has also been found in breastmilk; it now seems that some babies are infected by breastfeeding, although this is an uncommon mode of transmission (see Chapter 7). It is worth repeating here that a consensus statement from WHO and UNICEF in summary advises that in areas where infectious diseases and malnutrition are the main cause of infant deaths and where infant mortality rates are high, pregnant women, including those who are HIV-infected, should be advised to breast-feed their babies after delivery, because the risk of HIV infection through breast-milk is likely to be lower than the risk of death from other causes. Recent research indicates that pregnant HIV-infected women who consume adequate amounts of vitamin A are less likely to infect their infants than those whose vitamin A status is poor.

Another relationship between HIV and nutrition arises because AIDS in some African countries and elsewhere is creating many orphans whose parents have both died of the infection. Poor orphans have a high risk of malnutrition.

In some countries where AIDS has resulted in sickness of many people and many deaths, there is a shortage of able-bodied people to produce crops and to undertake other activities necessary for food production or food acquisition. In some rural communities this shortage is having a markedly negative impact on agricultural production and is threatening the food security of many families.

The AIDS epidemic in heavily infected countries also has demographic implications because of markedly increased mortality rates in very young children and in younger adults. This increased mortality is raising the dependency ratio, that is the ratio of dependents (old people, children, sick individuals) to able-bodied productive adults. The higher dependency ratio also negatively influences food security.

Some general principles for prevention are almost universal, but in other ways the epidemic in each country may be different, and there may be somewhat specific behaviours influencing transmission in certain groups in a community or nation. Almost everywhere some level of surveillance combined with epidemiological studies will be helpful if appropriate preventive strategies are to be mounted. Investigations that provide information on behaviours likely to be linked to transmission are important but seldom accomplished. Unless the most risky behaviours in a population are known, sensible preventive measures are difficult to design. Each population may have specific social and cultural practices, mores and norms of behaviour and even particular communication channels that may influence prevention measures.

As the main strategy for prevention is likely to focus on preventing, reducing or modifying risky behaviours that may influence the spread of HIV, it is important to know which of these behaviours are most prevalent and who practises them in each society. For example, in the United States one risky behaviour that has been

greatly reduced is blood transfusion using untested blood. A second behaviour, which has not been adequately addressed, is use of contaminated needles among drug addicts. These two behaviours probably have a relatively small role in the spread of AIDS in, for example, Brazil, India and Uganda.

There are only three known ways in which HIV is transmitted from person to person: through sexual intercourse; through blood; and from mother to infant. In each country educational efforts should consider these three modes of transmission and local behaviour patterns that influence activities at the national, local and individual level. Educational messages may need to inform people not only of how the virus is transmitted but also of how it is not transmitted. It has been reported that 25 percent of people in the United States believe that AIDS can be spread by mosquitoes or by eating food cooked by a person who has the HIV virus, and many think that donating blood puts a donor at risk. These are not methods of transmission, and it is worth educating the public on this subject. In some African societies AIDS, like some other diseases, is blamed on bewitchment or a curse from the gods because of some moral transgression. Education should be culturally sensitive and should conform with societal norms. The educators need to have credibility with the groups of persons most at risk of infection. This is often ignored.

Perhaps the most prominent obstacle to the prevention of AIDS in Africa is widespread fatalism. In East Africa when a baby dies, the roof of a house collapses or the harvest fails, it is said in Kiswahili to be *"shauri ya Mungu"*, translated as "the will of God". This kind of fatalism has a useful function. Poor people have little control over many events that impinge importantly on their lives. It may be soothing then to accept adversity by saying, "this is the will of God". Many people shrug off risky behaviour either with this fatalism or by self-assurance that "other people get AIDS but not me". These commonly held views constitute a major obstacle to prevention of AIDS using educational methods.

Many infections are difficult to prevent. What can a person do to avoid contracting the common cold or pneumonia? AIDS, however, is generally spread by human behaviour, and if individuals avoid risky behaviours they reduce the likelihood of contracting the infection. Unless people can be made to understand this, AIDS will continue to spread. Thus the key to AIDS prevention is AIDS education using a wide variety of channels: community organizations and women's groups; the mass media and health services; appropriate religious organizations and social clubs; schools and colleges; and also entertainers, artists and politicians. Educational efforts should not await social science research of the kind discussed above, but would benefit from it.

The only certain way to avoid getting AIDS is, of course, to be sexually abstinent and to avoid contact with blood products. The next level of prevention is to have sexual intercourse only with a single partner known to be HIV-free and monogamous. Risk can be reduced by always properly using a condom during sexual intercourse, a practice often rejected by men from all continents. In many places, especially rural areas in Africa, condoms are not widely available and their cost is very high relative to income.

A more sustainable strategy to reduce the spread of AIDS in some societies lies in actions to endow females with much more control than is now common over sexual behaviour and in decisions related to their own health. Women must have rights to protect themselves from infection by promiscuous husbands or other partners. Education of females, more job opportunities and higher incomes would help.

Certain Asian countries such as India, the Philippines and Thailand are now experiencing rapid increases in AIDS cases. It is predicted that by the middle of the next decade Asia will have more HIV-positive people than Africa.

In the health sector much more widespread and vigorous treatment and prevention of other sexually transmitted diseases, including syphilis, chancroid and gonorrhoea, would help reduce the spread of AIDS. Early recognition of HIV infection and early diagnosis of AIDS, with appropriate counselling of both the infected person and his or her partner, is important. This requires more available testing in developing countries, and those who test positive must understand that they are likely to infect their partners and that they should either abstain from sex or practise "safe sex". However, this conduct is not usually realistic for prostitutes, unless programmes allow alternative sources of income for them. Widespread testing is relatively expensive for poor developing countries.

AIDS has a particular impact on women, not only because the disease will probably kill 2 million African women before the year 2000, but also because women bear the brunt of the consequences of the epidemic. It is usually women who look after sick individuals and orphans in the community; many already overburdened women are taking over the duties of husbands who have died of AIDS; and it is women who have to deal with the negative socio-economic and agricultural consequences of the AIDS epidemic. Women need to be in key positions in the design and implementation of AIDS programmes, and they also need to be a central focus of them. Women need to be provided with the facts and knowledge, the resources and the skills to deal better with the disease and its consequences in a less demanding, more effective and more humane way.

Support is needed for social science research so that action can be based on sound knowledge.

It is important to remember that although AIDS is a terrible scourge and will require large health and other resources, developing countries still have other health problems that may be more important or more prevalent than AIDS and that deserve more attention. Malaria remains a much greater killer, and worm infections and malnutrition are much more prevalent diseases than AIDS. New resources for AIDS control should not lessen health expenditures on other diseases, but should preferably come from reduced military expenditures or increased foreign assistance.

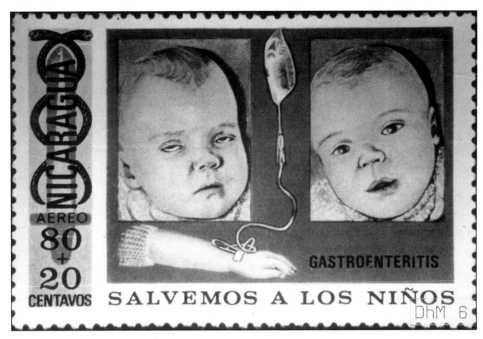

PHOTO 73
Nicaraguan stamp showing dehydration from gastro-enteritis and rehydration

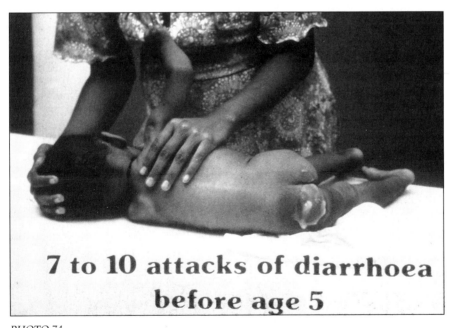

PHOTO 74
Indonesian poster indicating importance of diarrhoea

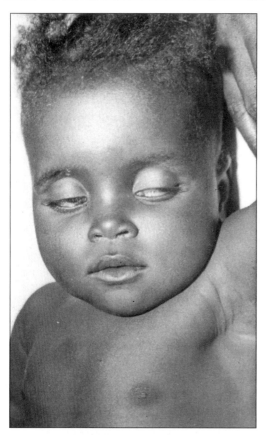

PHOTO 75
Child with signs of dehydration resulting from
diarrhoea

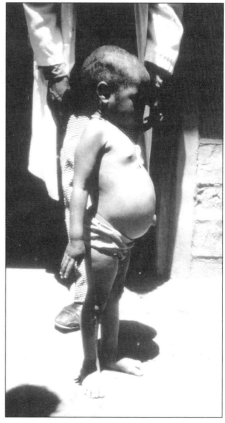

PHOTO 76
Moderately malnourished Kenyan
girl with pot-belly

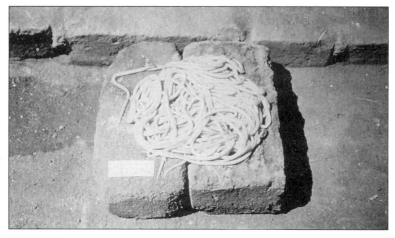

PHOTO 77
Roundworms passed by the girl in Photo 76 after she had received one
dose of anthelmintic

Chapter 38
Promoting appropriate diets and healthy lifestyles

The major nutritional problems in the world can be divided into two general categories:

- those caused by insufficient intake of nutrients, which may be related to food insecurity, disease (especially infections) and/or lack of care;
- those caused by excessive or unbalanced intake of food or of particular dietary constituents.

These types of nutritional problems, their underlying causes, their clinical manifestations and some aspects of their prevention have been discussed elsewhere in this book.

The prevention of malnutrition in both categories is greatly assisted if the people affected have accurate information on what constitutes a healthy diet and how they may best meet their nutritional needs. Education at all levels is important in the promotion of healthy diets and lifestyles (Photo 78). For those who have poor diets or nutritional problems, nutrition education and health education are strategies to influence behaviour change. Behaviour change requires motivation and efforts to recognize personal preferences, lifestyles and perhaps time constraints. Nutrition education and communication are described in this chapter.

PROTECTING AND PROMOTING HEALTHY LIFESTYLES

Almost all governments in Asia, Africa and Latin America are advocating and working to enhance and improve development, and many international, bilateral and non-governmental organizations (NGOs) are assisting with development in general or with specific development projects. Development involves change: cultural, social, economic and political change, and even changes in values. Any individual or group suggesting or implementing changes should consider carefully whether the outcome will be better for those affected by the change. Too often programmes and actions introduced from the outside foster change for the sake of change, or individuals or countries try to promote change to make others more like themselves, or agencies implement projects that involve change without considering the implications in terms of quality of life and with a naive assumption that all new structures are automatically better than the old ones.

Eight strategies for promoting appropriate diets and healthy lifestyles are given below. Some of these strategies do suggest changes. Where malnutrition is rampant and infectious diseases are prevalent, where these result from widespread food insecurity and a very unsanitary environment, and where the people (particularly women) lack knowledge regarding appropriate child feeding and do not understand the germ concept of disease, then clearly change is necessary if nutrition and health are to improve. There is a need for improved knowledge, improved resources and better standards of living.

In some groups of the population in the non-industrialized countries very rapid change has already taken place in the last 50 years: lifestyles have changed, age-old social practices are disappearing, and Western diets and modern ways are replacing traditional ones. Some of these changes have contributed to improvements in health, improved infant mortality rates and a reduction in certain forms of serious malnutrition such as xerophthalmia; but not infrequently these changes have also led to a new set of nutrition and health problems and to a less caring society. As described in Chapter 23, a steep rise in diet-related non-communicable diseases such as arteriosclerotic heart disease, obesity, certain cancers, stroke, dental caries, diabetes and others is occurring in many developing countries. Some of these problems have resulted from changing lifestyles including changed diets. Parallel with these changes there has also often been an increase in the prevalence of abandoned children, delinquent youths, child prostitution, elderly sick people not receiving proper care, and mental illness.

Not all change and not all westernization is for the good. Many poor societies possess social values that are superior to those found in many modern Western societies. Examples include emphasis on the extended family, better treatment of the elderly and infirm at home rather than in institutions, greater tolerance of the insane and more community spirit. Of course it is dangerous to glamorize life in the villages of developing countries. For many poor people life is extremely difficult; much of their day is spent doing hard manual labour, and they may lack sufficient food, housing or health care. There is no doubt that good health, a variety of social activities and, of course, enough food to eat are needed by all people everywhere. The argument here is not to oppose modernization or development, but rather to recognize, first, that all modernization and development efforts do not automatically provide benefits to the poor; and second, that some of those actions thought

to be benevolent may actually downgrade the quality of life of poor people.

Adoption of so-called modern habits and lifestyles sometimes has mixed blessings. Transfer and application of modern food production technologies and food preservation and processing practices have resulted in better quality, more variety and greater safety of food available for consumption. At the same time, adoption of certain food habits and behaviours such as overconsumption of saturated fats, decline in breastfeeding and concomitant increase in bottle-feeding and cigarette smoking may be detrimental to good health and nutrition. It is therefore necessary that the potential ill effects of undesirable practices be offset by taking suitable preventive measures.

It is not suggested that change is necessarily bad. Change is inevitable and is necessary for the improvement of nutrition and health. Modern knowledge can be harnessed for the good of the poor, and each country should freely choose its actions. When change is encouraged, however, either by outsiders or by governments, it is important to consider the possible adverse effects of the changes. The question everyone should ask is: "Will the change improve the quality of life of most affected people?" Perhaps a nutrition and health impact statement should be required of all new projects before implementation, in the same way that environmental impact statements are now required in the United States.

As non-industrialized countries plan for the beginning of a new century, special attention is needed to prevent the adoption of lifestyles and dietary patterns that will lead their people into epidemics of heart disease, lung cancer, stroke, obesity, diabetes and other chronic diseases. Countries in their impatience for modernization should not neglect protecting those aspects of traditional lifestyles that are conducive to good health and nutrition. A high priority should be given to protecting good traditional eating habits and good national diets; protecting good caring practices for children, the sick and the old; and protecting good moral, social and religious values. The rush to modernity and to westernization could pose a major health and nutritional threat to the populations of developing countries.

Healthy lifestyles are implicit in the strategies described below, whether they refer to dietary guidelines or goals which should ensure a balanced, healthy diet or to areas such as training, education, extension or communications conducted by ministries of agriculture, education, health, women's affairs, community development, etc.; workers in these strategies should be trained and employed to promote healthy lifestyles and better diets. In all cases the aim should be to reduce undernutrition and infections and also to prevent the risks of non-communicable chronic diseases and health problems associated with inappropriate diets and lifestyles.

It is not possible to prescribe a healthy lifestyle; in this book it is considered more appropriate to suggest strategies to promote appropriate diets with the aim of reducing diet-related health problems. It is clear that:

- almost every society has a cuisine that with proper selection and little change can provide good balanced diets and that accordingly deserves protection;
- immediate action to prevent non-smokers, especially young people and women, from becoming addicted to tobacco or from becoming users of cigarettes is vital;
- traditional good caring practices for children deserve protection and support;
- the traditional family, and sometimes the extended family, often provides a

lifestyle conducive to the well-being of children;

- priority needs to be given to avoiding risky behaviours that may lead to infection with acquired immunodeficiency syndrome (AIDS) or with other sexually transmitted diseases;
- families and communities need to provide a support system for children, the sick and the elderly and to improve activity levels of those who lead a sedentary life through active recreation and sports.

Lifestyles can be improved in many countries, especially for the poor, with:

- attention to hygiene, including food hygiene;
- improved sanitation and disposal of human excreta and garbage;
- safer and more plentiful water supplies;
- greater knowledge and awareness of health risks and avoidance of risky health behaviours;
- improved health services, including primary health care and public health measures;
- agricultural improvements in rural areas, including land reform in some countries, elimination of sharecropping, better access to credit, improvements in animal husbandry and greater availability of agricultural inputs such as fertilizers, irrigation and tools.

Cutting across many of these areas, lifestyles of the poor would improve if there were more equity, and those of women and children would improve if there were no discrimination against females and if there were more empowerment of women.

EIGHT STRATEGIES TO INFLUENCE BEHAVIOUR FOR IMPROVED NUTRITION

Several strategies besides education are available and have been used to influence behaviour change to improve nutrition.

Eight of them are discussed here:
- dietary guidelines and food goals,
- food and nutrition labelling,
- food advertising,
- institutional meals,
- food industry involvement,
- ensuring a consistent message,
- protecting traditional diets,
- nutrition training.

One important topic beyond these eight strategies needs special attention and is discussed in a separate section concluding the chapter: public nutrition education.

Dietary guidelines and food goals

Dietary guidelines are usually produced by governments but may also be provided by other groups. Chapter 23 discussed dietary guidelines mainly in relation to chronic diseases and described a set of suggested goals to help ensure food consumption for optimal health. These goals are somewhat unorthodox in that they were designed to be applicable both to poor countries where undernutrition is prevalent and to affluent countries where chronic diseases related to overconsumption or inappropriate modern diets are prevalent; in the past most national dietary guidelines were produced in industrialized countries and therefore addressed mainly problems of chronic disease, not undernutrition.

The dietary guidelines issued in the United States in 1990, which address mainly chronic health problems, have been augmented with an educational tool called the food guide pyramid (Figure 21). The pyramid, designed for nutrition educators and the public, replaces the concept of food groups. A pyramid is used because its base is wide, suggesting that most of the diet should come from carbohydrate-rich foods (the bread, cereal, rice and pasta group). The next broadest swath is the fruit and vegetable group. The pyramid may be appropriate for industrialized countries,

but it is much less so for developing countries. The top of the pyramid suggests that fats, oils and sweets be used sparingly, but this may be appropriate only where the population tends to have excessive intakes of energy.

Revised dietary guidelines for the United States were published in 1995 which are simple and easily understandable by the general public.

Food and nutrition labelling

Literate people who are interested in selecting a nutritious diet can be greatly assisted by clear and accurate labelling on food products. Food labelling that gives information on nutrient content has been used more in industrialized than in developing countries. It can be useful in almost all countries and is particularly helpful if used with a set of dietary guidelines. Other useful information on the label may include an expiry date.

The FAO/WHO Codex Alimentarius Commission has produced guidelines on nutrition labelling which deserve serious consideration by governments, especially those that do not have nutrient labelling regulations or that are dissatisfied with their existing situation. These Codex guidelines deal with pre-packaged foods and foods for catering purposes.

Nutrition labelling is often criticized for being too detailed and therefore too difficult to use. It is true that labels often list the content of some vitamins and minerals that are not causes of serious deficiencies and are not of public health importance in the country where the product is consumed. In addition to data on the nutrient content of the food and perhaps the percentages of Recommended Dietary Allowances, food labels sometimes also provide other nutritional information, for example, dietary claims such as "cholesterol-free", "low-calorie", "high-fibre" or "sugar-free". Countries need to

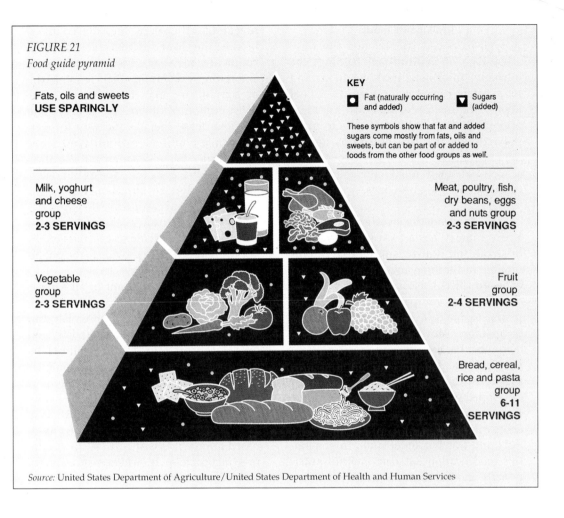

FIGURE 21
Food guide pyramid

Fats, oils and sweets
USE SPARINGLY

KEY

◻ Fat (naturally occurring and added)   ▽ Sugars (added)

These symbols show that fat and added sugars come mostly from fats, oils and sweets, but can be part of or added to foods from the other food groups as well.

Milk, yoghurt and cheese group
2-3 SERVINGS

Meat, poultry, fish, dry beans, eggs and nuts group
2-3 SERVINGS

Vegetable group
2-3 SERVINGS

Fruit group
2-4 SERVINGS

Bread, cereal, rice and pasta group
6-11 SERVINGS

Source: United States Department of Agriculture/United States Department of Health and Human Services

examine these claims, to determine their accuracy and perhaps to evaluate their effectiveness. It may be more important to draw up enforceable criteria for nutritional claims. Countries moving to develop guidelines or regulations for food labelling would be wise to consult the FAO/WHO Codex Alimentarius Commission and its publications.

Food advertising

Commercial advertising can serve to promote healthy eating, but it can also contribute to poor diets. Advertising, including food advertising, is difficult to control. Most countries expect advertising

to be truthful, and truth in advertising is a basic expectation. Concerns regarding dietary claims on food labels also apply to claims made in advertisements for products and services. Advertising, particularly television advertising, of inappropriate foods to children has been the subject of much criticism and has been discussed in many reports. Most nations have agreed to the principle of regulating the advertising of breastmilk substitutes, and many have adopted appropriate legislation. However, advertising can also have a good impact on nutrition, and the food industry has an important part to play as indicated below.

Institutional meals

A well-balanced diet is not the only advantage of institutional feeding; the introduction of new, healthier foods and food habits can also be a result. School meals, for example, provide an ideal opportunity to introduce pupils to unfamiliar foods that are nutritious and to demonstrate to children what constitutes a well-balanced meal consistent with dietary goals and guidelines.

Food industry involvement

Every country has a food industry, large or small, and it always has a role in promoting and influencing the consumption of healthy diets. Clearly the main objectives of industrial companies are to market foods, to make a profit and to outsell competitors. However, this can only be achieved by responding positively to public demand for particular foods. For example, the dairy industry in many developed countries has responded to the desire of people to reduce their fat and energy intakes by marketing more low-fat milk and less whole-fat milk. In general, this modification has been helpful nutritionally and has come about as consumers have become more nutritionally informed. However, changes that are beneficial to nutrition or health in the industrialized countries of the North may not be helpful in poor nations of the South. For example, where undernutrition and protein-energy malnutrition (PEM) are common and where mean intakes of fat in children are below 10 percent of total energy, a campaign to promote low-fat milk would be inappropriate.

Ensuring a consistent message

Nutrition education makes much more sense to the public if there is some degree of consistency in the main messages. This is not to suggest that there is a need for control or censorship; but regarding nutri-

tion and health, people are often confused because they hear different and sometimes conflicting messages. For example, many extension workers and others in ministries of agriculture may be promoting the consumption of diversified, energy- and nutrient-dense diets as the way to overcome micronutrient malnutrition, while others may be undermining these messages by advocating the widespread distribution of dietary supplements in the form of pills and capsules.

If nutrition educators can agree on the main nutritional problems and then on the appropriate advice to provide to the public, everyone's work becomes easier.

Consistency is important in all aspects of information, not just in content. Nutrition education must not distinguish four food groups according to one ministry and three according to another. Similarly, national agricultural and food policies need to address the nutrition problems of the country, and the ministry of health needs to promote sustainable solutions to the major deficiencies by advocating food-based approaches that address the fundamental problems of widespread poverty and food insecurity.

Protecting traditional diets

A neglected but important topic, protection of dietary tradition is especially relevant for those countries where diet-related chronic diseases (see Chapter 23) are not prevalent but where economic development permits at least some people to purchase a wide variety of foods, including animal food products.

In general, traditional diets in Asia, Africa and Latin America are based on cereals or root crops, with significant amounts of legumes, fruits and vegetables. Often poultry, meat and dairy products provide only a small proportion of total energy but are appreciated as side dishes or tasty additions to the staple foods.

Usually, these diets are protective against the chronic diet-related diseases described in Chapter 23. Relatively low in total fat, saturated fat and cholesterol, these diets are high in complex carbohydrates and fibre. If plenty of fresh vegetables and fruits are also consumed, these diets are often rich in carotene and vitamin C, which are antioxidants.

Protecting good traditional diets starts with protecting or enhancing the production and marketing of traditional foods. Working with the local food industry to help in safe food preservation and packaging is important, and making foods easier to prepare for the table would contribute much to their popularity. One obvious attraction of many Western dishes is their convenience; busy people are attracted to them and homemakers can save time using them.

Nutrition training

Most countries have far too few professionals who are expert in or knowledgeable about nutrition. Moreover, nutrition training is often a neglected topic for persons other than nutritionists and dietitians. A wide range of professionals could benefit from more and better training in nutrition: health professionals such as doctors, nurses, midwives, health assistants or auxiliaries; agricultural staff, including extension workers, research scientists and high-level ministry officials; teachers and others throughout the formal and non-formal education system; social and community development workers; workers in institutional feeding; staff in NGOs involved in development, health, agriculture, community development and other activities; professionals in the food and related industries; and many others.

A prerequisite for designing appropriate training at suitable levels is a review of the nutrition content of the curricula of training institutes of many kinds in various

fields such as health, education, agriculture and community development. Most institutes will be found to have inadequate coverage of nutrition. If this proves to be the case, a group of experienced persons might be formed to make recommendations regarding strategies for improving nutrition training, changes in the curricula and the means to make the changes.

The first need might be to train the trainers. In poor countries this may require external assistance. In designing the training several questions need to be addressed. What are the most important topics in training, taking account of the most important nutrition problems? What do those being trained need to know in order to integrate nutrition in their jobs? Can some progress be made in the near future with the organization of short courses?

NUTRITION EDUCATION AND COMMUNICATION

Nutrition education is a strategy that has been widely used for many years to promote healthy diets and thereby ensure proper growth of children and a reduction in all forms of malnutrition. The basis of any nutrition education programme should be to encourage the consumption of a nutritionally adequate diet, to promote healthy lifestyles and to stimulate effective demand for appropriate foods.

In the past, nutrition education was too often conducted in an unimaginative way. People were instructed to eat this or that food because it was "good for you". Attempts were sometimes directed at making radical rather than gradual changes in the diets of the people who were the targets of the nutrition education. As a result, very few of the nutrition education programmes were successful. They were frequently carried out by persons of a different culture or social class from those being educated. The lessons of history show clearly that nutrition educators should start from the premise that most mothers are doing their best to feed their families properly. If they are not managing to do so, the reasons may well be beyond their control.

In most circumstances the nutrition education content must be formulated on the basis of a problem analysis. The education must be relevant to the reality.

Inadequate total intake of food by young children (energy deficiency) is the main cause of malnutrition in Africa, Asia and Latin America. Therefore, initial advice might be to feed a malnourished infant with the same food as before but more frequently, or to provide just a little more of the food. This advice should be more acceptable to parents than an attempt to make major, often unrealistic, changes in the diet. Other recommendations for change should be simple and feasible for the family, consistent with its cultural habits and of course nutritionally sound.

Nutrition education has frequently failed because the advice did not conform with the above criteria. Throughout the world there have been examples of nutrition education messages that urged poor mothers to provide their children with meat or fish every day, or one egg per day or three cups of milk per day. This advice may have been nutritionally reasonable, but in all other respects it lacked sense. Except in very few communities and countries, poor families cannot afford to provide these foods to their young children so often, and it is now known that it is unnecessary to do so. As described elsewhere in this book, there are cheap alternatives, the legumes being particularly good examples.

Nationally, nutrition education may be carried out by several ministries (health, agriculture, education, social or community development, etc.) and also by various NGOs. All these bodies should agree on common objectives for a nutrition

education programme, and each ministry must decide how it plans to implement it. Factors that should be decided upon, which are rarely clearly defined, include the content of the message (discussed above), the target audience for the programme and the media to be used. This strategy may appear simple, but its application will require a change in both the philosophy and the operation of most nutrition education programmes.

The choice of media depends on the formal and informal information and communications infrastructure of the area in question. In general it is wise to use a combination of communications media in an integrated way. However, a concentrated radio campaign may often be the cheapest and most effective way of reaching the bulk of the population. In addition to stations controlled by the government, commercial radio and television should be used for nutrition education. Certain priority issues or areas of concern should receive concentrated effort.

As mentioned, the stress should be on small changes that will complement existing dietary practices and not on major changes. Failure has occurred in past campaigns that attempted to impart a mass of general information on nutrition, rather than hitting hard with a few well-designed messages in a limited number of priority areas.

The efforts of the various ministries and organizations involved in nutrition education should be closely coordinated so that the messages received from different sources will complement and reinforce each other.

Who should give nutrition education? When should it be offered? To whom should it be aimed? The answers to these questions are in general quite simple. Everyone who has the knowledge (for example, members of health teams, schoolteachers, agricultural extension workers) should provide nutrition education. They should do so at every possible opportunity (for example, the doctor when treating a patient, the midwife at the antenatal clinic, the health nurse when visiting a home, the extension officer at a farmers' meeting, the schoolteacher in a class or at a parents' meeting). Every person in the country should be the target of nutrition education. Even if the message concerns PEM in the preschool child, for example, the problem is so important that all people can benefit from being informed about it.

Perhaps the most persistent and frequent error that has been made in nutrition education has been the overriding atten-

tion given to animal protein. It is now generally agreed that protein deficiency is not the main dietary shortcoming to be overcome, and that even if it were, animal products do not offer a reasonable or feasible solution in most poor societies. PEM, which is the most important nutritional problem, is much more often the result of a low total intake of food by the child, who may then be deficient in both energy and protein. The solution is to increase the quantity of foods already eaten. If efforts are to be made to increase protein intake, then the stress should be on vegetable foods that are rich in protein, such as legumes, rather than on animal

---

Priority points for nutrition education

Priority points for nutrition education in many countries might include:

- suggesting that young children be fed more frequently with existing foods;
- suggesting that amounts of foods at each meal be increased for children during the weaning and post-weaning period;
- recommending increased consumption by children of any legumes that are available and commonly consumed by the family;
- promoting inclusion in the diet of foods such as groundnuts that are rich in protein and provide a concentrated source of energy;
- promoting increased consumption of foods rich in carotene (dark green leafy vegetables and yellow fruits and vegetables) by young children in areas where vitamin A deficiency is a problem;
- increasing availability of fruits and vegetables through promotion of home gardening;
- demonstrating the proper preparation, cooking and processing of home-grown fruits and vegetables to preserve their nutritional value (Photos 79 and 80);
- encouraging breastfeeding and discouraging

bottle-feeding (i.e. protection, support and promotion of breastfeeding);
- encouraging attendance by pregnant women at clinics where iron and other supplements are available and where the progress of pregnancy can be checked;
- encouraging families' attendance with their children at under-five and similar clinics for immunizations and growth monitoring of children;
- increasing knowledge about protecting the quality and safety of foods, and promoting sanitation, hygiene and safe water to reduce infectious diseases, which often contribute to malnutrition;
- informing parents about the importance of continuing breastfeeding and other foods when children have diarrhoea, and about the use of home fluids and oral rehydration solution (ORS);
- providing information on birth spacing and ways to limit family size.

These examples are not all applicable to all communities or countries, but each is practical and appropriate for many areas.

products. Nevertheless, in many nutrition education programmes of the past 40 years emphasis has been placed on increasing the consumption of meat, fish, milk, eggs and manufactured protein-rich foods. This education has totally failed because economic reasons have precluded the adoption of the advice and frequently the foods recommended have not been easily available.

Nutrition educators have much more to learn from commercial advertising, which has often been successful in changing food habits and attitudes (see the following section on social marketing). Commercial promotion uses the media skilfully. The talent available in commerce should be harnessed more often to assist with nutrition and health education.

Past nutrition education initiatives have had some successes but many failures in terms of improving dietary intake and reducing the extent of malnutrition in a community or a country. The failures have occurred not mainly because nutrition education is a wrong strategy, but rather because the methods used have not led to the desired behaviour change.

In the past 30 years new approaches have been used to elicit changes in behaviour with a nutrition objective, and there is evidence that some have been more successful than older, more traditional approaches. One approach, which has been termed "social marketing", uses some principles from commercial marketing. Other approaches using principles adopted from the behavioural sciences have also improved nutrition education efforts: nutrition educators seek to identify the nutrition problems and eating behaviours of people within the social context in which they live, taking cognizance of cultural factors; only then are the communication techniques chosen and appropriate messages formulated for specific or general audiences.

SOCIAL MARKETING

In recent years social marketing to promote improved health and better nutrition has been widely, and sometimes successfully, used. There have been some real success stories.

A major difference between traditional nutrition education and the newer social marketing approach is that the latter starts with what commercially would be called "consumer research". An attempt is made to discover, using various techniques such as surveys and focus group interviews, what the consumer or the public is doing and why. The older nutrition education approach started from the premise that malnutrition exists, that people's diets are bad and that people need to be told to eat a good diet providing foods in all four basic food groups. The new approach would be likely first to use consumer research to identify a few important problems such as decline in breastfeeding, infrequent meals or drinking of contaminated water, and would then address them. The results of the research regarding consumer views, perspectives and practices lead to decisions on appropriate messages, communication techniques and targeting.

In the commercial world test-marketing is nearly always done before launching a product. It may also be sensible in nutrition education using social marketing and modern communication techniques; the messages developed and the communication techniques chosen to tackle the problems assessed and analysed may be tried out in a limited way. They can then be reassessed, reanalysed and modified, changed or abandoned, before they are implemented for a larger audience.

These methods, if successful, could lead to a major national campaign or to more limited nutrition education activities in certain communities; they could lead to use of television time or to the use of communicators in the villages. The major difference between these and older methods is a recognition that people have reasons for their behaviour and that nutritionists need to respect and learn from people before they attempt to change their behaviour. It may be necessary to identify the resistance points that impede change. Any nutrition education approach that incorporates empowerment and respect for local culture is more likely to be successful than those that do not.

Those interested in using social marketing methods can obtain detailed information in publications included in the Bibliography.

Beyond social marketing, and sometimes including it, social mobilization has been successfully used in improving the nutrition and health of communities. This is a broader approach in which nutrition education plays a part. It is described in Chapter 40.

FAO and other United Nations organizations provide assistance for the development of appropriate nutrition education programmes. They maintain that nutrition education should be carried out broadly through schools, newspapers, television, radio and other mass media as well as through face-to-face contact. To be most effective, nutrition education needs to be integrated into broad nutrition improvement programmes like those described elsewhere in this book. Communication experts need to be involved in the design of programmes.

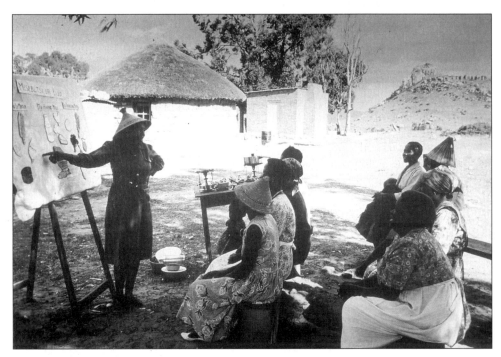

PHOTO 78
Nutrition education in Lesotho

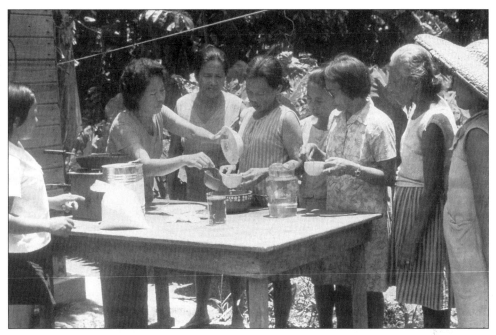

PHOTO 79
Food demonstration in the Philippines

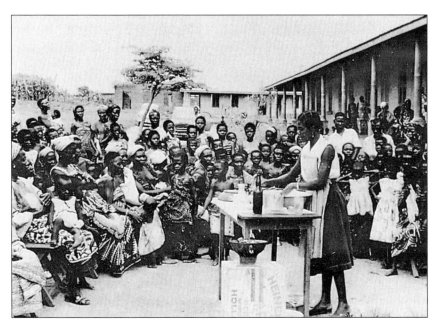

PHOTO 80
Cooking demonstration in a village

Chapter 39
Preventing specific micronutrient deficiencies

Over 30 micronutrients are essential for human health and for the proper growth and development of children. They are all vitamins and minerals available in foods. (See Chapters 10 and 11 for properties of micronutrients and Chapters 12 to 22 for deficiencies and disorders.) Micronutrient deficiencies are prevalent public health problems in many countries, especially developing countries. The micronutrient deficiencies that are most prevalent in the world are those of vitamin A, iodine and iron. Together with protein-energy malnutrition (PEM), these deficiencies constitute the "big four" nutritional problems. There is wide geographic variation in their prevalence.

In the early 1990s almost all countries pledged to devote major efforts to eliminating vitamin A and iodine deficiencies and substantially reducing iron deficiency by the year 2000. These tasks will be more difficult for some countries than for others, but all countries where these micronutrient deficiencies exist should have a policy and strategies to deal with them. However, the initiatives should not undermine, replace or reduce efforts to control PEM, which is often more prevalent and more important as a public health problem. In some countries some other micronutrient deficiencies may also constitute a public health problem and may perhaps be more important than the deficiencies of vitamin A, iodine or iron. In these countries appropriate attention needs to be devoted to the most important deficiencies based on their prevalence, the extent of the morbidity they cause, their contribution to mortality rates, their social and public health significance

and, finally, the feasibility and cost of control. See Chapters 16, 17 and 18 for discussions on thiamine, niacin and vitamin D deficiencies and their control.

Individual countries and communities can take many different strategies and actions to address these micronutrient deficiencies. It is important to make certain that the strategies and actions are coordinated and that consideration is given to strategic actions that address more than one nutrition problem simultaneously.

COMPREHENSIVE VERSUS TARGETED APPROACHES

Policies and programmes designed to control the three major micronutrient deficiencies are usually either comprehensive or targeted. A relatively comprehensive (or holistic) approach to deal with vitamin A deficiency might include public health measures, horticultural activities, treatment and control of infections, fortification of foods and judicious use of vitamin A supplements, allied with government activities to reduce poverty and improve food security. A narrowly targeted approach might be a distribution of high-dose vitamin A capsules to young children at high risk of vitamin A deficiency.

The comprehensive approach can be compared to firing a shotgun: many small pellets are fired, rather than a single bullet, and these may hit a wider area or different targets. The targeted approach, on the other hand, is analogous to using a rifle: there is one bullet, which is lethal, but only if it hits the target. Thus it has sometimes been termed the "magic bullet" approach.

For many public health problems and most types of malnutrition, the holistic approach is philosophically and politically preferable and is more likely to be sustainable than the narrow, targeted approach. In practice, the place for the magic bullet is in dealing with a single problem or individual.

Holistic approaches might appear to be more daunting, more difficult and perhaps slower for reaching the optimistic goals for micronutrient deficiency control. However, this need not be so, because the holistic approach can also embrace the magic bullet approach. A vitamin A deficiency control strategy, for example, can include targeting of high-dose vitamin A supplements along with initiatives for increasing production and consumption of carotene-rich foods, fortification, nutrition education and broad public health measures. Optimism that holistic approaches will be successful depends to some extent on a favourable political and social climate and some chance of social mobilization and community participation. Favourable economic development is a helpful but not necessary condition.

The goals of virtually eliminating vitamin A and iodine deficiencies and reducing iron deficiency substantially by the year 2000 are ambitious, but they are realizable in several countries. In all cases their realization will require a rather rapid and sustained increase in levels of appropriate activity. Achievement of the goals will depend not, as is often stated, primarily on political will, but more on government actions. Will is important, but actions are essential. Many international agencies, non-governmental organizations (NGOs) and others are poised to assist countries and their local experts in concentrating efforts to control micronutrient deficiencies. FAO, the United Nations Children's Fund (UNICEF) and the World Health Organization (WHO) are among the agencies concerned.

A MICRONUTRIENT DEFICIENCY CONTROL PLAN

The first requirement, which some countries have already met, is to formulate a national plan with defined strategies and actions and clear lines of authority to take action. In most cases an overall micronutrient plan is desirable. However, specific deficiencies may call for different control strategies, involving different professionals and perhaps necessitating separate plans of action.

The prevalence of each deficiency in different parts of the country and the underlying determinants may or may not be well known. Action should not await new comprehensive nutritional surveys, but more detailed assessment of the micronutrient deficiencies and their underlying causes may be desirable. This can also provide baseline information to judge the effectiveness of actions taken. Baseline information on the prevalence of the deficiencies is often usefully supplemented with specific information on food intakes; relevant social, cultural and economic factors; and data on the health situation.

FOUR CONTROL STRATEGIES

Four main strategies can be implemented to reduce or control micronutrient deficiencies. They operate in concert with broader strategies to improve the quality of life in particular countries and communities. Actions at all levels – international, local and family – to improve household food security, individual health and care can have an impact on micronutrient deficiencies and should always be taken into account in micronutrient deficiency control strategies.

The four basic micronutrient strategies are:
- improving diets, especially dietary diversity;
- public health actions;
- fortification or nutrification of foods;

• providing medicinal supplements.

These four strategies are listed in order of sustainability; clearly improved diets contribute to controlling a micronutrient deficiency in a much more sustainable way than medicinal supplements. Public health actions and fortification are of intermediate sustainability. Many public health measures, such as improved health knowledge, water supplies and hygiene, remain in place, whereas other measures, such as immunizations, require continuing action. Undoubtedly conferring the knowledge and ability to produce, procure and consume an appropriate diet is the most sustainable way to prevent micronutrient deficiencies.

Improving diets, especially through dietary diversity

Clearly the ultimate goal in attainment of micronutrient food security is to ensure that people consume a diversity of foods that provide them with the required quantities of all essential micronutrients on a continuing basis. This surely should be the basic long-term strategy of all governments addressing the problems of vitamin A and iron deficiencies. (As stated in other parts of this book, iodine deficiency often cannot be controlled in this way, and salt iodization is recommended.) For infants, the protection, support and promotion of breastfeeding and emphasis on the health and good nourishment of the mother offer the best protection. To prevent iron and vitamin A deficiencies in adults, stimulating the production and consumption of micronutrient-rich foods is vital.

Nutrition education is an important part of this strategy. However, it will be effective only if the appropriate foods are available. Education to improve production and especially consumption of appropriate micronutrient-rich foods must go beyond old nutrition education methods which exhorted people to consume certain foods because they were "good"; education programmes must be designed to elicit behaviour change that will be permanent. A programme in Thailand, for example, successfully used social marketing methods to raise dietary vitamin A intakes in the northeastern part of the country, and Bangladesh has seen some successes in increasing home or village production and consumption of carotene-rich foods.

Improving dietary diversity is best considered as an integral part of community actions to improve household, and then child, food security. The actions planned will often be cooperative and may include agricultural activities, school-based projects and assistance to families, both urban and rural.

This sustainable approach to the control of micronutrient deficiencies is often criticized as being too difficult or at best a very long-term strategy. Recent examples from many parts of the world, however, suggest that good results can be seen in a relatively short time. Critics of this strategy are often those who are philosophically tied to "quick-fix", medically oriented solutions that can be planned from outside the country or outside the community. But the food-based strategy is sustainable and is the only one that controls vitamin A deficiency permanently.

Public health actions

Clearly any measures that reduce infections and promote good health will also help to reduce most micronutrient deficiencies, especially vitamin A and iron deficiencies. The relationship of nutrition and infection has been discussed in Chapters 3 and 37.

Specific health actions in the control of micronutrient deficiencies include early diagnosis and treatment of deficiencies. When a deficiency is recognized early and properly treated it cannot lead to serious consequences. Thus recognition by health workers that preschool-age children in a community have night blindness or Bitot's spots, that schoolchildren have small enlargements of the thyroid gland or that women have low haemoglobin levels can prompt timely medical action and cure. This evaluation can be part of primary health care.

At the next level are public health actions, particularly those that control infections. They include immunizations against infectious diseases; mass deworming and measures to reduce the transmission of parasitic infections; and improvements in sanitation, household hygiene and availability of safe potable water. All can help in the control of micronutrient deficiencies. Good maternal and child health services, availability of family planning, health and nutrition education and household and environmental hygiene measures contribute to reducing malnutrition.

Some of these health interventions are highly sustainable and many will have an impact on nutrition and health beyond the micronutrient deficiencies.

Fortification or nutrification of foods

Food fortification, usually salt iodization, is widely recognized as the most important strategy for the control of iodine deficiency disorders (IDD). Fortification can also contribute to the control of vitamin A and iron deficiencies among populations who purchase food and can afford fortified ingredients. Many different foods in industrialized countries are fortified with iron and vitamin A. Many North Americans get more than their total daily requirement of vitamin A and iron from one large bowl of a fortified breakfast cereal and from a slice of toast liberally spread with margarine fortified with both carotene and vitamin A. It is believed that food fortification was responsible for the

control and often the virtual elimination of many serious micronutrient deficiencies that were prevalent in industrialized countries early in the twentieth century.

Food fortification has to be continued as long as there is a risk of people suffering from a particular micronutrient deficiency and dietary diversification or other steps are not removing the risk. The sustainability of a fortification programme depends on food industry cooperation, monitoring and legal enforcement.

Fortification, including salt iodization, has been successfully used for many years in industrialized countries, but in some developing countries there have been serious problems in introducing it. A national programme requires advocacy, political will and often multisectoral actions or involvement, with the participation of several ministries. It also requires cooperation from the food industry, whose opposition would make fortification difficult if not impossible. An early step to successful implementation is often the establishment of an interdisciplinary committee, including people from universities or research institutes who have conducted research on the problem; representatives of appropriate ministries including health, commerce and industry, finance and perhaps education and agriculture; and representatives of the food industry. Consideration can be given to fortifying more than one commonly eaten food. Chapter 34, which deals with ways to improve food quality and safety, includes an outline of the important factors to consider in a fortification programme.

Medicinal supplements

The provision of micronutrients taken orally or by injection is usually simply called "supplementation" rather than "medicinal supplementation", but in fact these supplements are generally provided as medicine or used in a medicinal sense.

Eight steps for successful food fortification

A food fortification programme to solve a micronutrient deficiency considered a national problem usually needs to follow a series of steps. These might include:
- justification on the basis of data showing the prevalence, distribution and seriousness of the problem;
- consideration of other methods to control the deficiency, such as food diversification;
- advocacy to educate government decision-makers, the food industry and the public and to obtain their feedback;
- selection of the food or foods to be fortified (based in part on criteria discussed in Chapter 34) and of the form of nutrient or nutrients to be added;
- actions related to implementation, including establishment of an interdisciplinary committee to work with the food industry involved and the micronutrient supplier and

determination of a time frame for implementation;
- consideration of budget and organizational aspects, not necessarily after the preceding step;
- development of legislation and other regulations;
- establishment of a system for evaluation and continuous monitoring.

In practice, the key to success in carrying out these steps has often been the dedication of an individual or a small group that is knowledgeable about the problem, committed to its solution by fortification and tireless in seeking and involving allies from international organizations such as FAO, UNICEF, WHO, the International Anaemia Consultative Group (INACG) and the International Council for Control of Iodine Deficiency Disorders (ICCIDD).

(The term "food supplementation", in contrast, refers to the addition of more nutritious foods to a simple diet, for example, the addition of dried skimmed milk to maize meal as a supplement to basic rations in emergency situations. In this case, the added food is a food supplement, not a nutrient supplement; it is given as a food intervention, not as a medical intervention.)

The major role of supplementation with iodine, vitamin A or iron is as a short-term measure. It may be used in the longer term for individuals at special risk of the deficiency. Programmes of medicinal supplementation should usually be introduced for rapid improvement while long-term, sustainable interventions are planned and readied for implementation.

In some instances medicinal supplements may be the only feasible intervention

to protect people. They are especially useful in the event of natural or civil disasters, when no alternative strategy may be immediately available.

Medicinal supplementation is the least sustainable strategy because it depends, first, on a delivery system that reaches almost all persons at risk of the deficiency and, second, on active participation, including behaviour change, by those at risk of the deficiency (or in the case of the children, by their families and guardians). These two essential components are very seldom fully realizable, and this is one reason for failure.

However, as indicated below, there is a good distance between a rejection of all supplementation and a decision to attempt a national programme to provide a medicinal micronutrient supplement (such as high-dose vitamin A capsules) to all children between six months and five years of age throughout the country. The middle ground is the usual choice and is most appropriate; this includes medicinal supplements for persons at special risk, as well as broader programmes, for example, provision of oral iodine to non-pregnant females of child-bearing age in IDD-endemic areas to protect their future foetuses from iodine deficiency while salt iodization is being introduced.

Micronutrient supplementation is more effective if it reaches people through existing delivery systems, for example, when iron is routinely given in antenatal clinics, vitamin A to malnourished children when they come for growth monitoring and oral iodine at school to female pupils 14 to 19 years of age. It has been suggested that high doses of vitamin A be given to infants at the time of immunization as part of WHO's Expanded Programme on Immunization (EPI), but this proposal should probably not be recommended. The infants would be "captive" subjects, but infants in their first six months of life are usually breastfed and at low risk of xerophthalmia, and there is evidence that high doses of vitamin A in young infants can cause undesirable reactions. Similarly, more and more projects have been aimed at providing schoolchildren perhaps once a year with an anthelmintic drug to rid them of intestinal worms, and vitamin A promoters have suggested that high doses of vitamin A be given at the time of deworming. However, school-age children usually do not have serious clinical manifestations of vitamin A deficiency. Targeted use of micronutrient supplements should aim at people at special risk of the deficiency, not at people who are easy to reach but who have little risk of the deficiency.

PREVENTING VITAMIN A DEFICIENCY

The reduction and eventual control of vitamin A deficiency in most poor coun-

tries where it is prevalent almost always requires a broad approach. Seldom will it be appropriate to use only one strategy.

The United Republic of Tanzania is one of several countries taking a broad approach. The country's interdisciplinary, interministerial national micronutrient committees have set actions in place to improve dietary intakes of vitamin A-rich foods. They include horticultural activities and nutrition education; public health actions of various kinds; an exploration of possible foods to fortify; and judicious use of high-dose vitamin A supplements, widely available through health services. At the same time, Tanzania is striving, by means of economic, agricultural and other policies, to improve the well-being of poor Tanzanians in a sustainable way, which if successful will also work to reduce vitamin A deficiency.

Each country needs to consider to what extent it will aim to use each of the four possible strategies described above. Communities and families also take their own actions, becoming participants to a greater or lesser extent in strategies planned nationally.

Improving the vitamin A intakes of at-risk people

In developing countries most people get most of their vitamin A from carotene in foods, not from preformed vitamin A, which is present only in foods of animal origin. Therefore endeavours to increase dietary diversity to improve intakes of vitamin A will focus mainly on raising the intakes of foods containing carotene. Certainly there is some place, if appropriate in view of incomes and availability, for modest attempts to increase intakes of foods of animal origin that contain vitamin A, but the main step is to promote the consumption of carotene-rich fruits and vegetables. Other sources of carotene in certain countries are red palm oil and

Justifying medicinal supplementation

FAO (1993a) has suggested a set of questions that need to be answered to justify supplementation. These questions include:

- Are there any population subgroups for which supplementation may be required as short-term assistance? Which? Why?
- How well defined are these subgroups (women of reproductive age, infants, young children, the elderly, refugees or displaced persons)?
- What are their specific needs? Have those needs been measured, or are they just presumed to exist?
- Are we sure that the problem is so acute and urgent that supplementation would be appropriate?
- Are we sure that we can match the acuteness and urgency requirements with appropriately massive and prompt interventions?
- Where would we get the necessary supplies from? How would they be delivered? How would they be distributed? How would we ensure that the target population (and only the target population) gets them?
- Is there sufficient support from the authorities (national, local) to ensure the success of the operation?

- Are the proposed beneficiaries aware of the problems? What are their likely attitudes to the proposed assistance?
- Are we confident that the assistance would continue for as long as needed? If this is not guaranteed, should we initiate the intervention, or not?
- What parallel measures are we introducing to reduce the period over which supplementation would be needed? Will we be creating an ongoing expectation for the supplements? Has an end-point to supplementation been defined and accepted by authorities?
- How can we ensure that supplementation does not prove counterproductive by giving the false impression that the basic causes of micronutrient deficiency are being tackled satisfactorily? How can we ensure that there is no consequent diversion of resources that might have otherwise been available for interventions which are either more sustainable or more long-lasting?

Answers to these questions will provide the basis on which to decide whether supplementation will be superior as a major strategy, feasible and likely to reach the objectives set.

yellow maize. It is also important that diets contain adequate fat, which assists with absorption of carotene, and enough protein for retinol transport.

To increase intakes of vitamin A- and carotene-containing foods, including breastmilk (see Chapter 7), it will often be necessary to stimulate changes, first in production and availability of these foods and second in consumption, especially by those who are at risk of vitamin A deficiency. Chapters 2 and 35, which discuss food production and household food security, and Chapter 38, which

discusses strategies for promoting appropriate diets including the use of nutrition education and communications to influence behaviour change, describe methods appropriate for influencing change in vitamin A intakes.

Several projects have led to improvements in knowledge, attitudes and practice relating to consumption of vitamin A-containing foods and in some cases to improvements in vitamin A nutritional status. In Thailand and Indonesia social marketing and other methods were successfully used to increase consumption of vitamin A-rich foods. In Bangladesh the emphasis was on home production of carotene-containing foods and the consumption by children of more green leafy vegetables and carotene-rich fruits. This project was allied with an endeavour to raise families' awareness of night blindness as a sign of vitamin A deficiency. Reductions in night blindness then illustrated the success of the project. In the Philippines and Indonesia projects in selected communities have attempted to increase children's complementary consumption of foods rich in vitamin A with foods containing adequate fat. A dietary approach in the United Republic of Tanzania involves a broad set of activities, including information, education and communication components aimed at creating public awareness of the vitamin A problem and stimulating increased production and consumption of vitamin A-rich foods. There is wide use of radio and newspapers. Special efforts are being undertaken to improve horticultural practices and to link these with control of vitamin A deficiency. Work is under way to increase the production and improve the marketing of red palm oil.

Breastfeeding is protective against vitamin A deficiency. Colostrum is also rich in vitamin A. The baby who is exclusively breastfed for four to six months is protected against xerophthalmia, and for babies six to 24 months of age breastmilk provides very important amounts of vitamin A. For these reasons protecting, supporting and promoting breastfeeding is a very important strategy in the control of vitamin A deficiency. Breastmilk will provide more vitamin A if the mother has an adequate intake of the vitamin. Therefore foods rich in vitamin A should be promoted not only for young children, but also for women of child-bearing age and those who are breastfeeding their babies.

At the community level the health worker, schoolteacher, extension officer or social worker needs to emphasize the importance of vitamin A-rich foods for children and pregnant and lactating women. Families need to know which local foods of those that they can afford to buy and that their children will willingly eat are rich in carotene. Often children will prefer mango, papaya, yellow sweet potato and pumpkin over green leafy vegetables. When red palm oil and liver are available, children should have priority in getting these. Families might be assisted in growing vitamin A-rich foods in urban or rural gardens and in preserving them. Another action is to inform families how to prepare vitamin A-rich foods for consumption by children (see Chapter 40). The foods prepared and served to children differ from society to society, but cooked green leaves put through a sieve or shredded with a little oil or with groundnuts, or mashed cooked pumpkin, sweet potato or carrots, will often be appropriate.

The strategy of improving production and consumption of vitamin A-rich foods is the only sustainable long-term solution for controlling vitamin A deficiency. In most countries it should be a high-priority strategy.

Public health actions

The first health-related action is to ensure that health workers, especially those who see children in out-patient and in-patient facilities within the primary health care system, easily recognize xerophthalmia and appreciate those conditions and illnesses that raise the risk of vitamin A deficiency. Having made their diagnosis or assessed the risk, they must also be in a position to provide appropriate treatment, usually a high dose of vitamin A given orally. Of particular importance is routine oral administration of high-dose vitamin A to all measles cases: 200 000 IU for children over two years of age, and half this dose for those under two.

The second health-related action is to treat, and more importantly to control, infectious diseases. Many infectious diseases exacerbate vitamin A deficiency and not infrequently push a vitamin A-deficient child into overt xerophthalmia. Prevention of measles by immunization is a vitamin A intervention. Vitamin A given to a child with measles greatly reduces the risk of death. Infections influence vitamin A status by reducing appetite, thus lowering food intake and vitamin A intake. Viral, bacterial and parasitic intestinal infections may also reduce vitamin A absorption or conversion of carotene to retinol. Infections are made worse by PEM, which almost always is present in children with xerophthalmia.

The third health-related action is to take steps to control disease and promote health, because these might influence vitamin A status. Deworming of children, treatment and control of diarrhoea and respiratory infections, immunizations and improved sanitation and water supplies can all have a role.

The health sector's support of breast-feeding will also help in the control of vitamin A deficiency. Health and nutrition education also contribute. At the community level, it is important that families be motivated to have their children immunized, to seek early treatment, to control infections and to improve personal, food and household hygiene.

Fortification with vitamin A

Fortification is an attractive strategy, especially when compared with medicinal supplementation, because the market system delivers the nutrient. When one or more commonly eaten foods are fortified with vitamin A, behaviour change is not required, and there is no need for a cadre of workers to take vitamin A capsules from house to house or for the major government expenditure that is required for supplementation. Fortification is usually a relatively low-cost intervention for governments. Once in place it needs to be maintained and perhaps mandated for the food industry by legislation. Thereafter it is a relatively sustainable intervention, unlike medicinal supplementation. Monitoring may be all that the authorities need to do.

The methodologies of vitamin A fortification are well tested. Hundreds of different foods have been fortified, mostly in industrialized countries without at-risk people especially in mind. Breakfast cereals of all types (based on maize, rice, wheat or oats), margarine, dairy products and other foods are fortified. Food technologists, who long ago developed methodologies for adding vitamin A to oils and fats, are now able to add the vitamin to many other foods. In developing countries the vehicles used for vitamin A fortification include monosodium glutamate (MSG), sugar, tea and margarine.

In the past, developing countries have tended to seek only one widely consumed food as the vehicle for vitamin A. Because the technology exists to fortify many foods, it now seems preferable to consider fortifying several foods simultaneously to achieve wider coverage. The risk of toxicity needs to be considered, especially where quality assurance is difficult to achieve. Industrialized countries such as the United States fortify many foods and do not report widespread cases of toxicity.

Fortification has not been an easy strategy to initiate and sustain in developing countries. In many countries the major problems of vitamin A deficiency are in children who may consume mainly local foods and very few foods that are centrally processed at a facility where vitamin A could be added. Another problem is the cost of the fortified foods and their affordability for the poorest, high-risk groups.

Nonetheless, national committees given responsibility for developing strategies to control micronutrient deficiencies to meet the goals of the World Summit for Children and the International Conference on Nutrition (ICN) need to give serious consideration to fortification for control of vitamin A deficiency. They may need the assistance of outside expertise, and United Nations agencies are often ready to provide it, but local food scientists and food technologists should be brought into the effort and should begin investigating the possibilities of fortification as a strategy. Thereafter it is necessary to consider the foods widely consumed by the poor that could be fortified. The conditions necessary for fortification described in Chapter 32 require consideration. Other decisions before a trial is undertaken include consideration of what form of vitamin A to use and at what levels, the cost and how and where the trial should be conducted. After the trial, it is necessary to consider whether legislation is needed, how monitoring will be conducted, how quality control will be ensured and who will bear the costs.

Often, if all of a particular food is to be fortified, consumers can bear the cost: if all sugar or all MSG sold in a country is fortified with vitamin A, the price of the product can be raised very slightly per amount purchased. This is usually the best option. In a trial in the Philippines vitamin A and a flow-enhancing substance were added to MSG. The public usually purchased 2.4-g packets of MSG to add to soups, stews or other foods. It was decided to add 0.1 g of the fortificant and to reduce the amount of MSG per packet to 2.3 g to maintain the same packet weight. As the MSG costs more than the fortificant, the packet could thus be sold at the old price. It does no harm if families consume very slightly less salt, sugar or MSG per day.

Fortification of foods with vitamin A has been difficult in several countries mainly because of political constraints or industrial opposition and sometimes because of misinformation by advocates opposed to the use of the food vehicle or to the principle of fortification. Fluoridation of water supplies has received similar opposition.

When vitamin A fortification is implemented consideration might be given to simultaneous fortification of the chosen foods with iron and perhaps other micronutrients.

Medicinal vitamin A supplements
Vitamin A is a fat-soluble vitamin; once absorbed, it is excreted slowly and a good proportion of a high dose remains for some time in the body. Therefore large doses of vitamin A can be given at long intervals.

About 30 years ago it was found that 200 000 IU of vitamin A given to children aged one to five years protects them from vitamin A deficiency for some weeks. Most programmes provide vitamin A every six months, but by then serum vitamin A levels may have returned to deficient levels, so dosing every four months is probably preferable.

Governments using medicinal vitamin A supplementation sometimes attempt universal supplementation to reach all children of a defined age group in the country or perhaps in certain regions of the country. However, this approach has usually failed to reach the objectives set, has proved expensive, has required a complex delivery system, has had coverage rates that have dropped off rapidly after the first dosing and has missed the children most at risk of xerophthalmia. Populous countries with serious vitamin A problems such as India, Indonesia and Bangladesh have attempted nearly universal supplementation at least in some regions of the country. These programmes have no doubt benefited some children, but in general continuing attempts at universal supplementation are not justified. In Indonesia, the major reduction in xerophthalmia undoubtedly resulted more from general improvements in the standard of living of poor people, better household and national food security, improved health services, general improvements in the economy and national attention to nutritional problems than from high-dose medicinal supplements. Major reductions in infant and young child mortality and lowered rates of nutritional marasmus occurred simultaneously with the reduction of xerophthalmia.

Many countries are now targeting vitamin A supplements to particular groups or, more commonly, making them available to those at risk of vitamin A deficiency when they come in contact with the health care system. Free or subsidized supplements are made available to health centres, dispensaries, clinics and hospitals. This strategy has advantages over universal supplementation.

Groups to be targeted for supplementation might include all cases with signs of xerophthalmia, measles, moderate or severe PEM, gastro-enteritis or other selected diseases and conditions. In some countries vitamin A supplements have been tied to other health interventions, for example, child immunizations. This approach should probably be confined to children over six months of age. Supplementation could be combined with regular deworming of young children and with growth monitoring for children who have poor growth. It is also important to give supplements to children in refugee camps or in times of drought or famine. Providing women before pregnancy with vitamin A supplements is not recommended because of the increased risk of birth defects.

When selective supplementation is first introduced it is important to follow the Tanzanian example and train the primary health care workers in the appropriate use of vitamin A supplements. One- or two-day courses, led by a travelling team of trainers, can provide simple literature (e.g. a short hand-out), educate health workers on signs of xerophthalmia and present an agreed list of conditions that warrant vitamin A doses.

In all supplementation programmes there is a need to establish a record system to reduce the possibility that children will get high-dose supplements too frequently and therefore risk toxicity.

Vitamin A supplementation programmes should be used in combination with activities to improve dietary intake of foods rich in vitamin A and with public health measures aimed to reduce vitamin A deficiency. The use of fortification should also be taken into consideration.

The provision of vitamin A supplements to reduce the risk of mortality in groups of children who have no evidence of vitamin A deficiency is not recommended.

PREVENTING IODINE DEFICIENCY DISORDERS

Iodine is the easiest of the three important micronutrient deficiencies to control. The strategy most strongly recommended is not dietary improvement but salt fortification, usually termed salt iodization. Public health measures are not an important strategy for the control of IDD, but medicinal supplementation can have a place in highly endemic areas, especially as a short-term measure while salt iodization is being introduced.

Iodine is an absolutely vital nutrient, but humans require it in tiny amounts. Adults should consume 100 to 200 µg of iodine per day; this amounts to less than a spoonful of iodine per person every 50 years.

Improving diets

Nutrition education and other methods to influence people to change their diets do not work as measures to control IDD because the iodine content of foods depends more on geography than on the foods. The iodine content of plants is much affected by the iodine content of the soil in which they are grown. Thus most foods grown in soils depleted of iodine, found most frequently in highland areas, are deficient in iodine. The vegetables, cereal grains, legumes and other foods grown in iodine-depleted soils high in the Andes or Himalayas have much less iodine than those grown in the lowlands near the mouth of the Amazon River or in the Ganges Delta. Influencing higher consumption of particular local foods is therefore not effective. Seafood and seaweed are rich sources of iodine, because sea water has high levels of the mineral. However, these foods cannot be promoted in areas far from the sea.

Nutrition education and other methods to influence behaviour change can be used to reduce consumption of foods containing goitrogens, such as cabbage and other vegetables of the genus *Brassica* and also some kinds of cassava. In countries where salt is available in both iodized and non-iodized forms, nutrition education and other means should be used to encourage people at risk to use the iodized salt. Nutrition education can also serve to explain the cause of the problem and to stimulate demand for government and other action.

Public health actions

No specific public health measures are used to control IDD. However, good health care and medical services are useful in the diagnosis of goitre and hypothyroidism and in the recognition of cretinism and of metabolic and neurological problems in children whose mothers were iodine deficient during pregnancy. Large nodular goitres that do not respond to iodine or other medical therapy may require surgical excision.

Fortification

It is almost unanimously agreed that fortification is the most effective strategy for the control of IDD. Iodine has successfully been added to water, bread, milk, various sauces and mixed foods, salt and other foods. Recently research has again focused on adding iodine to drinking-water as a means of controlling IDD, but iodizing salt is the major recommended strategy to control IDD by the year 2000.

In temperate climates potassium iodide has been most widely used, but in tropical countries potassium iodate is recommended. It mixes readily with salt at levels from 40 to 100 mg of iodine per kilogram of salt. It is more stable and less likely to be adversely affected by heat and humidity than potassium iodide. The level of fortification varies from country to country and should be based on two considerations: mean levels of salt intake by at-risk populations and other sources of iodine in the diet.

The technology for iodine fortification of salt has been known for a long time, and it is a simple, relatively inexpensive process. It does not change either the appearance (including the colour) or the taste of the salt.

It is believed that once a government manages to get the iodization of salt well established and supported by legislation, it provides by far the best solution to the control of IDD for those who consume the salt, and the control should be sustainable. Many of the industrialized countries have maintained salt iodization for decades and have controlled IDD.

For a variety of reasons, not all of which have been fully elucidated or publicized, iodization of salt in many developing countries, even when legislated, has not been successful. It has not failed because the technology is wrong, but because of other failures in the system. To work, the strategy requires not only political will,

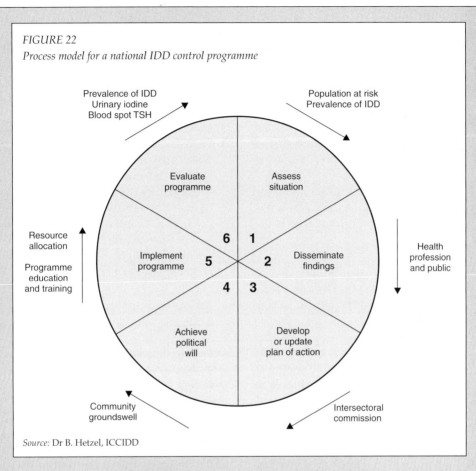

FIGURE 22
Process model for a national IDD control programme

Prevalence of IDD
Urinary iodine
Blood spot TSH

Population at risk
Prevalence of IDD

Evaluate
programme

Assess
situation

Resource
allocation

6 1

Health
profession
and public

Programme
education
and training

Implement
programme 5   2 Disseminate
findings

4 3

Achieve
political
will

Develop
or update
plan of action

Community
groundswell

Intersectoral
commission

Source: Dr B. Hetzel, ICCIDD

Six steps to a national programme of IDD control

Figure 22 illustrates the six steps needed for the development of a national programme of salt iodization.

- It is necessary first to assess the prevalence of goitre and cretinism and the population at risk of IDD, as well as the status of the salt industry and salt importations in the country.
- The findings from the assessment and from other sources must be disseminated to the public, to key government officials and to politicians. Communications should stress the effects of IDD on physical and psychological development of children and the possibility of adverse influence on school performance of children and on work

productivity of all affected people and should emphasize that the deficiency burdens the State with handicapped citizens. This step perhaps needs to go beyond simple dissemination of information and might include strong advocacy.

- The next step is the development of a plan. The plan is much more likely to be implemented if various actors are involved in the planning process: IDD experts, senior staff from the national nutrition institute and from research institutions and representatives from the salt industry and from consumer organizations. In many countries this effort should generate not only a plan

▶

but also an interdisciplinary committee, commission or implementation group with broad representation, a political mandate and proposals for funding (or ensured funding).

- A political decision to move forward to implement the plan is the next essential step. It requires the commitment of funds and perhaps the use of some external financing and expertise.

- Implementation of salt iodization follows, involving activities at the site where salt is prepared and distribution of the salt to the market, combined with education and training.

- Monitoring and evaluation is the last step in what is a continuous cycle. There should be national monitoring of the distribution of the iodized salt, and if possible assessment of the iodine content of the salt at all stages of the food chain from the factory, to the retailer, to the household. There should be attempts to show the effectiveness of the programme in terms of reduction in goitre prevalence, perhaps using sentinel sites which may correspond to those used in the first step. In some countries measurement of urinary iodine and determination of thyroid hormone levels may be feasible as part of the evaluation. Reduction in rates of cretinism may be more difficult to demonstrate because goitres are highly prevalent, whereas cretinism usually is not.

but genuine political and government action; honest and incorruptible people at all levels, from top government officials to lower-level technologists; well-trained personnel with knowledge and expertise; social support for the exercise; and finally adequate funding. Control of IDD is an intervention for which poor countries can usually quite easily get support from organizations such as FAO, UNICEF, WHO, the World Bank and bilateral aid agencies. At US$0.05 per person per year, iodization of salt is a very cheap intervention.

It should be noted that the availability of a solution that produces a colour if added to salt that contains iodine has made it much more feasible to monitor salt locally to make certain that it is iodized. This is, of course, more a qualitative than a quantitative test.

In countries where iodization has been tried but has not seemed to work or where implementation has been fraught with difficulties, it is vital to assess the problems and the resistance points. Salt is a profitable, commercially marketed product, and efforts to develop successful partnerships among governments, the salt industry, retailers and consumers can make salt iodization successful.

Medicinal iodine supplements

Iodine can be provided medicinally to cure IDD, to reduce goitre size and to prevent IDD, including cretinism. Widespread dosing with either oral or injectable iodine has been used in high-risk areas and may be a suitable strategy to reduce IDD quickly while salt iodization is being introduced. Unfortunately, often much more time passes than planned before iodized salt is generally available and consumed.

The preparation most widely available is Lipiodol, which provides 480 mg iodine in 1 ml of oil. It can be either given by injection or taken orally. The doses of iodine in oil, which are much higher than daily physiological needs, are designed to work prophylactically. They provide iodine that lasts for many months. Injections of iodized oil are claimed to prevent IDD for three to four years, and oral iodine capsules for one to two years. Good evaluations have not been done.

In children injections of iodine in oil should be given in the thigh or buttocks. In adults and older children the thigh or buttocks can be used, but the upper arm is better. Oral iodine is often provided in capsules which are swallowed or as a liquid given using a dispenser or syringe which gives a measured dose into the mouth, if possible without touching the lips or tongue.

Oral iodine has many advantages over injectable iodine. It can be given by persons who are not trained to give injections, and therefore it is cheaper to provide. More doses can be given per hour. Above all, there is no risk of spreading acquired immunodeficiency syndrome (AIDS) or other infections which can be spread by syringes and needles that are not sterile.

An alternative to high oral doses of iodine is to provide physiological doses much more frequently. The product usually used is called Lugol's iodine solution. One drop of Lugol's iodine, undiluted, contains about 6 mg of iodine. Lugol's iodine can be diluted so that perhaps 1 mg of iodine is consumed per person per week. If one drop of Lugol's iodine is put in 30 ml of water, then one teaspoonful of dilute solution will provide about 1 mg of iodine.

PREVENTING IRON DEFICIENCY

Iron deficiency anaemia is the most prevalent of the three major micronutrient problems. It is the only one common in both industrialized and developing countries, and it is the most difficult of the three to control. For this reason the goal for the year 2000 is to reduce its prevalence markedly and not to eliminate it. This goal is achievable.

Iron nutrition is more complex than that of some other nutrients (see Chapters 10 and 13). Dietary iron comes in two main forms, namely haem and non-haem iron,

which are not equally well absorbed and utilized; various dietary components adversely influence the absorption of iron from the intestine; and other substances such as vitamin C enhance the absorption of iron.

Unlike iodine and vitamin A deficiency, iron losses are caused by a highly prevalent parasitic infestation: hookworm disease. Some 800 million persons worldwide, mainly in developing countries, harbour hookworms and are therefore at risk of iron deficiency because the hookworms cause blood and iron loss. Schistosomiasis is another parasitic disease that causes loss of blood and therefore loss of iron in the urine or in the faeces. As in vitamin A deficiency, infections also contribute to iron deficiency, but they are not as prevalent or important as hookworm. Thus the treatment and control of hookworm infections and schistosomiasis constitute an important part of the strategy to combat iron deficiency in many tropical and subtropical countries. This tactic is considered below in the section on public health actions.

Improving diets

To reduce the likelihood of iron deficiency, dietary diversity with a good balance of foods is particularly important. A small amount of food of animal origin such as meat, poultry or fish (especially the liver of these animals) is very helpful. While not essential, intake of animal products can greatly improve iron status. Cereals (such as rice, maize and wheat) and legumes provide most of the iron for most people worldwide; however, the iron is in the non-haem form, and absorption of the iron may be relatively poor. Diets promoted to control nutritional anaemias will include increased consumption of iron, but also foods rich in folate and especially vitamin C, which increases iron absorption.

Several of the foods being promoted to help control iron deficiency are the same as those recommended to improve vitamin A status; thus in many countries steps to increase dietary diversity might aim at the same time to improve both iron and vitamin A nutritional status. The promotion of green leafy vegetables and fruits will help both. Green leafy vegetables are relatively rich sources of iron and vitamin C and very rich sources of carotene, so an increase in their consumption will provide more iron, will enhance iron absorption because of the vitamin C and will increase the intake of vitamin A.

Another dietary measure is to reduce the intake at mealtimes of substances such as tannin in tea which decrease iron absorption or utilization.

The iron in breastmilk is very well absorbed, especially when compared with the iron in cows' milk or in products such as infant formula or milk powder made from cows' milk. Thus protection, support and promotion of breastfeeding is a strategy to prevent iron deficiency while the baby is exclusively breastfed, as well as to maintain iron status after the child is put on home foods while breastfeeding continues perhaps for 18 to 24 months. Breastfeeding also delays the return of menstruation, often by eight or more months. Menstruation is a cause of blood and iron loss for women. Thus breastfeeding may help to protect some mothers against iron deficiency when more iron is lost in menstruation than in breastmilk.

Public health actions

A broad range of public health measures and hospital practices contribute to reducing iron deficiency and other nutritional anaemias. The first area is obstetric practices. The traditional midwife often delivers the baby so that after birth it is below, not above, the mother. Also, in traditional practice the umbilical cord is not cut until it stops pulsating, or at least not immediately after delivery as is the practice of Western-trained doctors and obstetricians. When these two traditional practices are followed, considerably more blood enters the baby and red blood cell and haemoglobin levels are increased. They should be standard practices. Putting the baby to the breast in the first 30 minutes after delivery stimulates the uterus to contract, and this also reduces blood loss. Blood loss for the mother means iron loss, and many women go into delivery in an anaemic state. Iron supplementation during pregnancy is discussed below.

Another public health measure of great importance in many countries is the control of hookworm infestations. Other parasites may also contribute to anaemia, and their control will reduce its prevalence. These include schistosomiasis, which is a cause of blood loss in urine if the infection is *Schistosoma haematobium* and in the faeces if the infection is *Schistosoma mansoni* or *Schistosoma japonicum*. Malaria also causes anaemia, mainly a haemolytic anaemia because the parasite destroys red blood cells.

Control of hookworm disease as a means of reducing anaemia has been a relatively neglected strategy until recently. Hookworm can be cured with a single dose of an anthelmintic drug such as albendazole, whereas curing anaemia may require 100 or more doses of iron using ferrous sulphate or some other compound. The delivery system is much simpler and problems of compliance do not exist. Deworming not only prevents chronic blood loss in the stools, but also improves the growth and appetite of children; if appetite improves, food intake including iron and vitamin C intakes may increase. In endemic areas treatment should be given at least once a year, while other public health measures are introduced to control transmission. These include health education and improved sanitation and water supplies.

The prevalence of nutritional anaemias is also influenced by the availability of birth spacing services. Pregnancy and childbirth increase iron needs and therefore contribute to anaemia. Some family planning methods that help prevent pregnancy such as abstinence, condoms or contraceptive pills thus contribute to control of iron deficiency. In contrast, intra-uterine devices (IUDs) in most women increase menstrual and other uterine blood losses and may thus contribute to anaemia.

Iron and folate supplementation, discussed below as a separate strategy, is usually considered a public health action. Nutrition and health education is also important in controlling iron deficiency.

Fortification of foods with iron

Fortification of a wide variety of foods with iron has been feasible and used for many decades. In industrialized countries many different purchased foods are enriched with iron, especially cereal-based products. Unfortunately, fortification is much less used in developing countries where iron deficiency is particularly prevalent.

Fortification offers a very important strategy for control of iron deficiency in almost all countries North and South. If iron deficiency is to be substantially reduced before the year 2000, much more attention needs to be given to fortification, usually combined with the other strategies discussed here. Studies and various dietary surveys may be needed to determine the extent to which iron intake, iron bioavailability and other factors are the major causes of anaemia and to determine which foods are widely consumed and lend themselves to fortification. Several foods may be fortified with iron (whereas it is recommended that iodine should be added only to salt), but careful monitoring and quality assurance are essential.

Iron is not an easy nutrient to add to foods in a form that is well utilized and does not alter the quality of the food. The difficulty is to find a form of iron that is adequately absorbed and yet does not adversely influence the taste, colour or other attributes of the food being fortified. Unfortunately, ferrous sulphate, which is cheap and well absorbed, will often react with food constituents and cause colour changes. Iron phosphate does not have these negative attributes, but it is poorly absorbed. Sodium iron EDTA (ethylenediaminetetraacetate) has recently been used successfully in Guatemala and elsewhere. It seems to lack the negative features of other preparations, and the iron is well absorbed. In Guatemala the vehicle for sodium iron EDTA has been sugar.

Many different foods have been fortified with iron and therefore offer possibilities for any country. These include wheat, wheat flour and bakery products, rice, maize flour, salt, sugar, condiments (such as fish sauce in Thailand) and processed foods. Chocolate-flavoured milk with added iron has been successfully used to control iron deficiency in children in Mexico.

Thirty years ago two research projects in Tanzania, one to investigate the causes of anaemia and the second to evaluate school feeding, used a powdered meat product manufactured in Kenya. This method was more or less abandoned until very recently, when animal haemoglobin was again suggested as a food additive or fortificant. Its advantage is that small amounts of haem iron will greatly increase the absorption of the good quantities of non-haem iron provided by a cereal-based diet.

Nutritionists and public health workers interested in the reduction of iron deficiency should advocate the fortification of foods with iron and perhaps also with vitamin C, folate and vitamin A. Iron fortification in Latin America has been estimated to cost US$0.20 per person per year.

Medicinal iron supplements

In many countries the main strategy for reducing iron deficiency is medicinal iron supplementation. The most common supplementation programmes provide or prescribe iron only for pregnant women. The coverage is sometimes extended to lactating women, but usually only at one postnatal visit soon after delivery. These programmes miss pregnant women who do not attend antenatal clinics, pregnant women before their first visit to the antenatal clinic, most breastfeeding mothers, females at risk prior to their first pregnancy and between pregnancies and all other iron-deficient people (or those at risk of iron deficiency) including children and adult males. Research in Kenya showed that 50 percent of primary school children and 40 percent of adult male road workers had low haemoglobin levels. Clearly iron deficiency is not confined to pregnant women.

Most iron supplementation programmes worldwide use ferrous sulphate, which is very cheap and provides iron in a form that is well absorbed. It is usually given in tablets providing 60 mg of elemental iron, and women are advised to take three tablets per day throughout pregnancy. Sometimes the use of this regime in antenatal clinics is allied with health and nutrition education to influence clinic attendance, in part to reduce anaemia. Ferrous sulphate is often combined with folate; such a product is often supplied to countries by UNICEF.

Problems have been encountered with compliance. It is reported that many women do not take the tablets because of perceived adverse reactions such as constipation, abdominal pain and black stools. Antenatal centres, clinics and health centres often run out of tablets, or health workers fail to give them out even if they are included in essential drug supplies.

There is a need to expand the use of iron supplements beyond pregnant women to include lactating women, females before pregnancy and between pregnancies, premature infants or those with low birth weight and, depending on the circumstances, certain preschool- and school-age children and some male adults.

Two important recent developments may change the way in which iron supplements are recommended. The first, and the less important, of these is the development and availability of slow-release iron capsules or spansules. These are made so that the iron, often ferrous sulphate, is slowly released in the intestine. Their advantages are that one rather than three doses is taken daily and some of the adverse reactions are reduced.

The second change is based on limited studies reported in 1993 which suggest that iron taken once per week is as effective as iron taken three times per day. Therefore it may soon be recommended that pregnant women and all others who can benefit from medicinal iron supplements be advised to take their iron supplement once per week, not three times per day. If one ferrous sulphate tablet providing 60 mg of elemental iron taken each week or every five days proves to be sufficient, iron supplementation will be easier, more acceptable to the public and much cheaper.

The control of malaria will also reduce anaemia, but it is not discussed here because it is not strictly a nutrition intervention. For many tropical countries malaria is the most important health problem, and it is a major cause of child deaths. Malaria does cause anaemia, but unlike the anaemia resulting from hookworm infection, it is not strictly a nutritional anaemia. In heavy infections, with massive parasitaemia, malaria parasites rupture millions of red blood cells. This causes haemolysis, the haemoglobin being released into the blood serum. Treatment of cases of malaria and the control of malaria transmission deserve a very high priority. Textbooks of tropical medicine discuss malaria and its control in detail.

SIMULTANEOUS ATTENTION TO SEVERAL MICRONUTRIENT DEFICIENCIES

There is great merit in combining actions to deal with several deficiencies at the same time. In particular, basic action to improve household access to and consumption of varied and adequate diets will help to control all micronutrient deficiencies. The fact that multiple benefits are achievable through food-based strategies is another reason why such interventions as home gardening, improved local food processing and nutrition education are the approaches of choice.

The following three topics also deserve further consideration.

Relationship of vitamin A to iron

For a long time it has been known that vitamin A deficiency is associated with anaemia and that it causes anaemia in animals. Now there is overwhelming evidence from many developing countries that vitamin A deficiencies are an important cause of anaemia in humans. In societies where vitamin A deficiency is prevalent, iron deficiency is almost always prevalent as well. Research suggests that where both are prevalent it is necessary to provide both iron and vitamin A supplements to achieve good rises in haemoglobin levels. Therefore in many developing countries provision of vitamin A supplements should be included in programmes to provide iron supplements for pregnant women and others.

Parasitic infections and iodine utilization

A recent study showed that subjects with intestinal parasitic infections given oral iodized oil absorbed the iodine less efficiently. It is suggested that in areas with a high prevalence of intestinal parasites, deworming should precede the provision of oral iodine supplements.

Supplementation with several micronutrients

In industrialized countries prevalent micronutrient deficiencies were generally controlled by a combination of improved food supplies and rising incomes and levels of education. However, some conditions, such as rickets, were also improved through the use of cod-liver oil and similar supplements. Many of these contained dietary vitamins D and A and other micronutrients. Parents either obtained them through the health services or purchased them in pharmacies or in grocery stores. Then at home children were regularly dosed with the supplement. It is possible, and trials are being initiated, to produce a nutrient mixture as a flavouring for milk or to be mixed with water. These mixtures, given daily or weekly, could provide approximately the recommended dietary allowances for iron, vitamin A, iodine and other nutrients known to be deficient in a community. If these flavourings, like cod-liver oil 60 years ago, can be made available through both the health services and the market, parents could be empowered to prevent micronutrient deficiencies in their children by regular dosing at home.

Chapter 40

Family feeding, group feeding and street foods

Most of the food that people consume in rural areas is eaten at home. This is also true in many urban areas, although street foods or foods eaten in stalls are providing an increasing percentage of food for urban dwellers. Inadequate family diets and family feeding are the fundamental causes of malnutrition in Africa, Asia, Latin America and elsewhere. For those who live away from home, particularly in institutions such as boarding schools, prisons or refugee camps, malnutrition or undernutrition may result from poor institutional diets.

This chapter deals briefly with food procurement, group feeding of different kinds and street foods. More information is available in books and meeting reports on each of the different methods of feeding described here (see Bibliography).

Food procurement refers to people's means of gaining access to the food they consume. Chapters 2 and 35, dealing with food production and food security, discuss the major methods by which humans in normal life obtain the food that they consume in their households. Also discussed are difficulties that make people food insecure and suggestions for improving food security at the national and household levels.

In households, the two most important ways of procuring food are own food production, most commonly on small farms in rural areas, and purchase of food using money earned from work at home or outside the home or from sale of farm-produced products (termed cash crops,

although they may be food crops such as cereals, fruits and vegetables put up for sale). These two methods of food procurement are not discussed here because they have been covered in Chapters 2 and 25 and elsewhere in this book. Families or households may also procure food in other ways; these include take-home food donations, rations provided in exchange for work (food-for-work) and provision of supplementary foods to vulnerable groups. Foods may also be provided to households by friends or families as gifts or donations.

This chapter first deals with home feeding and then describes situations in which people obtain food other than through home production, food purchases or gifts or consume food outside the household or home. Many of these situations are characterized as "group feeding". The general and most important categories covered here are:

- home feeding;
- institutional feeding, including school feeding;
- vulnerable group feeding;
- food-for-work and take-home rations;
- emergency feeding;
- street foods and related feeding outside the home.

FEEDING THE FAMILY

Earlier chapters have discussed the prevalent problem of household food insecurity, both temporary and chronic. Food-insecure households are those where there is often an insufficient amount of food to satisfy the energy requirements, and also the energy wants or desirable allowances, of family members. There are other households, perhaps the majority, where for most of the year there is adequate food to assuage hunger, to fill everyone's stomach and at most times to satisfy energy wants. However, this "sufficient" food may comprise predominantly bulky, carbohydrate-rich foods and be very low in micronutrient-rich foods. As described elsewhere, bulk and insufficient frequency of feeding may result in energy intakes too low for requirements of young children, even if the food is available. In addition, poor appetites may reduce intake. These problems are discussed in other chapters.

Different family members have different nutrient requirements which depend to some extent on age, gender, size, activity and other factors (see Annex 1). Meals should provide adequate food to ensure that each family member receives all that is necessary to meet his or her nutrient requirements.

Cereals such as maize, rice, millet or wheat, if lightly milled, will usually provide both sufficient energy and B vitamins, although in the case of maize not enough to prevent pellagra. Foods other than the staple must provide the extra protein, fat, calcium, iron and vitamins A and C required. Africans, Asians and Latin Americans usually obtain adequate vitamin D from the action of sunlight on the skin. Iron may be almost sufficient in quantity from staple foods but is not in an easily utilizable form (see Chapters 10 and 13).

The extra protein required may come from protein-rich vegetable foods such as beans, groundnuts, cowpeas, soybeans, lentils or other legumes. Some may come from animal products such as meat, fish, milk and eggs. If the main foodstuff in the diet is cooking bananas, cassava, sweet potatoes or some other starchy food, then an even greater quantity of additional protein is necessary than in a diet based on a cereal grain.

A mixture of vegetable foods eaten at one meal, such as a cereal and a legume (e.g. maize or millet and cowpeas) or a root, a cereal and a legume (e.g. cassava, sorghum and groundnuts), provides better-quality protein than larger quantities of a single vegetable food would; the mixture usually contains all the essential amino acids, whereas a single cereal, root or legume is usually deficient in one or more of the essential amino acids.

A diet containing good quantities of legumes and occasional animal protein foods in addition to a cereal, banana or root staple probably satisfies the family's requirements for energy, iron, protein and B vitamins. It also provides fat if the legumes include good quantities of groundnuts or soybeans or if the animal protein consists of fatty meat, fish, milk or eggs.

Such a diet is lacking only in vitamins A and C, which can best be supplied by fresh fruit and vegetables. Dark green leaves also provide much iron and some calcium.

Every family should be advised to put the above principles into practice so that all its members have a satisfactory diet. The variety so important for a balanced diet (Photo 81) can be achieved if family members consume daily, or better still at every meal, a reasonable quantity of food from each column in Table 40, with the main bulk of the diet provided by the staple food. A certain amount of fat is also essential. This may be cooking oil (Photo 82) or solid fat, or it may be obtained in the diet from milk, groundnuts, etc. If the main staple of the diet is a highly refined cereal, as opposed to a home-pounded or lightly milled one, then extra vitamin B-containing foods should be consumed. Figure 23, taken from FAO's *Food and nutrition in the management of group feeding programmes* (FAO, 1993b), illustrates how to make balanced meals.

TABLE 40

Categories of foods needed for a balanced diet

Staple foods	Energy-rich foods	Protein-rich foods	Foods containing vitamins and minerals
Cereals	Butter	**Vegetable origin**	**Fresh fruits and**
Maize	Ghee	Beans	**vegetables**
Millet	Lard	Peas	Dark green leafy
Rice	Margarine	Groundnuts	vegetables
Wheat	Oil	Soybeans	Orange- and yellow-
Teff	Sugar	Lentils	coloured fruits and
		Cowpeas	vegetables
Starchy foods			Citrus fruits
Bananas		**Animal origin**	Guavas
Cassava		Meat	
Potatoes		Fish	
Yams		Eggs	
		Milk and milk products	
		Insects	

Note: Appropriate spices, herbs, onion and salt can be added to increase the flavour and palatability of the diet.

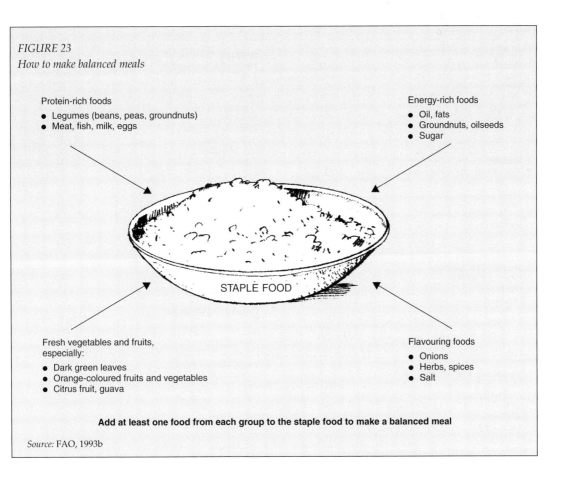

FIGURE 23

How to make balanced meals

Protein-rich foods
- Legumes (beans, peas, groundnuts)
- Meat, fish, milk, eggs

Energy-rich foods
- Oil, fats
- Groundnuts, oilseeds
- Sugar

STAPLE FOOD

Fresh vegetables and fruits, especially:
- Dark green leaves
- Orange-coloured fruits and vegetables
- Citrus fruit, guava

Flavouring foods
- Onions
- Herbs, spices
- Salt

Add at least one food from each group to the staple food to make a balanced meal

Source: FAO, 1993b

Table 41 gives seven examples of family diets based on the above information. In each instance the amount given is that which should be eaten by an average man. The amounts can be varied for women and children by using the tables in Annexes 1 and 3. Extras such as spices, tea and other beverages are not included, since, although they make the diet more palatable, they add little of nutritive value. The localities refer to places where this type of diet might be eaten; the diets are not average diets in these areas, but are suggestions as to what would constitute a satisfactory diet.

Where foods of animal origin are not often available, the quality of the protein in the diet can be improved by providing a mixture or variety of vegetable products at each meal. Thus if a household has maize and beans available it is far better nutritionally to eat some of both at each meal rather than to eat maize for two weeks and then beans for two weeks. Mixtures of vegetable products are frequently eaten by many people in Africa and Latin America. Examples, of which some are traditional dishes, include:

• rice and bean stew;

TABLE 41

Seven examples of reasonably balanced diets (quantities for an adult male)

Food	Amount (g/person/day)	Food	Amount (g/person/day)
Philippines		**Santiago, Chile**	
Rice	500	White wheat bread	400
Fish	100	Rice	100
Beans	150	Eggs	30
Green leafy vegetables	100	Meat	100
Mango	100	Carrots	100
Coconut	50	Green leaves	50
Oil	15	Butter or margarine	25
Salt	15	Fresh bananas	100
		Milk (in coffee)	60
Uganda		Sugar	30
Plantains (cooking bananas)	1 000	Salt	10
Sweet potatoes	200		
Meat	50	**Rural Mozambique**	
Beans	150	Millet	400
Sweet potato leaves	150	Cassava	200
Tomatoes	50	Sour milk	150
Oil	15	Tomatoes	100
Salt	10	Cassava leaves	100
		Groundnuts	50
Mexico City, Mexico		Bambara nuts	75
Maize (as tortillas)	500	Baobab fruit	30
Meat	50	Salt	10
Beans	100		
Tomatoes	100	**Coastal village, India**	
Oranges	100	Rice	500
Onions	50	Fish	100
Oil	15	Lentils (dhal)	150
Salt	10	Papaya	150
		Vegetables (mixed)	200
Masailand, East Africa		Groundnuts	75
Milk	2 000	Oil	20
Animal blood	100	Salt	10
Maize	150		
Wild leaves	100		
Wild fruit	100		
Bananas	200		
Salt	15		

- maize tortillas and beans;
- maize, beans and green leafy vegetables;
- baked sweet potatoes served with peas or beans and amaranth leaves;
- rice and lentil dhal;
- sorghum gruel and bananas with groundnut paste;
- millet served with onion, yam, peas and tomato relish;
- baked beans on wheat toast;
- plantains with beans and vegetables.

The various foods do not have to be physically mixed together, but can just as well be eaten separately at the same meal.

Family feeding of infants and young children

The role of various nutrients in the diets of infants and young children has been described elsewhere in this book. The importance of introducing foods to supplement breastfeeding when an infant is six months of age has been stressed. Table 42 gives some examples of dishes suitable for infants and young children. There are of course innumerable other recipes. For each family the foods used will depend on local customs, food preferences, food availability and cost.

As can be seen from the recipes in Table 42, a wire sieve is useful in preparing infant foods. It serves to transform a solid or lumpy food into one of fine, soft consistency suitable for a child with few or no teeth. If a sieve is not available, one can easily be made by punching 20 to 30 holes in the bottom of an empty tin with a medium-sized nail (Figure 24). This makes a perfectly adequate sieve, but it should be carefully washed after each use.

Many adult dishes, after being put through a sieve, are suitable and good for young children. It must be remembered, however, that spices, especially those that have a burning hot taste, are unsuitable. Dishes containing curry powder, hot peppers, etc. should be avoided.

In this book no attempt is made to produce a weaning chart or daily menus for children of different ages. Tables of this kind tend to be too dogmatic and may prevent both teachers and mothers from deciding for themselves what is the desirable food in a particular instance. It is better that each family and each infant be treated individually as long as the diet is based on sound nutritional principles. Advice on diets should always be realistic and adapted to the foods most commonly used and most easily available.

As has been stated, breastfeeding should, under most circumstances, continue for as long as possible. An infant who has developed satisfactorily should begin supplementary feeding by the sixth month. A gruel of the local staple with added milk is an excellent food on which to start mixed feeding. If milk is not available, then any legume can be used instead. The supplementary food should at first be given in one feeding a day using a spoon and cup. After a week or two, when the child has become accustomed to semi-solid food, other dishes can be introduced. Next might come mashed fruit (e.g. mashed papaya) or vegetables, or possibly tomato or orange juice. A week or two later, some different foods, such as groundnut soup or bean mush (see Table 42), can be tried while the others are continued. At this stage, semi-solid food might form part of two feedings a day.

By the end of the first year, all or any of the types of food in the recipes can have been tried, while breastfeeding continues. The infant should also by this time have been given the experience of trying many of the adult dishes of the family, with the exception only of obviously unsuitable foods such as peppery curries and alcoholic beverages.

During the period from 12 to 24 months,

TABLE 42

Dishes suitable for weaning and for toddlers and young children

Dish	Ingredients	Method
Gruel with beans or groundnuts	Flour made from maize, millet, cassava or rice Bean mush or groundnut soup (see recipes below)	Prepare a gruel in the customary way. While it is simmering in the pot, add bean mush or thick groundnut soup. Stir vigorously. Cook for 2 to 5 minutes. Remove the gruel from the fire or stove. Cool.
Gruel with sour (or fresh) milk or dried skimmed milk (DSM)	Flour from maize, millet, cassava, rice, etc. 1/2 cup sour (or fresh) milk or 1 tablespoon DSM powder	Prepare a gruel in the customary way. While it is simmering in the pot, add sour (or fresh) milk or DSM. Stir and serve when sufficiently cool. (Include salt and/or sugar if desired.)
Papaya mush or banana mush	1 papaya or 1 banana 4 tablespoons fresh or sour milk or 1 tablespoon DSM (optional)	Take a slice of ripe papaya, or a peeled banana. Mash it in bowl or on plate. Add milk or DSM powder, if available. Mix and serve.
Amaranth or other green leafy vegetables with lentils	Handful of amaranth or other edible leaves 1 tablespoon family dhal (lentils) 1/2 teaspoon oil (optional)	Wash amaranth leaves and remove stalks. Boil until leaves are tender (about 5 minutes). Cut up leaves finely. Mix heated dhal and leaf mush together, adding 1/2 teaspoon oil, if available. Serve alone or mixed with gruel.
Vegetable mush	Handful edible leaves 1 carrot (optional) 1 tomato (optional)	Take some cooked green leaves and a cooked carrot, if available, from family pot. Rub through sieve. Take ripe tomato, if available, and rub through sieve. Mix and serve alone or mixed with cooked mashed potato or cereal gruel.
Groundnut soup	1/2 cup groundnuts Pinch of salt	Roast groundnuts until pale brown. Remove skins. Crush groundnuts with pestle and mortar (or on a stone). Add salt. Mix with water to form paste. Cook for 10 minutes in small quantity of water. Serve alone or mixed with gruel.
Bean (or other legume) mush	50 g beans (or other legume)	Soak beans overnight. Boil in the usual way. Mash with fork or spoon. Force through sieve, removing skins. Feed with maize or other gruel.
Groundnut and banana mush	1 banana 1 handful groundnuts	Roast groundnuts and remove skins. Boil or roast banana. Put groundnuts and banana in mortar and pound until mush has a fine, smooth consistency.
Rice and lentil gruel	50 g lentils (or other legume) 120 g rice	Boil lentils or beans, or take a portion of beans cooked for adults. Remove skins and crush through sieve. Take cooked rice from adult meal. Mash with wooden spoon until soft and creamy. Add beans and mix.
Millet with beans or cowpeas	120 g millet (or other cereal) flour 50 g beans or cowpeas Pinch of salt	Cook finely ground millet flour into gruel or thin porridge. Soak beans overnight and simmer in water with salt. Crush through sieve. Mix with millet gruel and serve.

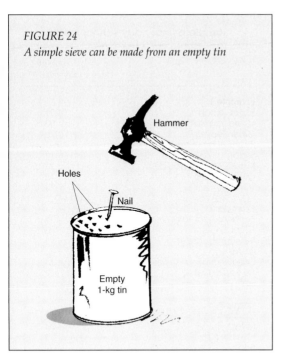

FIGURE 24
A simple sieve can be made from an empty tin

Hammer

Holes

Nail

Empty
1-kg tin

the infant can cope with many family dishes, but he or she should receive more frequent meals than adults and should have proportionately larger quantities of dietary fat, proteins and some other nutrients (see Annex 1). A number of the suggested recipes can continue to supplement the family food and breastmilk that the toddler receives.

After the second year breastfeeding has usually ceased and extra energy- and nutrient-rich foods are important. The child is now able to cope with most of the family food but must get more than would appear to be the child's fair share. Extra dishes such as some of those suggested in Table 42 are highly desirable during this preschool period. The young child may need more frequent feeding (four or more meals a day) than the adult members of the family. Meals consisting mainly of starchy foods can be made more energy dense by the addition of a little oil or fat.

INSTITUTIONAL FEEDING

There are many types of institutions where people receive food. The most important of these are schools, because at any one time many hundreds of millions of children worldwide are attending school. Most attend for part of the day at primary and secondary schools, where meals may or may not be provided. At boarding schools, where children sleep overnight, meals should be provided to supply all the nutrients needed for health and growth. Nutrition of school-age children and ways in which children acquire food at school have been discussed in Chapter 6.

In the examples of institutional menus given below (Tables 43 to 48), the amounts of food are roughly designed to meet the likely minimum energy and micronutrient needs of the particular group in the institution. Thus, for example, larger amounts of food are suggested for older than for younger children. The quantities of the more expensive protein-rich foods of animal origin and of some other items such as sugar, fat and tea are not based mainly on nutrient requirements. These amounts may reflect the likely budget of the institution and the level in society of the usual participants. For example, the nutrient requirements of a 50-kg male adult in a prison and a man of the same weight in an army camp may be identical, but the sample diets suggest more meat for the army trainee than for the prisoner, as the former is likely to be given a more expensive, more "luxurious" diet.

Clearly, in institutional feeding the main dish should be based on what is normally eaten in the country. This may be boiled rice, maize tortillas, *ugali* (maize porridge similar to grits, eaten in Africa) or wheat pasta.

In all of the institutional diets for which examples are given below, small additions of beverages or foods that are locally liked or traditionally eaten can be added. In many parts of the world such additions might include tea, coffee or other beverages. Another addition might be a particular relish, spice or other product to make the food more tasty or palatable, such as salsa, chutney, jam, honey or tomato sauce. Many dishes made in particular countries need or benefit from certain additional foods such as tomato paste, garlic, green peppers or relish. These items, as far as availability and cost allow, should be included.

Nursery schools, day-care centres and kindergartens

Many countries have an increasing number of nursery schools, day-care centres and kindergartens which are established as pre-primary schools or where children from one to six years of age can be left while their mothers work. Children attending such institutions should receive a daily meal consisting of food rich in those nutrients likely to be deficient in the home diet. Toddlers could with advantage be supplied with any of the protein-rich dishes given in Table 42.

Older preschool children should be given a properly balanced midday meal similar to those suggested below for children in primary schools.

Every effort should be made to provide nutrition education for the mothers who bring their children to these institutions. Mothers could be asked to help with meal preparations and would thus get first-hand experience in preparing nutritious dishes for young children.

Day schools

The importance of a midday meal at day schools (Photo 83) and of a good balanced diet at boarding schools has been discussed in Chapter 6. Some suggestions or examples for a suitable midday meal at a primary day school are given in Table 43.

For a secondary day school the same

TABLE 43
Sample primary day school meals

Food	Amount (g/person/meal)
Example 1	
Maize or rice	200
Mixed vegetables	50
Green leaves	25
Beans or groundnuts	100
Sugar	10
Milk (full-cream powder)	10
Oil (red palm)	10
Salt	5
Example 2	
Bananas (plantains) or potatoes	400
Groundnuts	50
Mixed vegetables	50
Beans	50
Dried skimmed milk powder (DSM)	20
Oil (red palm)	10
Salt	5
Example 3	
Cassava flour	150
Millet	100
Meat or fish	50
Beans	100
Green leaves	75
Fruit	100
Oil (red palm or other)	10
Salt	5
Example 4	
Bread	150
Potatoes	150
Tomatoes	75
Onions	50
Beans	100
Fruit	75
Oil	10
Salt	5

foodstuffs could be provided, but the amount of each item should be increased by about 25 percent because older, taller and heavier children have increased nutrient requirements (see Annex 1).

It is not true that for a school lunch to be nutritious it must include a hot dish. Heat has nothing to do with nutritive quality. A cold lunch may be as nutritious as a hot lunch. It is the food served that determines the nutritive value of the meal.

School feeding or a midday school meal or snack can be linked with supporting activities. In some feeding programmes parents can have a role, either a minor one in supporting school meals or a major one in organizing and managing school feeding. In Chapter 6 the link between school feeding and small-scale food production activities was mentioned. These activities are usually organized around school gardens which can produce nutritious foods for school meals or for sale. Other activities might include raising small animals (poultry, rabbits, pigeons, guinea-pigs, etc.) or keeping a school orchard or school fish pond.

School feeding and school food production can be linked very usefully with classroom activities relating to biology, health, home economics, geography, mathematics and agriculture. For example, practical lessons such as how to weigh and calculate amounts of foods in school meals and how to determine area and crop yields of school gardens can link mathematics to nutrition.

School feeding can be associated with school health services, which do not exist for many primary schools. It is useful to provide health examinations, some level of primary health care and first aid, to follow children's height and weight and to test their sight and hearing. A way should be found to make certain that children are immunized. There is also now beginning to be a movement to see that schoolchildren if necessary are regularly dewormed (where intestinal parasites are prevalent) and are provided with nutrient supplements such as iron, vitamin A and iodine.

There are many different reasons for and benefits of school feeding. These include preventing children from feeling hungry, which also helps them concentrate and benefit from classes; providing extra nutrients to improve children's nutritional status; improving attendance; and perhaps making it easier for mothers to work away from home, to be more productive in their fields or to increase their income.

Increasing data from research suggest that short-term hunger in schoolchildren who are not fed adequately before or at school adversely influences school performance, including learning and performance on psychological development tests.

Schoolchildren, even quite young ones, can assist school feeding in a number of ways. They can help bring water to the feeding site if there is no running water at the school; carry wood or other fuel to the school; help in food preparation, in maintaining good food hygiene and in keeping the feeding area and utensils clean; and participate in school garden or small animal production activities.

Boarding schools

Four examples of suitable boarding school diets are given in Table 44. The quantities of food given are suitable daily amounts for a secondary school pupil; these quantities should be divided up and served as three meals. Items such as meat, for which small daily amounts are indicated, may be given perhaps twice a week in larger amounts. For example, 20 g of meat per day make 140 g per week, which can be given in two equal portions of 70 g on Sunday and Wednesday.

In a primary boarding school, the same foods could be provided but with an overall reduction in quantity of about 25 percent because younger children have lower requirements than older children.

Hospitals

Hospital patients usually spend most of their time in bed. Their needs for energy are therefore lower than those of active persons of the same sex, age and weight. However, some may have increased nutritional requirements. These include patients who entered hospital undernourished; those who are pregnant or lactating or have recently had a baby; and those with diseases that require a special diet or extra nutrients. A generally suitable diet is shown in Table 45.

TABLE 44
Sample secondary boarding school diets

Food	Amount (g/person/day)
Example 1	
Maize, rice or wheat (or mixture)	600
Beans	150
Groundnuts	100
Meat	20
Dried fish	20
Leafy vegetables	150
Fruit	100
Sugar	30
Dried skimmed milk (DSM) powder	20
Oil (red palm)	20
Salt	10
Example 2	
Bananas (plantains)	600
Potatoes	400
Rice	150
Meat	20
Beans	150
Groundnuts	50
Mixed vegetables	150
Fruit	100
Sugar	50
DSM powder	50
Oil (red palm)	10
Salt	10
Example 3	
Cassava flour	300
Millet	150
Green leaves	150
Fruit	100
Cowpeas	150
Groundnuts	100
Fish	50
DSM powder	50
Oil (red palm)	10
Salt	10
Example 4	
Rice	300
Potatoes	150
Maize	100
Bread	150
Meat	50
Eggs	30
Vegetables (mixed)	150
Margarine	50
Sugar	50
Fruit	150
Lentils	75
Groundnuts	50
Jam	30
Oil (red palm)	20
Milk (fresh)	0.5 litre
Salt	10

Agricultural estates and industrial enterprises

In some cases large numbers of agricultural and industrial workers spend six to ten hours working some distance from eating establishments. Where possible, a midday meal should be made available. The employer should decide, in consultation with the workers, whether the meal should be provided free, at subsidized prices or in a canteen where foods are sold more or less at cost. Free or subsidized meals will encourage as many workers as possible to partake. Canteen meals for workers may be expected to result in a higher output of work, a healthier, more contented labour force and reduced absenteeism. It is therefore often an economic advantage for an employer to provide such a meal.

Other institutions

A prison should provide a completely balanced diet suitable for persons doing heavy work. The diet should be cheap and simple. In some countries the scale of prison rations is laid down by law. In the United Republic of Tanzania each prisoner receives one 50-mg tablet of niacin per week in addition to the prescribed diet, to prevent the occurrence of pellagra. A suitable prison diet is shown in Table 46.

TABLE 45
Sample hospital diet

Food	Amount (g/person/day)
Bread	100
Maize	200
Rice	150
Meat or fish	100
Vegetables	150
Fruit	150
Legumes	100
Milk (full-cream powder)[a]	75
Oil	20
Salt	10

[a] Or 0.5 litre fresh milk.

A diet that might be served in the army is shown in Table 47, and a diet for a training college of health, agriculture or police work is shown in Table 48.

VULNERABLE GROUP FEEDING

Throughout this book there are examples of groups within the population who are especially vulnerable to malnutrition and particular deficiencies. In general, the vulnerable are usually defined as children aged six months to six years who are undernourished and women who are pregnant and lactating. The term "vulnerable" is better used, however, if it is applied to those at special risk of malnutrition.

Thus vulnerable children may include those who do not have evidence of malnutrition but are at risk for any of numerous different reasons; for example, they may include children from very poor families, children from large families with narrow birth spacing and in some cultures female children from a low caste. Similarly, it might be better to say that women of child-bearing age, rather than just pregnant and lactating women, are at risk, and then again to find criteria such as poverty, female-headed households and other factors that place them at risk. Other vulnerable groups include older people if not cared for by an extended family, individuals with mental illness and orphans who are not cared for by relatives. Some chronic diseases such as tuberculosis and acquired immunodeficiency syndrome (AIDS) make subjects very vulnerable to malnutrition.

Supplementary feeding of young at-risk children may be done at feeding centres to which mothers take the children or by providing take-home food supplements or even rations for a complete diet. Research

TABLE 46
Sample prison diet

Food	Amount (g/person/day)
Maize, rice, wheat or millet	750
Beans	150
Vegetables	150
Groundnuts	100
Meat	20
Sweet potatoes	50
Fruit	100
Salt	10
Oil	5

TABLE 47
Sample army diet

Food	Amount (g/person/day)
Maize, rice or wheat products	400
Bread	100
Potatoes	400
Beans	100
Vegetables (mixed)	150
Onions	25
Groundnuts	100
Fruit (fresh)	200
Fruit (dry)	50
Meat	250
Milk (fresh)	0.5 litre
Sugar	60
Oil	50
Salt	10

TABLE 48
Training college (health, agriculture, police) diet

Food	Amount (g/person/day)
Rice	250
Bread (whole-meal)	200
Maize	200
Potatoes	200
Beans	100
Groundnuts	50
Onions	25
Green leaves	50
Vegetables (mixed)	75
Fruit (mixed)	100
Sugar	60
Meat	100
Fish	25
Eggs	30
Butter	25
Milk (full-cream powder)	25
Oil (red palm)	25
Salt	10

Food substitutions

In the parts of this chapter dealing with home and institutional feeding, examples are given of specific diets or suggested menus. In each of the diets or menus, specific foods are mentioned as examples. They can be substituted, in many instances, by foods of equivalent nutritive value. Substitution may be desirable if the alternative food is preferred, is cheaper or is more easily available. Tables 49 to 51 give equivalents to suggest how much in weight of a particular food can be consumed to provide nutrients equivalent to those provided by a given amount of another food.

Table 49 suggests the amount in grams of some common foods to provide 1 000 kcal of energy. Table 50 gives the amount to provide 10 g of protein, and Table 51 to provide 200 µg of vitamin A.

To find equivalents for other nutrients or the nutrient content of an institutional diet described here, readers can make the calculations themselves using the table of nutrient content of selected foods given in Annex 3.

TABLE 49
Amount in grams to provide approximately 1 000 kcal

Food	Amount (g)
Rice	325
Maize meal	325
Millet meal	350
Wheat flour	350
Dried cassava	350
Bread	500
Plantains	800
Yams	1 000
Sweet potatoes	1 000
Potatoes	1 350

TABLE 50
Amount in grams of selected uncooked foods to provide approximately 10 g of protein

Food	Amount (g)
Dried fish	16
Dried skimmed milk (DSM)	27
Soybeans	28
Winged beans	30
Dried groundnuts	32
Fish (sea- or freshwater)	40
Meat (beef, mutton, goat or poultry)	40
Kidney beans	42
Cowpeas	45
Chickpeas or pigeon peas	50
Eggs	75
Cereals (rice, wheat or maize)	100
Potatoes	500
Plantains	1 000
Cassava	1 200

TABLE 51
Amount in grams of selected foods to provide approximately 200 µg of vitamin A

Food	Amount (g)
Vegetables	
Carrots	6
Leaves, dark green (spinach)	30
Pumpkin	124
Tomatoes	160
Leaves, light green (cabbage)	330
Fruits	
Mango	25
Papaya	99
Lemon	6 600
Animal products	
Beef liver	7
Human breastmilk	310
Cows' milk (whole)	646
Beef flesh	1 100

on supplementary feeding has shown that often some of the food taken home is consumed by others and not all by the target child. If the household is food insecure, however, this food may help all members. Consideration might be given to providing for more than just the nutritional needs of the child.

Supplementary feeding has been used in growth monitoring programmes where the food is provided only to children under five years of age who have evidence of malnutrition. This approach has been used in Tamil Nadu, India. When the children show a defined degree of growth improvement, they become ineligible for further feeding. The approach is claimed to be very successful in rehabilitating children. However, feeding only malnourished children, rather than children at risk, constitutes a curative approach, whereas a preventive one would in general be preferable.

Supplementary feeding of children is much more likely to have an impact on nutritional status of populations if combined with sustainable agricultural development and efforts to reduce poverty, allied with primary health care, immunizations, education about treatment for diarrhoea and deworming.

Supplementary feeding has possible disadvantages which need to be appreciated. Families who receive food for their children may become overly dependent on free food and may not make adequate efforts to improve home food security. If rations are used as an incentive to motivate attendance at growth monitoring centres, then if supplements are not available, attendance might decline.

The same general principles apply to supplementary feeding of women or any other group. Some programmes provide dietary supplements to all pregnant and lactating women. Foods likely to reduce anaemia are of particular importance. Medicinal supplements of iron, or iron and folate, are often also provided. If women are to be selected on the basis of risk, then the first criterion should be the level of poverty. Other risk factors include teenage pregnancy; death or malnutrition of a previous child; chronic disease such as tuberculosis or AIDS; low weight for height

in small women; and poor social support, especially in female-headed households.

Supplementary feeding should not be done in isolation. Primary health care needs to be offered and must be easily accessible; nutrition and health education should be provided; and consideration needs to be given as to whether to refer mothers to family planning services.

FOOD-FOR-WORK AND TAKE-HOME FOOD RATIONS

Food-for-work, where food allocations are made in return for work rather than as free donations, is often used in food emergencies such as drought or famine. It was discussed in Chapter 24 in reference to starvation, famine and refugees. Food-for-work can also be used in development programmes and other situations.

Increasingly food-for-work has been used as full or partial payment of wages, often for work done on public works programmes planned by a government; as an incentive for voluntary labour; and sometimes as a budgetary support for a developing country. Food-for-work is a strategy often used by the World Food Programme (WFP).

The kinds of work undertaken have usually involved labour-intensive road building projects; environmental projects, including tree planting and forestry; and projects to open up new land. Usually these projects are carried out in areas with food shortages. They have both nutritional and non-nutritional objectives: to help prevent food insecurity, hunger and malnutrition, and to get good public work done. The internationally supported food-for-work programmes are usually also seen as economic assistance to developing countries.

Where food is given in exchange for work, it is highly desirable to provide some level of primary health care for workers and to give advice on nutrition, on how to prepare foods not normally eaten by those receiving the food and on what other foods besides the donated rations would help balance the diet.

Each programme establishes the amounts and kinds of foods to be given. These decisions should be based on sensible criteria and concern for local food habits. Often 2 100 kcal are provided per person, but food needs to be provided to satisfy family needs, not just the workers' needs. Often five daily rations of 2 100 kcal per day worked are provided as a family ration.

A typical ration would provide 400 to 500 g of cereal flour or rice, 25 to 50 g of legumes or pulses and 25 to 35 g of oil or fat. If available, about 20 g of meat or fish might be added. Fresh perishable foods are not usually included in the rations, and it is important that workers and their families supplement the ration with fruits and vegetables. There is some debate about the energy level; a higher level than 2 100 kcal may sometimes be advocated.

EMERGENCY FEEDING

Emergency feeding in conditions of famine and civil disturbances and in refugee camps is described in detail in Chapter 24.

STREET FOODS

Although the term "street foods" has only recently become widely used, the sale and consumption of food on city streets goes back many centuries. Now street foods (Photos 84 to 86) are recognized as having a very large role in urban food consumption, especially in developing countries and for the poor and middle classes. FAO studies have shown that in some countries street foods provide a very significant proportion of total food intake for many people. It is surprising that the nutritional, health, social and economic impact of street foods has not been studied or appreciated until relatively recently. FAO has had a leading role in drawing attention to the importance of street foods; the Organization has held conferences on the topic and provided advice to countries on appropriate measures to make these foods safer for the consumer. Because of its expertise in this area, FAO can provide very useful advice and assistance to member countries. A good deal of the following discussion has drawn on FAO publications and papers relating to street foods (see especially FAO, 1990a; Dawson and Canet, 1991).

FAO has defined street foods as follows: "Street foods are ready-to-eat foods and beverages prepared and/or sold by vendors especially in streets and other similar public places". This definition is now widely accepted. Street foods are mainly sold in urban areas, but they are also prepared and sold by vendors under similar circumstances in rural areas, and not strictly on the street. As mentioned in Chapter 6, it has become increasingly common for entrepreneurs to set up simple facilities or stalls adjacent to rural schools or to work under a nearby tree to prepare and sell ready-to-eat foods and drinks to schoolchildren and other passers-by. These foods have the same advantages and risks as urban street foods.

In developing countries the street food phenomenon has greatly mushroomed in recent years, in parallel with the huge increase of people living in urban areas, including the vast and ever-expanding megalopoli in Asia and Latin America and rapidly expanding cities everywhere. Street foods are also sold extensively in industrialized countries; it is not unusual for the New York banker or the London journalist to purchase a hot dog and a soft drink or a bag of fish and chips, respectively, on the street.

In cities in developing countries street foods provide a significant percentage of the total food intake of millions of people, have an important economic role and employ many persons, yet these activities are largely unregulated and create risks to health.

Even though authorities in many countries, North and South, regard food vendors on the street as generally undesirable and a cause of problems for the cities, the fact is that street vending has a vital role: urban workers and dwellers depend on it, it is a major employer, it contributes to the city economy and it is a major source of food for many people. Food vendors have also become an important part of urban social life and are not infrequently an attraction to the city.

City officials concerned about problems or potential problems caused by street food vendors should seek to resolve the problems, not drive the vendors off the streets. There are ways to improve the safety of street foods. Authorities should recognize that street foods are generally popular because they provide an accessible source of relatively cheap food of a kind desired by busy urban people such as factory and office workers, students, shoppers and travellers. Especially in the middle of the day, very few people can return home to eat. Street foods are also convenience foods: they save the home-maker or single person from cooking and perhaps from fuel gathering. Many poor people in crowded housing do not have proper cooking facilities, so the food vendor may provide breakfast, lunch and dinner. An FAO study revealed that in Bangkok street foods contributed 88 percent of the daily energy, protein, fat and iron intake of children aged four to six years.

In most countries the street food industry, even though very extensive and important economically, is considered part of the informal economy. It usually does not get much official or positive recognition. Consequently, governments and cities have not taken the necessary steps to improve the quality and safety of foods sold or generally to regulate the practice. The street food industry requires recognition, as it is often very large, involves large amounts of money, employs huge numbers of people and provides a real service to many citizens. Regulations should come at the same time as recognition. The industry is one of the few that can be entered with very little capital, relatively little education and only a small amount of expertise. Success requires hard work, ingenuity and street wisdom. These are characteristics of many unemployed people and of some who enter illegal parts of the informal economy. In many countries such as Nigeria and Indonesia, the majority of persons employed as street vendors are women, so the sector contributes to empowerment and economic gains for females.

Before the year 2000, there is surely a need for governments to recognize that street food vending is not a temporary phenomenon that will be replaced when development is successful. It may have undesirable features, but there are many positive aspects for cities and nations. What is now needed is recognition, legalization and improvement.

Regulation and control of street foods

The objectives of regulation and control are to improve the quality and safety of foods consumed and to let the industry have a positive role in city life. The difficulty is the risk that overregulation could drive the industry underground, force up prices and cause loss of jobs. Sensible steps must recognize the service provided by the industry. A prescription cannot be provided for the regulation and control of street foods in all countries. Appropriate regulatory activities must take cognizance of national differences, culture, local law and current street food practices.

In countries that do not have any regulations, the first step might be to recognize publicly the existence of street food vendors and to issue statements on the importance of the industry and its problems. The second step might be to map out and count the vendors and to classify them using some locally appropriate system. The third step might be to provide each vendor with an official licence. Usually a fee would have to be paid to obtain the licence. The fee should not be so high as to drive vendors away or underground, but it could go towards funds to assist in upgrading the hygiene and other practices of vendors.

It is necessary also to decide on certain minimum standards to help reduce health hazards. These standards will depend on local circumstances and probably should be established after consideration by a committee on which vendors and consumer associations have some representation. Regulations need to be appropriate and to fit in with national and city policies and legislation, and they must be aimed at improving the wholesomeness and safety of food sold without greatly raising the prices. They must have no negative impact of any significant degree either on employment or on the economy, and they must not greatly reduce the availability of street foods enjoyed by the public.

In some countries the first regulations introduced have been unnecessarily stringent health requirements for vendors which have contributed little to protection of the public. Regulations that should be considered might address the cleanliness of the facility, the quality and quantity of water used and the training of vendors regarding appropriate food handling practices in order to reduce the risk of contamination.

Regulations are only effective if there is some monitoring system and some surveillance. Inspections are useful and should

be used not entirely for punitive purposes, but also for educational opportunities. Trained inspectors should be able to record violations and possibly to threaten or take action, but they should also be used to make constructive suggestions for improvement of vendor practices or for upgrading the stall or facility. Guidelines for the design of control measures for street-vended foods in Africa are being developed by the Codex Alimentarius Commission along these lines.

An advantage of recognition, licensing and regulations is that they move the street food industry out of the strictly informal sector and into the formal sector. This may make it possible for vendors to get credit or loans to improve their operations. A disadvantage, especially if licence fees are high and regulations strict, is that many vendors will attempt to evade licensing while continuing to practise their trade. There is also a strong possibility that inspectors will be bribed to close their eyes both to non-licensed vendors and to contraventions of the regulations.

Singapore, a highly regulated country with a strong economic base, chose to resettle its food vendors into particular market areas or centres and to issue licences dependent on health standards. Singapore street foods are undoubtedly cleaner than those elsewhere in Asia, but they are perhaps less convenient for the public, less amenable as social meeting places and more likely to be run by persons not in the lower strata of society.

Food hygiene and sanitation

It does not take knowledge of tropical medicine or epidemiology to appreciate that foods prepared and offered for sale on the streets of many cities in developing countries present a health hazard. Anyone who appreciates that germs cause disease can realize that food that has been touched by dirty hands and utensils, that is not served very hot and that has been covered with flies may be unsafe.

Foods may be contaminated not only with pathogenic organisms such as viruses, bacteria and parasites which cause human disease, but also by dangerous levels of food additives, toxins, residues of pesticides used in food production or preservation or other poisonous substances such as heavy metals, e.g. lead, which is toxic.

There have been reports of deaths or disease from consumption of street foods from many countries; instances have included 14 deaths in Malaysia from consuming rice noodles, 300 people becoming ill in Hong Kong from consuming food that apparently contained a toxic pesticide, and a cholera outbreak in India.

Contamination results from unhygienic practices in the preparation, cooking, serving and storage of food. Food vendors, unlike well-run restaurants, often lack refrigeration, good storage facilities and efficient stoves. Bacteria may be in the food when it is purchased, but they are likely to multiply if the food is not refrigerated or properly stored. Organisms in food may be destroyed by the heat of cooking, but if the food is not thoroughly heated and well cooked they may infect the person who eats the food. Some organisms produce toxins in food. The problems are usually related either to lack of coldness or refrigeration for food storage or lack of heat to cook the food. The other risk factors contributing to food contamination are lack of cleanliness of the premises, the utensils and the food handlers. After preparation and cooking, foods may be contaminated by unwashed hands; by flies, cockroaches, rodents and dust; and by holding at temperatures that encourage explosive bacterial reproduction.

A major problem for street vendors which then produces a health risk for the client is water. Ice can also be a source of infections; vendors may use ice made from contaminated water. In some countries it is rare for street food vendors to have running water, and it is common for vendors to have to fetch water from a considerable distance from their point of operation. Then there is a temptation to use the water sparingly, because getting water takes time and energy. The water carried to the stall or other facility may be clean and safe, or it may be contaminated. Some food sellers on the street may have water that is not potable, and they very frequently have an inadequate supply of water. Water is essential for cooking many foods, for washing foods, for making some beverages or for drinking, for cleaning cooking vessels and utensils and for vendors to wash their hands. Vendors may not have hot water for washing utensils. Not infrequently an operator will rinse off utensils for hours in one bucket of water which becomes increasingly dirty and contaminated. All of these practices greatly enhance the likelihood that organisms such as salmonella, shigella and *Escherichia coli* will be transmitted and that certain parasitic infections such as giardia and ascariasis will be spread.

The food hygiene problem is made worse by the fact that most vendors have very little knowledge or appreciation of the importance of safe, hygienic food handling. City authorities may not take steps to control the unhygienic practices of food vendors because the officers who have authority on the streets may not themselves be aware of the risks. Many of the consumers of street foods also have little knowledge of or interest in food hygiene. This compounds the problem, because they may not, for example, insist on foods being well heated or select food stalls that appear cleaner.

Another health risk to the public is that street food vendors are often unable to dispose properly of waste water and refuse. Often there is no good system for disposal of garbage, which may end up in the street or gutter. Similarly, used water may not go into a drain but may accumulate around the stall or in puddles on the street, where it may attract flies and mosquitoes which may breed and spread disease. Singapore has strict regulations requiring vendors to use plastic garbage bags and provides metal bins near to where hawkers sell food.

Precautions that an informed purchaser can take are to insist that the food be very hot, that it come from the heating area to the customer very quickly and that it be served on a clean plate. Food taken straight off the grill is likely to be safe. It is wise to select fruits that can be peeled just before eating, such as bananas, and to order a beverage from a bottle that can be opened just prior to drinking.

Nutritional quality of street foods

Relatively little research has been published on the nutritive value of street foods sold in different countries. If large numbers of people get 50 to 80 percent of their nutrients from street foods, then it is important that the foods be nutritious and provide a good proportion of the essential nutrients. The nutritional quality of street foods obviously varies enormously from country to country, but also from vendor to vendor in a large marketplace. On city streets around the world it is possible to choose a meal that is nutritious and well balanced, as well as very tasty.

People naturally select foods or dishes for purchase more on the basis of preference, price and affordability than on the nutrient content of the meal or on nutritional quality criteria. Clearly anything that can be done to improve the nutritional quality of foods sold on the street will be helpful.

Recommendations

The street food industry now has a very important role in the cities and towns of many developing countries. It feeds millions of people daily with foods that are relatively cheap and easily accessible. It offers a very significant amount of employment, often to persons with little education and training who might otherwise be difficult to employ. Taken as a whole, it is a big business with major economic and social implications. As described above, the industry can prevent risks to consumers. As cities expand worldwide, the numbers of street food vendors will also greatly expand. In the past authorities have tended to ignore street vendors or even to obstruct them or to attempt to rid cities of them. A better policy is to recognize them and to take action to improve their practices.

The recommendations made here are largely based on the FAO publications mentioned above, and some of them have been adopted in FAO member countries. It is recommended that the following should be considered by most countries.

- Street food vendors or establishments should be recognized, registered and perhaps licensed for a given fee.
- Regulations to improve the practices of food vendors should be drawn up by a committee or other body with representation both from the vendors and from consumer organizations.
- Once regulations appropriate to the situation in each country have been drawn up, then legislation should be considered to help ensure food safety.
- A means to enforce the regulations and legislation should be implemented, involving trained inspectors to monitor especially the hygiene of street food stalls or outlets, and if feasible, inspectors should provide advice to vendors on how to improve their hygienic practices.
- If feasible, a food microbiology laboratory should be contracted or established to allow the monitoring of food

contamination and conducting of appropriate determinations.

- Training should be offered, or even required, for those who handle street foods.
- Steps should be taken to educate the public about food safety and to encourage the public to insist on hygienic food and to demand cleanliness at food stalls.
- Authorities should attempt to help street food vendors obtain access to potable water, electricity in some circumstances and ways to dispose properly of refuse and waste water.
- Countries should be encouraged to use available outside resources, such as FAO and the Codex Alimentarius Commission and their documentation, to provide assistance with the proper adoption of these recommendations. International assistance needs to be available and international publicity must be given to the importance of street foods.
- Research on street foods should be encouraged and supported so that sound information will be available to assist in improving the nutritional quality and hygiene of street foods.

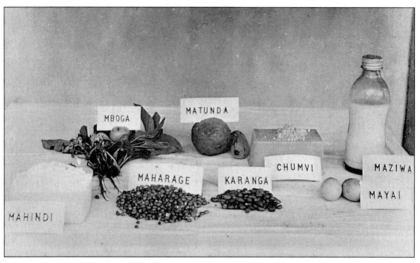

PHOTO 81
A balanced diet for one person for one day contains foods from each column in Table 40: maize (mahindi) for carbohydrate, beans (maharage) and groundnuts (karanga) for vegetable protein, milk (maziwa) and eggs (mayai) for animal protein, fruits (matunda) and vegetables (mboga) for vitamin C and carotene; groundnuts provide fat and, together with beans and maize, B vitamins; salt (chumvi) is also desirable

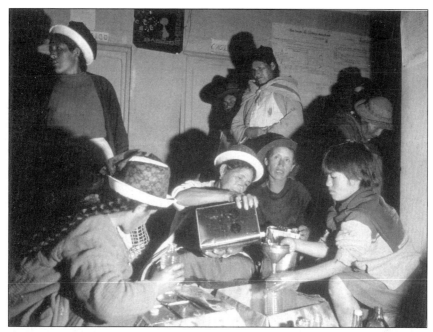

PHOTO 82
Oil distribution in Peru as part of food assistance

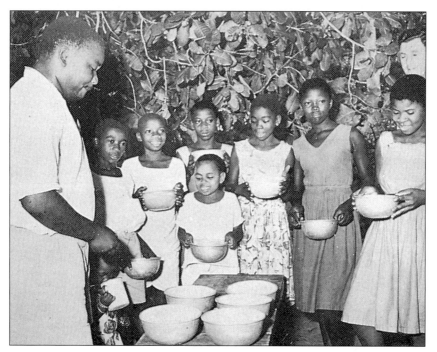

PHOTO 83
School feeding

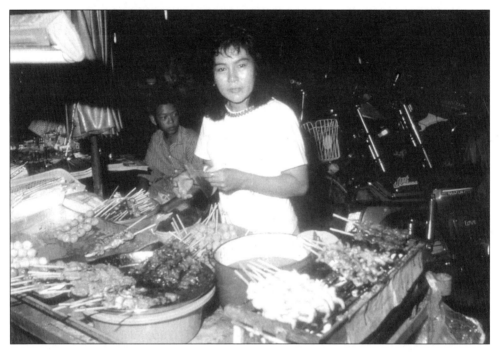

PHOTO 84
Sale of grilled meat and fish on the street

PHOTO 85
Typical fixed vending stall

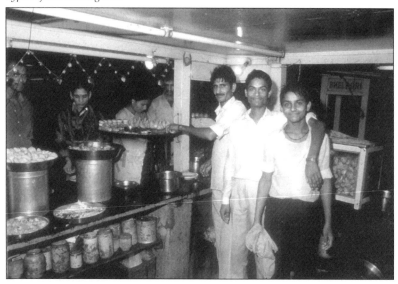

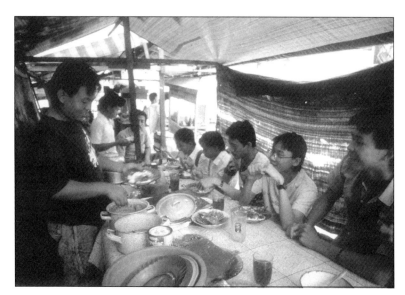

PHOTO 86
Eating street food

Chapter 41

Incorporating nutrition objectives into development policies and programmes at the national and local levels

Prevalent malnutrition in a country is clear evidence of poor development, and poor development is also an underlying cause of malnutrition and hunger. Economic growth and development that do not lead to substantial reductions in malnutrition are growth and development that are wrongly conceived. Even undirected economic growth and development can lead slowly to reduced rates of malnutrition, but the improvement is often unacceptably slow, and as a result many poor people suffer unnecessarily. There is a need for well-conceived policies for sustainable economic growth and social development that benefit the poor and the undernourished. This approach to development has been termed "development with a human face". Its goal is to ensure stable and safe food supplies for everyone, adequate protection from disease, available health services for all and an environment that encourages and assists good caring practices for those who need care. Accomplishing these aims is not easy for poor countries struggling out of poverty. Nonetheless promoting growth with equity is possible, and this is the only moral strategy to adopt.

At the same time every effort should be made to reduce malnutrition, irrespective of the rate of economic growth. Several countries have shown that this is possible. Nutrition interventions directed at the major forms of malnutrition, such as protein-energy malnutrition (PEM), vitamin A

deficiency, nutritional anaemias and iodine deficiency disorders (IDD), are usually needed, since they will help reduce malnutrition more quickly than economic growth alone is likely to do, even if it does have a human face. It is tempting to aim only or mainly at quick-fix solutions to micronutrient malnutrition while ignoring the more difficult actions needed to reduce PEM. This neglect is not desirable, because PEM is usually the leading form of malnutrition and steps to reduce PEM have other benefits.

The solutions to malnutrition can be assisted by governments, but in the end communities will often have the leading role in reducing malnutrition and promoting social development. People's participation is essential. It is necessary to recognize that the poor will be the principal actors in their own development and to foster policies and programmes that empower the underprivileged. Empowerment and participation of women are particularly important.

To succeed in reducing malnutrition it is important to strengthen technical and managerial capacities at all levels, from community to national; to address the problem of human resource development and training because most developing countries lack well-trained people in nutrition and related fields; and to pay particular attention to the status of women in society, not only because this is due, but also because women have the most important role in food security (and often in food production), in child care and in family health.

Undernutrition and malnutrition are an important part of the complex, widespread problem of poverty and deprivation that affects millions of people, perhaps the majority, in Africa, Asia and Latin America. The poor, the hungry and the malnourished are unable to live a normal life, are less likely to fulfil their potential as human beings and cannot contribute fully to the development of their own countries. In the last two decades the number of malnourished persons has declined moderately in Asia and Latin America. However, as indicated in Chapter 1, South Asian countries have a greater percentage of malnourished people than countries in Africa or the Americas. The numbers of persons who are poor or malnourished or both appear to be increasing in some African countries. One reason for the increase is that in many nations the population is increasing more rapidly than the services and goods necessary to relieve malnutrition and poverty. It is also clear that economic gains are slow and are not reflected in improvements in the quality of life of the majority of people. In many cases the gap between the rich and the poor is widening.

The challenge of malnutrition is so daunting and broad that it needs to be tackled by involving many different sectors, including governments, non-governmental organizations (NGOs), the private sector, international funding agencies and United Nations organizations such as FAO, the United Nations Children's Fund (UNICEF) and the World Health Organization (WHO). Of particular importance is good cooperation and coordination among government ministries and their staff; this applies particularly to ministries of agriculture and health, but also to other ministries such as those for education, community development and finance. Cooperation is also needed at the provincial, district and local levels.

THE INTERNATIONAL CONFERENCE ON NUTRITION AND ITS FOLLOW-UP

Greatly reducing malnutrition and providing human beings with their right to good nutrition is not an impossible dream, and is within the reach of humankind. Political actions, more than political will, to implement well conceived policies and programmes at the national level, while simultaneously acting internationally, can serve to greatly reduce nutrition problems worldwide.

Over 100 nations endorsed the World Declaration on Nutrition and the Plan of Action for Nutrition at the International Conference on Nutrition (ICN) in Rome in 1992. Section V of the Plan of Action describes the responsibility for action. This section is quoted here, as it is believed that it can influence the work of many people at many levels in the next decade.

NATIONAL FOOD AND NUTRITION POLICIES

As stressed and reiterated at the ICN in 1992, food and nutrition policies should be an integrated and important part of national development plans. The general objectives of food and nutrition policies should be to improve the quantity, quality and safety of food eaten by the population, with the aim of ensuring an adequate diet for all people, and to try to ensure good health and adequate care for all. In nutrition there exists the paradox that overconsumption of food or of certain dietary items also carries a risk to health. For example, consumption of more food than is needed for energy expenditure leads to obesity, and the high intakes of cholesterol and saturated fats typical of Western diets that are high in animal products increase the risk of heart disease. A more equitable distribution of food

Excerpt from the Plan of Action for Nutrition

V. Responsibility for action

The recommendations of the Plan of Action need to be translated into priority actions in accordance with the realities found in each country and must be supported by action at the international level. Taking these into account, governments should prepare national plans of action, coordinated as appropriate with follow-up activities related to the World Summit for Children, establishing priorities, setting up time-frames and, where appropriate, identifying the resources needed and those already available. The strategies to reach the objectives may vary from country to country, and the responsibilities rest with a variety of agents from government institutions to the individual.

1. At national level

(a) Within the context of the national plans of action, governments should formulate, adopt and implement programmes and strategies to achieve the recommendations of the Plan of Action, taking into account their specific problems and priorities. In particular, in countries where it is appropriate to do so, ministries of agriculture, food, health, social welfare, education, and planning, as well as other concerned ministries, should formulate concrete proposals for their sectors to promote nutritional well-being. Governments at the local and provincial levels should be encouraged to participate in the process, as well as NGOs and the private sector.

(b) All governments should establish appropriate national mechanisms to prioritize, develop, implement and monitor policies and plans to improve nutrition within designated time-frames, based on national and local needs, and provide appropriate funds for their functioning.

(c) All sectors of society should be encouraged to play an active role and to assume their responsibility in implementing related components of the national plan of action. Households, communities, NGOs, private institutions – including industry, small-scale producers and women farmers, trade and services as well as social and cultural associations – and the mass media should be mobilized to help individuals and population groups to achieve nutritional well-being in close association with government and technical service sectors.

(d) Programmes aimed at improving the nutritional well-being of the people, in particular of the groups at the greatest risk, should be supported by allocation of adequate resources by the public and the private sector so as to ensure their sustainability.

(e) Governments, academic institutions and industry should support the development of fundamental and applied research directed towards the improvement of the scientific and technological knowledge base against which food, nutrition and health problems can be analysed and solved, giving priority to research concerning disadvantaged and vulnerable groups.

(f) In most countries, high priority should be given to the development of human resources and training of personnel needed in all sectors to support nutrition-related activities.

(g) National governments, in cooperation with local authorities, non-governmental organizations and the private sector, should prepare periodic reports on the implementation of national plans of actions with clear indications of how vulnerable groups are faring.

2. At international level

(a) International agencies – multilateral, bilateral and non-governmental – are urged to define in the course of 1993 steps through

▶

which they can contribute to the achievement of the goals and strategies set up in the Declaration and the Plan of Action, including promotion of new partnerships in economic and technical cooperation among the countries.
(b) The Governing Bodies of FAO, WHO, UNICEF, the World Bank, UNDP, Unesco, ILO, WFP, UNHCR, and other concerned international organizations should, in the course of 1993, decide ways and means to give appropriate priority to their nutrition-related programmes and activities aimed at ensuring, as soon as possible, vigorous and coordinated implementation of activities recommended in the ICN Declaration and Plan of Action. This would include, as appropriate, increased assistance to the member countries. FAO and WHO, in particular, should strengthen within available resources their programmes for nutritional improvement, taking into account the recommendations in this Plan of Action.
(c) Regional Offices of UN organizations and regional intergovernmental organizations, are requested to collaborate and facilitate the implementation and monitoring of the Plan of Action.
(d) Regional institutions for research and training, with appropriate support of the international community, should establish or reinforce collaborative networks in order to foster the human resource development

needed, particularly at national level, to implement the Plan of Action; to promote inter-country collaboration; and to exchange information on the food and nutrition situation, technologies, research results, nutrition programmes' implementation and resource flows.
(e) As leading agencies of the United Nations system in the fields of food, nutrition and health, FAO and WHO are requested to prepare jointly, [every three years], in close collaboration with member countries and the relevant specialized agencies and other UN organs, consolidated reports on the implementation of the ICN Declaration and Plan of Action by Member States and international organizations for review by their Governing Bodies.
(f) UN agencies have a special responsibility for follow-up. All concerned agencies and organs of the UN system are urged to strengthen their collaborative and cooperative mechanisms in order to fully participate at international, regional, national and local levels in the achievement of the objectives of the Plan of Action. The ACC/SCN should facilitate coordination of these efforts and, in close collaboration with its participating agencies, prepare periodic reports on their activities in implementing the Declaration and the Plan of Action for consideration by the ACC for submission, through ECOSOC, to the UN General Assembly.

between the poor and the affluent might thus improve the health of both groups.

As described elsewhere in this book, nutrition actions in most of the poorest developing countries are mainly addressed to reducing PEM and some important micronutrient deficiencies. Increasingly, however, the middle-level developing countries undergoing increasing urbanization and some industrialization are witnessing a very significant increase in non-communicable chronic diseases related to

nutrition such as obesity, arteriosclerotic heart disease, high blood pressure, non-insulin-dependent diabetes and some forms of cancer (see Chapter 23). This problem also needs to be addressed.

FOOD PRODUCTION AND DEMAND

Adequate and stable availability of food at the national and household levels is one vital ingredient for good nutritional status. Most agricultural policies aim to increase overall production of food and non-food products. To improve nutrition this increased production needs to lead to increased food consumption by poor non-food secure households. Ensuring the poor with jobs or livelihoods on a sustainable basis will also contribute to lowering rates of malnutrition. Without adequate food production or regular and adequate incomes, nutritional status will often be compromised. Agricultural policy with nutrition objectives needs to address not only how much food is produced, but what foods are grown, where and by whom.

Cash crops sometimes compete with food crops and result in low food availability for human nutrition. However, crops sold for cash (which may be food or non-food products) may provide income to farming families and enable them to purchase more food for family consumption than could be produced on the same area of land. Cultivation of cash crops may also provide more stable income for regular food purchase, but only if the money obtained is used to acquire enough food rather than for other expenditures. It has been shown that if income from sale of farm-produced items is controlled by women rather than men, more will usually be spent on food and less on unnecessary items and children will benefit more.

In many countries much of the agricultural activity is carried out by persons who do not own the land on which they work. Land reform may improve equity and nutrition. In rural areas employment in agriculture, forestry, animal husbandry, fisheries, etc. is important for providing income and contributing to food intakes. New labour-saving technologies may sometimes reduce employment opportunities and contribute to food insecurity. Labour-intensive activities, provided wages are reasonable, will contribute to good nutrition. Other agriculture-related factors that can also influence food security include control of post-harvest food losses, storage of food crops, transport and marketing.

GOVERNMENT ORGANIZATION FOR NUTRITION POLICY FORMULATION AND IMPLEMENTATION

The need for coordination of nutrition policies and programmes has already been stressed. The main nutrition activities are almost always undertaken by government departments and ministries because nearly all countries are governed under a system that divides the functions of government in this way. Therefore, unless a separate ministry of food and nutrition is established, there needs to be some other mechanism to promote the proper development and coordination of national food and nutrition policies and programmes. It is necessary to ensure that policies within the various ministries are compatible, coordinated and, if possible, harmonized. The implementation of programmes, however, should remain the responsibility of the existing ministries, departments and agencies. As stressed below, many of the actions may depend on community mobilization.

In many cases there is no unit or organization that identifies, appraises and recommends in a systematic and comprehensive manner the measures and strategies that a government might use to meet the objectives of an adequate diet for the population. Similarly, there is seldom a structure or unit that analyses the nutritional implications of the national development plan and other programmes of government ministries. There is clearly a need to provide the function of overview and at least to have an identified focal point for nutrition.

In some countries various institutions or committees have been established to coordinate nutrition activities. In Zambia a national food and nutrition commission was set up soon after independence. In the United Republic of Tanzania the Tanzanian

Food and Nutrition Centre has been established as a parastatal body with responsibility to the Ministry of Health. In Indonesia the National Development Planning Agency (Bappenas) quite successfully coordinates nutrition activities and ensures the inclusion of sound nutrition policy objectives in each five-year development plan (Repelita). Many other countries have interministerial committees to discuss nutrition matters that concern several ministries. During the preparations for the ICN, national focal points for nutrition were established in 159 countries.

In the 1990s nutrition planning is less in vogue than in the 1970s. Even so, some mechanism is needed to formulate national food and nutrition policies and to ensure intersectoral cooperation in their implementation. The ICN document *Nutrition and development – a global assessment* (FAO/WHO, 1992b) states:

"Implementation of nutrition-related policies by ministries such as agriculture and health can be made more effective if there is intersectoral collaboration."

The Plan of Action for Nutrition includes the recommendation (see the preceding box for full text of the section) that:

"All governments should establish appropriate national mechanisms to prioritize, develop, implement and monitor policies and plans to improve nutrition within designated time frames, based both on national and local needs, and provide appropriate funds for their functioning.... In particular, in countries where it is appropriate to do so, ministries of agriculture, food, health, social welfare, education and planning, as well as other concerned ministries, should formulate concrete proposals for their sectors to promote nutritional well-being."

Food and nutrition policies are too important a part of national development to be ignored or only to be broken down into separate components of the activities of several ministries. All those concerned with nutrition can play a part, first by coordinating their activities with those of colleagues in other ministries and second by influencing the government to establish a suitable nutrition policy, planning and coordination mechanism. Sustained nutrition improvement is not usually achieved by implementation of vertical programmes. The benefits will come mainly from integrating nutrition considerations into various sectoral plans and policies of key government departments or ministries. Thus a mechanism to foster integration may be needed.

Beyond the need for national cooperation of ministries and departments, cooperation is vital at the district and village levels, with active participation of the stakeholders, if plans to improve nutrition are to be really effective. Community mobilization and community participation are of great importance.

EVALUATION AND MONITORING OF NUTRITION PROGRAMMES

Public health and nutrition programmes are frequently conducted without any plans for their evaluation. Campaigns to increase household food resources, to construct more toilets, to triple the number of under-five clinics, to establish new school feeding programmes or to give increasing emphasis to nutrition education may be important activities in a country or community, but such activities are seldom adequately evaluated.

Monitoring and evaluation are important activities in programmes and projects to improve nutrition. In general, monitoring is mainly done by the project workers themselves, preferably with the participation of the communities whose members are the beneficiaries of the actions being taken. Monitoring usually consists of the periodic collection and analysis of appropriate data.

UNICEF (1991) in its *Guide for monitoring and evaluation* has defined evaluation as "a process which attempts to determine as systematically and objectively as possible the relevance, effectiveness, efficiency and impact of activities in the light of specified objectives. It is an action oriented management tool and organizational process for improving both current activities and future planning, programming and decision making". This comprehensive definition is appropriate and relevant to nutrition evaluation in developing countries.

Evaluation consists of efforts to appraise, measure or judge the progress made by a programme or activity towards its stated objectives. The government that supports a programme, the workers who implement it and the beneficiaries should all be interested to know how effective the programme is. An integral part of all applied nutrition activities should therefore be some form of evaluation.

Because evaluation includes a determination of progress towards certain objectives, it has two basic prerequisites. First is the need to have the objectives of the programme stated, preferably in writing. Second is the need for some baseline data, however simple. In other words, it is necessary to know the position before the programme begins and the changes that are expected to occur as a result of the programme. Evaluation sometimes consists of a measurement before initiation and after completion of the action. The difference between the two measurements indicates the change that occurred during the period of the action; it may or may not have been entirely produced by the action.

Evaluation is useful in several different ways. It helps the worker to know how he or she is getting on with the job and may suggest ways of improving the work or accelerating progress. It may suggest that certain actions produce good results and others do not. Evaluation is useful for the programme planners; by analysing the evaluation reports they can obtain a measure of overall progress and of the relative contribution of each component of the programme. This information facilitates logical planning and may lead to revision of the programme's operations or to new actions.

Evaluation should also provide the beneficiaries of the programme with an indication of what has been achieved. Because community support is essential to the success of programmes, it is incumbent on the workers to let those receiving help know how the programme is progressing, much as a company or business must from time to time let its shareholders know how the business is doing. Unless people are shown and made to understand the changes that are occurring and their own role in the change, much of the value of a programme may be lost. If the people understand the results achieved, they might well be encouraged to cooperate more fully and to assist in programme activities. Evaluation might also convince them and their leaders that an aspect of the programme about which they were sceptical is producing results. For example, in an area where there is little enthusiasm about school feeding, parents might be greatly influenced to support it financially and with self-help activities if they are provided with clearly understandable evidence showing that children who received meals grew better, learned more and were less prone to absenteeism.

Evaluation is therefore a constructive process that can gain more support for the programme from the government, outside agencies and the public. It can also encourage the workers and help them to be more effective and efficient.

It is often suggested that evaluation should be carried out by persons external to, and not associated with, the programme being evaluated. That view is not universally accepted. Although outside evaluators can be presumed to be unbiased and impartial while programme workers cannot, it is sometimes an advantage to have persons who work on a project serve on an evaluation team because of their deep knowledge and understanding of the project and of the community where it is being implemented. The responsibility for objectivity and for ensuring that data are unbiased in an evaluation report then rests with the outsiders.

There is increasing interest in the use of rapid appraisal procedures as tools for evaluation. This method often relies mainly on qualitative data. There is often a place for the use of both quantitative and qualitative methods.

Chapter 33, on nutritional assessment, analysis and surveillance, refers to data that might be used in monitoring, evaluation or both. The reader desiring more information is advised to seek out publications that provide details about monitoring and evaluation (see Bibliography).

CRUCIAL ELEMENTS OF SUCCESSFUL COMMUNITY NUTRITION PROGRAMMES

The fifth International Conference of the International Nutrition Planners Forum (USAID, 1989) analysed major successful community nutrition programmes for Bolivia, Brazil, India, Indonesia, Thailand and the United Republic of Tanzania and concluded that the nutritional status of poor population groups in developing countries can be significantly improved through nutrition-oriented community development programmes if certain critical elements are built into the programmes from their inception. It also pointed out that nutrition projects and programmes cannot substitute for a country's and government's political commitment to sustainable and equitable economic growth and social development. A comprehensive strategy that either incorporates nutrition elements into development programmes or uses a community development approach in nutrition programmes was recommended. The conference also suggested that institutional and individual commitment to community self-reliance in a broad development context is crucial to promoting nutritional improvement. The conference identified the following six critical elements for programme success.

Political commitment

Firm and consistent political commitment reflected in concrete nutrition financing and action is crucial. Political commitment can be generated from the community needing nutrition services, as well as through advocacy by the technical and scientific community and/or by international organizations.

Community mobilization and participation

Effective community mobilization for active participation is essential for nutrition programmes to succeed. It is best achieved by involving the community in all phases of programme planning and implementation, including needs assessment, decision-making and programme supervision, monitoring and evaluation. Decentralization of power to the community facilitates organization and enables the community to identify its own needs, to search for solutions and to participate actively in programme implementation. Women's groups are key resources for community mobilization and participation.

Human resources development

The quality of human resources is an important element. Commitment to community work and strong leadership qualities are basic criteria for staff selection. These traits are also expected in volunteer workers and in staff paid by the community. Relatively large investments are needed in basic training and frequent in-service retraining. A combination of centre-based and field-based training may be the most effective. Skills-oriented, competence-based, comprehensive, multidisciplinary training is recommended, with special attention to the training of trainers.

Targeting

Appropriate targeting improves the efficiency and cost-effectiveness of nutrition intervention programmes by focusing resources on groups or individuals at highest risk and most likely to benefit from the intervention. When malnutrition is widespread, geographic targeting may be enough, but as the level of malnutrition decreases it is necessary to use a combination of geographic, household, family, economic and individual criteria. In targeting the poorest regions or communities, development of a minimum service delivery infrastructure is often required.

Monitoring, evaluation and management information systems

A functional management information system (MIS) for ongoing monitoring, evaluation and decision-making at the local and higher levels is an important element of programme success. A two-way (bottom-up and top-down) flow of information and decision-making should be established, with regular collection of reliable data, timely analysis and interpretation and immediate feedback. The MIS need not be highly sophisticated. It should not exceed the programme's data handling capacity or overload community workers as data collectors. A basic MIS includes a minimum set of data and indicators to be collected, analysed and used by the community, programme managers and policy-makers for decision-making.

Replicability and sustainability

Replicability and sustainability are inter-related elements of successful programmes. Replicability is contingent upon the extent to which programme elements, methodologies and implementation processes are suitable to particular contextual features found in other settings. For nutrition programmes to make a difference in the long term, sustainability of positive outcomes is crucial. Sustainability is enhanced by consistent political commitment, active community participation, development of a trained resource base and programme cost-effectiveness *vis-à-vis* resources available in the country. Sustainability is built in from the planning stage when nutrition interventions are designed within the context and capacity of a country's local resources. Effective technology transfer or the creation of cost-effective locally developed technologies can increase a programme's sustainability.

PRACTICAL SOLUTIONS TO NUTRITION PROBLEMS

The earlier part of this chapter has been rather general, dealing mainly with the processes necessary for actions and implementation. Presented below are some suggestions of actions that might be considered. This list is not a series of prescriptions, but rather a menu or catalogue of possible options. It is a summary of possible practical solutions to nutrition problems and is by no means complete. Some of the ideas may or may not be suitable for adaptation and adoption by a nation, a village or individuals in a community. Each area and each community has its own problems that must be tackled at the local level. The suggestions made here can therefore not be expected to do more than stimulate thought. Many of them may already be in practice.

Many of the solutions are educational, for again and again it has been stressed that one of the main causes of poor nutrition is a lack of knowledge about food, health and care. Many other suggestions are basically agricultural. This publication is not designed to give details on either teaching methods or agricultural practices. Information on increasing and improving food production must be sought in manuals of agriculture, horticulture, animal husbandry, fisheries and poultry keeping.

Improving nutritional knowledge
Lack of knowledge is an important cause of malnutrition. Nutrition knowledge can, for example, be improved by:
- nutrition education in schools, literacy classes, farmer training centres and village meetings;
- personal example, e.g. government ministers and respected local leaders including the topic of nutrition in their speeches or consuming controversial but nutritionally desirable foods in public;
- distribution of pamphlets and posters featuring material on nutrition and publicizing of nutrition facts through newspapers, radio and television and at agricultural and other shows;
- demonstration of the preparation and cooking of food, especially food suitable for children, by nurses in health centres and clinics, by community development workers and by home economics teachers in schools;
- a team approach for coordination of efforts to disseminate nutrition knowledge through district, village and other local committees;
- encouraging nutritionally good traditional food habits, e.g. the eating of amaranth and fermented soy products;
- discouraging undesirable food habits;
- teaching mothers good practical weaning habits, e.g. the use of sour milk in gruel, pounded groundnuts for infants and vegetable mixtures;
- use of social marketing methods to promote and protect breastfeeding, to

suggest appropriate prevention and treatment of diarrhoea and to encourage parents to immunize their children.

Improving and increasing food production
Increasing and improving food production is mainly an agricultural problem. Aims should be:
- to promote an overall increase to ensure a sufficient energy supply, with emphasis on having enough food available for times of intense agricultural activity at the end of the season, i.e. during the usual "hungry period";
- to increase production of plants that are good sources of protein, encouraging households to consider growing more beans, groundnuts, cowpeas, etc.;
- to increase vegetable and fruit production, especially to ensure adequate intakes of vitamins A and C, by
  - a policy of encouraging home gardens,
  - allocation of land allotments for growing food in towns,
  - establishment of school, village and community orchards and gardens,
  - wider growing of papaya, guava and other fruit-trees,
  - encouraging the production and use of edible dark green leafy vegetables such as amaranth,
  - encouraging planting of yellow- and orange-coloured vegetables such as pumpkins and carrots;
- to increase and improve production of animal foods, by
  - better animal husbandry,
  - use of goats' milk,
  - improving and increasing poultry keeping and use of eggs, especially as a food for toddlers and young children,
  - increasing and improving methods of catching and preserving fish,
  - construction of village and household

fish ponds in all areas that have perennial water,[1]

- wider use of dams, rivers and ponds as sources of fish production,
- extensive use of small animals for food, especially pigeons, guinea-pigs and rabbits,
- greater use of sea urchins, locusts, lake flies, etc., as food,
- wider use of meat from game animals, including controlled cropping and game farming where this is ecologically sound.

Improving food distribution

Food should be equitably distributed but often is not, even where sufficient food is available. More equitable distribution can be achieved by:

- improving communications to ensure that excess stocks in one area reach another area that is short of the commodity;
- better trading facilities, i.e. more food markets and shops, better stocks of nutritionally valuable manufactured and preserved foods in village shops at reasonable prices, improved marketplaces and more cooperative-type food shops;
- promoting equitable distribution within the family to ensure a fair share of food, especially nutritious foods, for children and increased supplies of food for pregnant and lactating women;
- instituting midday meals in day schools, encouraging children to take food to school and improving meals in boarding schools;
- making available special foods for young children and developing special recipes for toddlers;
- paying wages weekly instead of monthly and encouraging better family budgeting;
- ensuring availability of midday meals, subsidized canteens or rations for labourers.

Improving food and crop storage

In some developing countries an estimated 25 percent of all food produced is never consumed by humans. Instead it spoils or is eaten by insects, rats and other pests. Measures to correct this situation can be taken in fields, households, shops and warehouses. These may include:

- control of rats by trapping, poison, rat-proofing grain stores, etc.;
- control of insects by use of insecticides, better food stores and airtight food containers;
- control of fungi and food rot by storage of food in as dry a state as possible and by use of better containers;
- control of birds by destruction, especially in millet and wheat areas;
- protective measures against monkeys, baboons, porcupines, wild pigs and other destructive animals, even elephants;
- educating people about safe and hygienic food storage at home.

Improving food processing and safety

Proper food processing can ensure that nutrient values of food are maintained at the highest possible levels, that food surpluses are utilized and that food is safe. Suitable measures are:

- better methods of food preservation in the home and the village, e.g. drying or smoking of meat and fish, preservation of fruits and vegetables, home or village production of cheese and use of solar drying methods;
- better cooking, e.g. less prolonged

---

[1] Improperly maintained fish ponds can lead to an increase in malaria and schistosomiasis (bilharzia). Public health advice should be sought and steps taken to prevent mosquitoes and snails from breeding.

boiling of vegetables containing vitamin C, use of the minimal quantity of water for cooking rice and preparation of special dishes for infants;
- increased use of processes for preservation of local foods and/or for making them more palatable – e.g. drying or canning of food products, commercial fish drying and processing to make edible products from local soybeans – which requires more small-scale commercial enterprises;
- ensuring a supply of well-processed milk products at reasonable cost;
- enrichment of highly milled cereals with vitamins and iron (best achieved by legislation);
- iodization of salt to prevent IDD;
- fluoridation of community water to reduce dental caries in areas where this is feasible and where the water contains less than 0.5 parts per million (ppm) of fluoride;
- fortification of commonly eaten foods with vitamin A, iron and possibly other nutrients if feasible;
- education on food hygiene for households;
- improving the safety of street foods by educating vendors and establishing and enforcing regulations to reduce the possibility of disease resulting from eating these foods;
- promoting the use of more energy-dense staple foods by children, including where feasible the use of "power flour" (see Chapter 6) to make gruels thinner and more energy dense.

Improving health care
The following health measures could be considered to improve the nutritional status of local communities:
- ensuring the availability of immunizations and achieving very high coverage against common childhood infectious diseases;
- educating families about diarrhoea prevalence and treatment, including the home use of appropriate fluids and foods;
- organizing regular deworming of children;
- taking preventive measures against gastro-intestinal disease, infections and other diseases that predispose to malnutrition by encouraging good personal, household and food hygiene and helping to provide safe, clean water;
- providing good curative services to treat malnutrition and other diseases linked with malnutrition;
- teaching about the importance of a balanced diet in both in- and out-patient departments of hospitals and clinics, stressing the special needs of children, pregnant women and lactating mothers;
- weighing children regularly and maintaining proper weight charts of children;
- demonstrating food preparation at maternal and child health clinics and other suitable places, concentrating especially on suitable weaning-food mixtures for young children and always encouraging the use of foodstuffs that are locally acceptable and available, and inviting participation by the mothers;
- organizing the efficient distribution of supplementary foods where these are available and necessary for young children;
- protecting, promoting and supporting breastfeeding and discouraging bottle-feeding;
- encouraging supplementation of breast-milk with other foods when infants reach six months of age;
- organizing proper antenatal and postnatal clinics for women, providing both curative and prophylactic treatment for anaemia;
- providing health education for the general public.

Annexes

Annex 1
Recommended intakes of nutrients

The tables in this annex provide a basis on which advice can be given regarding recommended intakes of nutrients in diets for groups of people, particularly in developing countries. They also provide a yardstick by which to gauge the adequacy of institutional diets or food provided for refugees or in other feeding programmes. The tables give safe levels of intake for protein and micronutrients for different gender and age groups in a sample low-income country. These values are not necessarily appropriate for every low-income country because body weights and activity levels may be different from those used here. When possible, requirements, particularly energy requirements, should be calculated using national body weight data and local activity levels.

Safe levels of intake are the levels that maintain health and nutrient stores in almost all healthy individuals within a group. No allowance is made for food losses before consumption.

The tables, like similar tables of requirements or recommended dietary allowances for specific countries, apply to groups of persons and not to individuals. They refer to healthy people; for example, they do not take account of possible chronic iron loss in a population where hookworm infections may be prevalent. These recommended intakes, in normal circumstances, provide sufficient amounts of the nutrients for prevention of deficiency disease, for growth and healthy maintenance of the body and for optimum levels of activity.

TABLE A1

Average individual energy requirements and safe levels of intake for protein and iron

(values rounded)

Sex and age group	Weight[a] (kg)	Energy[b] (kcal)	Protein[c] Diet A (g)	Diet B (g)	Fat[d] (g)	Iron[e] Diet 1 (mg)	Diet 2 (mg)
Children							
6-12 months	8.5	950	14	14	–	21	11
1-3 years	11.5	1 350	22	13	23-52	13	7
3-5 years	15.5	1 600	26	16	27-62	14	7
5-7 years	19.0	1 820	30	19	30-71	19	10
7-10 years	25.0	1 900	34	25	32-74	23	12
Boys							
10-12 years	32.5	2 120	48	33	35-82	23	12
12-14 years	41.0	2 250	59	41	38-88	36	18
14-16 years	52.5	2 650	70	49	44-103	36	18
16-18 years	61.5	2 770	81	55	46-108	23	11
Girls[f]							
10-12 years	33.5	1 905	49	34	32-74	23	11
12-14 years	42.0	1 955	59	40	33-76	40	20
14-16 years	49.5	2 030	64	45	34-79	40	20
16-18 years	52.5	2 060	63	44	34-80	48	24
Men - active							
18-60 years	63.0	2 895	55	47	48-113	23	11
>60 years	63.0	2 020	55	47	34-79	23	11
Women - active							
Not pregnant or lactating	55.0	2 210	49	41	37-86	48	24
Pregnant	55.0	2 410	56	47	40-94	(76)	(38)
Lactating	55.0	2 710	69	59	45-105	26	13
>60 years	55.0	1 835	49	41	31-71	19	9

Sources: For energy figures: FAO, 1990b. For protein figures: WHO, 1985. For iron figures: FAO, 1988.
[a] Body weights are the thirtieth percentile of reference weights (i.e. United States National Center for Health Statistics [NCHS] data in FAO, 1990b), which are similar to those in many low-income countries but which give smoother curves.
[b] Energy requirements were calculated using the methodology described in FAO, 1990b. Adult requirements are based on body weights from a sample low-income country (Cameroon) and assume a physical activity level (PAL) for a rural population (i.e. 1.78 for men and 1.69 for women). Where values are grouped for tables in the text it has been assumed that 13 percent of women aged 18 to 59 years are pregnant and 13 percent are lactating. Children's requirements (to ensure enough energy for growth) were calculated using reference (NCHS) weights for Cameroon heights for age and energy allowance factors which allow for the energy needs of frequent infection and desirable levels of activity. These energy values are averages for groups of people; because of individual variation they will not necessarily satisfy the requirements for each individual in a group.
[c] Diet A represents a diet containing a great deal of cereals, starchy roots and pulses (and therefore high in fibre) and little complete (animal) protein. The digestibility factor used was 85 percent and the amino acid scores were 100 for ages six months to one year (assuming breast milk would be part of the diet), 70 for ages one to five years, 80 for ages 5 to 17 years and 100 for adults. Diet B represents a mixed balanced diet with little fibre and plenty of complete protein. The digestibility factor used was 100 and the amino acid score was 100 for all ages. For both diets A and B the requirements were plotted and the curves smoothed.
[d] Fat requirements were calculated at the recommended range of 15 to 35 percent of average energy requirements.
[e] Diet 1 represents a diet containing mainly cereals, starchy roots and legumes and very little meat, fish or vitamin C-rich foods and it is assumed that 5 percent of the iron in the diet is absorbed. Diet 2 contains small amounts of meat, fish and some vitamin C-rich foods and it is assumed that 10 percent of the iron is absorbed. The values given are for the basal requirement and allow for individual variation; safe levels of intake are not available for iron. The iron requirements during pregnancy are an estimate of the minimum needs over the whole nine months. In reality iron needs may increase to about five times the pre-pregnancy requirements in the second semester and about eight times the pre-pregnancy requirements in the third semester. Supplements are usually needed to cover these requirements.
[f] If a girl is pregnant, her energy requirements increase by 200 kcal, her protein requirements by 7 g for Diet A and 6 g for Diet B and her fat requirements by 4 g, while her iron requirements are at least doubled.

TABLE A2

Safe levels of intake for various micronutrients

Sex and age group	Iodine (μg)	Vitamin A (μg retinol)	Riboflavin (mg)	Niacin (mg)	Folate[a,b] (μg)	Vitamin C[b] (mg)
Children						
6-12 months	50	350	0.5	5.4	32	20
1-3 years	70	400	0.8	9.0	50	20
3-5 years	90	400	1.0	10.5	50	20
5-7 years	90	400	1.1	12.1	76	20
7-10 years	120	400	1.3	14.5	102	20
Boys						
10-12 years	150	500	1.6	17.2	102	20
12-14 years	150	600	1.7	19.1	170	30
14-16 years	150	600	1.8	19.7	170	30
16-18 years	150	600	1.8	20.3	200	30
Girls						
10-12 years	150	500	1.4	15.5	102	20
12-14 years	150	600	1.5	16.4	170	30
14-16 years	150	550	1.5	15.8	170	30
16-18 years	150	500	1.4	15.2	170	30
If pregnant	175	600	1.6	17.5	420	30
Men – active						
18-60 years	150	600	1.8	19.8	200	30
>60 years	150	600	1.8	19.8	200	30
Women – active						
Not pregnant or lactating	150	500	1.3	14.5	170	30
Pregnant	175	600	1.5	16.8	420	30
Lactating	200	850	1.7	18.2	270	30
>60 years	150	500	1.3	14.5	170	30

Sources: For iodine, vitamin A and folate figures: FAO, 1988. For riboflavin, niacin and vitamin C figures: FAO, 1982.
[a] Supplements may be needed to cover folate needs during pregnancy.
[b] There is evidence that higher levels of intake of vitamin C and folic acid may be beneficial and protective to health. Some countries have already adopted higher levels of intake of these nutrients as desirable.

Annex 2
Anthropometric tables for assessment of nutritional status and dentition ages

Anthropometric measurements (weight, height, arm circumference and skinfold thickness) are widely used to help assess the nutritional status of populations and of individuals. The values for weight and height (or length) presented in the following tables are derived from United States National Center for Health Statistics (NCHS) reference values as recommended by the World Health Organization (WHO). Some derived measurements such as weight for length are provided.

TABLE A3
Weight for age, both sexes, birth to 60 months

Age (months)	Weight (kg)			Age (months)	Weight (kg)		
	Median	80% of median	70% of median		Median	80% of median	70% of median
0	3.2	2.6	2.3				
1	4.1	3.3	2.9	31	13.5	10.8	9.5
2	4.9	4.0	3.5	32	13.6	10.9	9.6
3	5.7	4.6	4.0	33	13.8	11.0	9.7
4	6.4	5.1	4.5	34	14.0	11.2	9.8
5	7.0	5.6	4.9	35	14.1	11.3	9.9
6	7.5	6.0	5.3	36	14.4	11.5	10.0
7	8.0	6.4	5.6	37	14.5	11.6	10.2
8	8.5	6.8	6.0	38	14.7	11.8	10.3
9	8.9	7.1	6.2	39	14.9	11.9	10.4
10	9.2	7.4	6.4	40	15.0	12.0	10.6
11	9.6	7.6	6.7	41	15.2	12.2	10.6
12	9.8	7.9	6.9	42	15.4	12.3	10.8
13	10.1	8.1	7.1	43	15.5	12.4	10.9
14	10.3	8.3	7.3	44	15.7	12.6	11.0
15	10.6	8.4	7.4	45	15.9	12.7	11.1
16	10.8	8.6	7.6	46	16.0	12.8	11.3
17	11.0	8.8	7.7	47	16.2	12.9	11.3
18	11.1	8.9	7.8	48	16.3	13.1	11.5
19	11.3	9.1	8.0	49	16.5	13.2	11.6
20	11.5	9.2	8.1	50	16.6	13.3	11.6
21	11.7	9.4	8.2	51	16.8	13.4	11.8
22	11.9	9.5	8.3	52	16.9	13.6	11.9
23	12.1	9.7	8.5	53	17.1	13.7	12.0
24	12.2	9.8	8.5	54	17.2	13.8	12.1
25	12.4	9.9	8.7	55	17.4	13.9	12.3
26	12.6	10.1	8.8	56	17.6	14.0	12.3
27	12.8	10.2	8.9	57	17.7	14.2	12.4
28	13.0	10.4	9.0	58	17.9	14.3	12.5
29	13.1	10.5	9.2	59	18.0	14.4	12.6
30	13.3	10.6	9.3	60	18.2	14.5	12.7

Source: FAO, 1982.

TABLE A4
Weight for age, girls, 12 to 60 months

Age (months)	Weight (kg)			
	-2 SD	Median	80% of median	70% of median
12	7.4	9.5	7.5	6.7
13	7.6	9.8	7.8	6.9
14	7.8	10.0	8.0	7.0
15	8.0	10.2	8.2	7.1
16	8.2	10.4	8.3	7.3
17	8.3	10.6	8.5	7.4
18	8.5	10.8	8.6	7.6
19	8.6	11.0	8.8	7.7
20	8.8	11.2	9.0	7.8
21	9.0	11.4	9.1	8.0
22	9.1	11.5	9.2	8.1
23	9.3	11.7	9.4	8.2
24	9.4	11.8	9.4	8.3
25	9.6	12.0	9.6	8.4
26	9.8	12.2	9.8	8.5
27	9.9	12.4	9.9	8.7
28	10.1	12.6	10.1	8.8
29	10.2	12.8	10.2	9.0
30	10.3	13.0	10.4	9.1
31	10.5	13.2	10.6	9.2
32	10.8	13.4	10.7	9.4
33	10.8	13.6	10.9	9.5
34	10.9	13.8	11.0	9.7
35	11.0	13.9	11.1	9.7
36	11.2	14.1	11.3	9.9
37	11.3	14.3	11.4	10.0
38	11.4	14.4	11.5	10.1
39	11.5	14.6	11.7	10.2
40	11.6	14.8	11.8	10.4
41	11.8	14.9	11.9	10.4
42	11.9	15.1	12.1	10.6
43	12.0	15.2	12.2	10.8
44	12.1	15.4	12.3	10.8
45	12.2	15.5	12.4	10.9
46	12.3	15.7	12.6	11.0
47	12.4	15.8	12.6	11.1
48	12.6	16.0	12.8	11.2
49	12.7	16.1	12.9	11.3
50	12.8	16.2	13.0	11.3
51	12.9	16.4	13.1	11.5
52	13.0	16.5	13.2	11.6
53	13.1	16.7	13.4	11.7
54	13.2	16.8	13.4	11.8
55	13.3	17.0	13.6	11.9
56	13.4	17.1	13.7	12.0
57	13.5	17.2	13.8	12.0
58	13.6	17.4	13.9	12.2
59	13.7	17.5	14.0	12.3
60	13.8	17.7	14.2	12.4

Source: FAO, 1990c.

TABLE A5
Weight for age, boys, 12 to 60 months

Age (months)	Weight (kg)			
	-2 SD	Median	80% of median	70% of median
12	8.1	10.2	8.2 ·	7.1
13	8.3	10.4	8.3	7.3
14	8.5	10.7	8.6	7.5
15	8.7	10.9	8.7	7.6
16	8.8	11.1	8.9	7.8
17	9.0	11.3	9.0	7.9
18	9.1	11.5	9.2	8.1
19	9.2	11.7	9.4	8.2
20	9.4	11.8	9.4	8.3
21	9.5	12.0	9.6	8.4
22	9.7	12.2	9.8	8.5
23	9.8	12.3	9.8	8.6
24	10.1	12.4	9.9	8.7
25	10.2	12.5	10.0	8.8
26	10.3	12.7	10.2	8.9
27	10.4	12.9	10.3	9.0
28	10.5	13.1	10.5	9.2
29	10.6	13.3	10.6	9.3
30	10.7	13.5	10.8	9.5
31	10.9	13.7	11.0	9.6
32	11.0	13.9	11.1	9.7
33	11.1	14.1	11.3	9.9
34	11.2	14.3	11.4	10.0
35	11.3	14.4	11.5	10.1
36	11.4	14.6	11.7	10.2
37	11.5	14.8	11.8	10.4
38	11.7	15.0	12.0	10.5
39	11.8	15.2	12.2	10.6
40	11.9	15.3	12.2	10.7
41	12.0	15.5	12.4	10.9
42	12.1	15.7	12.6	11.0
43	12.3	15.8	12.6	11.1
44	12.4	16.0	12.8	11.2
45	12.5	16.2	13.0	11.3
46	12.6	16.4	13.1	11.5
47	12.8	16.5	13.2	11.8
48	12.9	16.7	13.4	11.7
49	13.0	16.9	13.5	11.8
50	13.1	17.0	13.6	11.9
51	13.3	17.2	13.6	12.0
52	13.4	17.4	13.9	12.2
53	13.5	17.5	14.0	12.3
54	13.7	17.7	14.2	12.4
55	13.8	17.9	14.3	12.5
56	13.9	18.0	14.4	12.6
57	14.0	18.2	14.6	12.7
58	14.2	18.3	14.6	12.8
59	14.3	18.5	14.8	13.0
60	14.4	18.7	15.0	13.1

Source: FAO, 1990c.

TABLE A6

Length for age, both sexes, birth to 24 months

Age (months)	Length (cm)		
	Median	90% of median	80% of median
0	50.2	45.2	40.1
1	54.1	48.7	43.3
2	57.4	51.7	45.9
3	60.3	54.3	48.2
4	62.8	56.5	50.2
5	65.0	58.5	52.0
6	66.9	60.2	53.5
7	68.5	61.7	54.8
8	70.0	63.0	56.0
9	71.4	64.3	57.1
10	72.7	65.4	58.2
11	74.0	66.6	59.2
12	75.2	67.7	60.2
13	76.4	68.7	61.1
14	77.5	69.8	62.0
15	78.5	70.7	62.9
16	79.7	71.7	63.8
17	80.7	72.8	64.8
18	81.7	73.5	65.4
19	82.6	74.4	66.1
20	83.6	75.2	66.9
21	84.4	76.0	67.6
22	85.4	76.8	68.3
23	86.2	77.6	69.0
24	87.1	78.4	69.7

Source: Cameron and Hofvander, 1983.

TABLE A7

Length for age, girls, 12 to 23 months

Age *(months)*	Length *(cm)*			
	-2 SD	Median	90% of median	80% of median
12	68.6	74.3	66.9	59.4
13	69.8	75.5	68.0	60.4
14	70.8	76.7	69.0	61.4
15	71.9	77.8	70.0	62.2
16	72.9	78.9	71.0	63.1
17	73.8	79.9	71.9	63.9
18	74.8	80.9	72.8	64.7
19	75.7	81.9	73.7	65.5
20	76.6	82.9	74.6	66.3
21	77.4	83.8	75.4	67.0
22	78.3	84.7	76.2	67.8
23	79.1	85.6	77.0	68.5

Source: FAO, 1990c.

TABLE A8

Length for age, boys, 12 to 23 months

Age *(months)*	Length *(cm)*			
	-2 SD	Median	90% of median	80% of median
12	70.7	76.1	68.5	60.9
13	71.8	77.2	69.5	61.8
14	72.8	78.3	70.5	62.8
15	73.7	79.4	71.5	63.5
16	74.6	80.4	72.4	64.3
17	75.5	81.4	73.3	65.1
18	76.3	82.4	74.2	65.9
19	77.1	83.3	75.0	66.6
20	77.9	84.2	75.8	67.4
21	78.7	85.1	76.6	68.1
22	79.4	86.0	77.4	68.8
23	80.2	86.8	78.1	69.4

Source: FAO, 1990c.

TABLE A9
Height for age, girls, 24 to 60 months

Age (months)	Height (cm)			
	-2 SD	Median	90% of median	80% of median
24	78.1	84.5	76.1	87.6
25	78.8	85.4	76.9	68.3
26	79.6	86.2	77.6	69.0
27	80.3	87.0	78.3	69.6
28	81.0	87.9	79.1	70.3
29	81.8	88.7	79.8	71.0
30	82.5	89.5	80.6	71.6
31	83.2	90.2	81.2	72.2
32	83.8	91.0	81.9	72.6
33	84.5	91.7	82.5	73.4
34	85.2	92.5	83.3	74.0
35	85.8	93.2	83.9	74.6
36	86.5	93.9	84.5	75.1
37	87.1	94.6	85.1	75.7
38	87.7	95.3	85.8	76.2
39	88.4	96.0	86.4	76.8
40	89.0	96.6	86.9	77.3
41	89.6	97.3	87.6	77.8
42	90.2	97.9	86.1	78.3
43	90.7	98.6	88.7	78.9
44	91.3	99.2	89.3	79.4
45	91.9	99.8	89.8	79.8
46	92.4	100.4	90.4	80.3
47	93.0	101.0	90.9	80.8
48	93.5	101.6	91.4	81.3
49	94.1	102.2	92.0	81.8
50	94.6	102.8	92.5	82.2
51	95.1	103.4	93.1	82.7
52	95.8	104.0	93.6	83.2
53	96.1	104.5	94.1	83.6
54	96.7	105.1	94.6	84.1
55	97.1	105.6	95.0	84.5
56	97.6	106.2	95.6	85.0
57	98.1	106.7	96.0	85.4
58	98.6	107.3	96.6	85.8
59	99.1	107.8	97.0	86.2
60	99.5	108.4	97.6	86.7

Source: FAO, 1990c.

TABLE A10
Height for age, boys, 24 to 60 months

Age (months)	Height (cm)			
	-2 SD	Median	90% of median	80% of median
24	79.2	85.6	77.0	68.5
25	79.9	86.4	77.8	69.1
26	80.6	87.2	78.5	69.8
27	81.3	88.1	79.3	70.5
28	82.0	88.9	80.0	71.1
29	82.7	89.7	80.7	71.8
30	83.4	90.4	81.4	72.3
31	84.1	91.2	82.1	73.0
32	84.7	92.0	82.8	73.6
33	85.4	92.7	83.4	74.2
34	86.0	93.5	84.2	74.8
35	86.7	94.2	84.8	75.4
36	87.3	94.9	85.4	75.9
37	87.9	95.6	86.0	76.5
38	88.6	96.3	86.7	77.0
39	89.2	97.0	87.3	77.8
40	89.8	97.7	87.9	78.2
41	90.4	98.4	88.6	78.7
42	91.0	99.1	89.2	79.3
43	91.6	99.7	89.7	79.8
44	92.1	100.4	90.4	80.3
45	92.7	101.0	90.9	80.8
46	93.3	101.7	91.5	81.4
47	93.9	102.3	92.1	81.8
48	94.4	102.9	92.8	82.3
49	95.0	103.6	93.2	82.9
50	95.5	104.2	93.8	83.4
51	96.1	104.8	94.3	83.8
52	96.6	105.4	94.9	84.3
53	97.1	106.0	95.4	84.8
54	97.7	106.6	95.9	85.3
55	98.2	107.1	96.4	85.7
56	98.7	107.7	96.9	86.2
57	99.2	108.3	97.5	86.6
58	99.7	108.8	97.9	87.0
59	100.2	109.4	98.5	87.5
60	100.7	109.9	98.9	87.9

Source: FAO, 1990c.

TABLE A11
Weight for length, both sexes, length 50 to 109 cm

Length (cm)	Weight (kg)			
	-2 SD	Median	80% of median	70% of median
50	2.6	3.4	2.7	2.4
51	2.7	3.5	2.8	2.4
52	2.8	3.7	3.0	2.6
53	2.9	3.9	3.1	2.7
54	3.1	4.1	3.3	2.9
55	3.3	4.3	3.4	3.0
56	3.5	4.6	3.7	3.2
57	3.7	4.8	3.8	3.4
58	3.9	5.1	4.1	3.6
59	4.1	5.3	4.2	3.7
60	4.3	5.6	4.5	3.9
61	4.6	5.9	4.7	4.1
62	4.8	6.2	5.0	4.3
63	5.1	6.5	5.2	4.6
64	5.4	6.7	5.4	4.7
65	5.6	7.0	5.6	4.9
66	5.9	7.3	5.8	5.1
67	6.1	7.6	6.1	5.3
68	6.4	7.9	6.3	5.5
69	6.7	8.2	6.6	5.7
70	6.9	8.5	6.8	6.0
71	7.2	8.7	7.0	6.1
72	7.4	9.0	7.2	6.3
73	7.6	9.2	7.4	6.4
74	7.8	9.5	7.6	6.6
75	8.1	9.7	7.8	6.8
76	8.3	9.9	7.9	6.9
77	8.5	10.1	8.1	7.1
78	8.6	10.4	8.3	7.3
79	8.8	10.6	8.5	7.4
80	9.0	10.8	8.6	7.6
81	9.2	11.0	8.8	7.7
82	9.4	11.2	9.0	7.8
83	9.6	11.4	9.1	8.0
84	9.7	11.5	9.2	8.0
85	9.9	11.7	9.4	8.2
86	10.1	11.9	9.5	8.3
87	10.3	12.1	9.7	8.5
88	10.5	12.3	9.8	8.5
89	10.7	12.6	10.1	8.8
90	10.8	12.8	10.2	9.0
91	11.1	13.0	10.4	9.1
92	11.3	13.2	10.6	9.2
93	11.5	13.5	10.8	9.4
94	11.7	13.7	11.0	9.6
95	11.8	14.2	11.4	9.9
96	12.0	14.5	11.6	10.2
97	12.2	14.8	11.8	10.4
98	12.4	15.0	12.0	10.5
99	12.6	15.3	12.2	10.7

TABLE A11 *(continued)*

Length (cm)	Weight (kg)			
	-2 SD	Median	80% of median	70% of median
100	12.8	15.5	12.4	10.8
101	13.0	15.8	12.6	11.1
102	13.3	16.1	12.9	11.3
103	13.5	16.4	13.1	11.5
104	13.7	16.7	13.4	11.7
105	14.0	16.9	13.5	11.8
106	14.2	17.2	13.8	12.0
107	14.5	17.5	14.0	12.2
108	14.7	17.8	14.2	12.5
109	15.0	18.2	14.6	12.7

Source: FAO, 1982.

TABLE A12
Weight for length, girls, length 65 to 95 cm

Length (cm)	Weight (kg)			
	-2 SD	Median	80% of median	70% of median
65	5.5	7.0	6.5	4.9
66	5.8	7.3	5.8	5.1
67	6.0	7.5	6.0	5.3
68	6.3	7.8	6.2	5.5
69	6.5	8.1	6.5	5.7
70	6.8	8.4	6.7	5.9
71	7.0	8.6	6.9	6.0
72	7.2	8.9	7.1	6.2
73	7.5	9.1	7.3	6.4
74	7.7	9.4	7.5	6.6
75	7.9	9.6	7.7	6.7
76	8.1	9.8	7.8	6.9
77	8.3	10.0	8.0	7.0
78	8.5	10.2	8.2	7.1
79	8.7	10.4	8.3	7.3
80	8.8	10.6	8.5	7.4
81	9.0	10.8	8.6	7.6
82	9.2	11.0	8.8	7.7
83	9.4	11.2	9.0	7.8
84	9.6	11.4	9.1	8.0
85	9.7	11.6	9.3	8.1
86	9.9	11.8	9.4	8.3
87	10.1	11.9	9.5	8.3
88	10.3	12.2	9.8	8.5
89	10.5	12.4	9.9	8.7
90	10.7	12.6	10.1	8.8
91	10.9	12.8	10.2	9.0
92	11.1	13.0	10.4	9.1
93	11.3	13.3	10.6	9.3
94	11.5	13.5	10.8	9.5
95	11.8	13.8	11.0	9.7

Source: FAO, 1990c.

TABLE A13
Weight for length, boys, length 65 to 95 cm

Length (cm)	Weight (kg)			
	-2 SD	Median	80% of median	70% of median
65	5.7	7.1	5.7	5.0
66	6.0	7.4	5.9	5.2
67	6.2	7.7	6.2	5.4
68	6.5	8.0	6.4	5.6
69	6.8	8.3	6.6	5.8
70	7.0	8.5	6.8	6.0
71	7.3	8.8	7.0	6.2
72	7.5	9.1	7.3	6.4
73	7.8	9.3	7.4	6.5
74	8.0	9.6	7.7	6.7
75	8.2	9.8	7.8	6.9
76	8.4	20.0	8.0	7.0
77	8.6	10.3	8.2	7.2
78	8.8	10.5	8.4	7.4
79	9.0	10.7	8.6	7.5
80	9.2	10.9	8.7	7.6
81	9.4	11.1	8.9	7.8
82	9.6	11.3	9.0	7.9
83	9.6	11.5	9.2	8.1
84	9.9	11.7	9.4	8.2
85	10.1	11.9	9.5	8.3
86	10.3	12.1	9.7	8.5
87	10.5	12.3	9.8	8.6
88	10.6	12.5	10.0	8.8
89	10.8	12.8	10.2	9.0
90	11.0	13.0	10.4	9.1
91	11.2	13.2	10.6	9.2
92	11.4	13.4	10.7	9.4
93	11.6	13.6	11.0	9.6
94	11.9	13.9	11.1	9.7
95	12.1	14.1	11.3	9.9

Source: FAO, 1990c.

TABLE A14
Weight for height, girls, height 75 to 135 cm

Height (cm)	Weight (kg)			
	-2 SD	Median	80% of median	70% of median
75	7.7	9.7	7.8	6.8
76	7.9	10.0	8.0	7.0
77	8.1	10.2	8.2	7.1
78	8.3	10.4	8.3	7.3
79	8.5	10.6	8.5	7.4
80	8.7	10.8	8.6	7.6
81	8.9	11.0	8.8	7.7
82	9.1	11.2	9.0	7.8
83	9.3	11.4	9.1	8.0
84	9.5	11.6	9.3	8.1
85	9.7	11.8	9.4	8.3
86	9.9	12.0	9.6	8.4
87	10.1	12.3	9.8	8.6
88	10.3	12.5	10.0	8.8
89	10.5	12.7	10.2	8.9
90	10.7	12.9	10.3	9.0
91	10.8	13.2	10.6	9.2
92	11.0	13.4	10.7	9.4
93	11.2	13.6	10.9	9.5
94	11.4	13.9	11.1	9.7
95	11.6	14.1	11.3	9.9
96	11.8	14.3	11.4	10.0
97	12.0	14.6	11.7	12.2
98	12.2	14.9	11.9	10.4
99	12.4	15.1	12.1	10.6
100	12.7	15.4	12.3	10.8
101	12.9	15.6	12.5	10.9
102	13.1	15.9	12.7	11.1
103	13.3	16.2	13.0	11.3
104	13.5	16.5	13.2	11.6
105	13.8	16.7	13.4	11.7
106	14.0	17.0	13.6	11.9
107	14.3	17.3	13.8	12.1
108	14.5	17.6	14.1	12.3
109	14.8	17.9	14.3	12.5
110	15.0	18.2	14.6	12.7
111	15.3	18.6	14.9	13.0
112	15.6	18.9	15.1	13.2
113	15.9	19.2	15.4	13.4
114	16.2	19.5	15.6	13.7
115	16.5	19.9	15.9	13.9
116	16.8	20.3	16.2	14.2
117	17.1	20.6	16.5	14.4
118	17.4	21.0	16.8	14.7
119	17.7	21.4	17.1	15.0
120	18.1	21.8	17.4	15.3
121	18.4	22.2	17.8	15.5
122	18.8	22.7	18.2	15.9
123	19.1	23.1	18.5	16.2
124	19.5	23.6	18.9	16.5

TABLE A14 *(continued)*

Height (cm)	Weight (kg)			
	-2 SD	Median	80% of median	70% of median
125	19.9	24.1	19.3	16.9
126	20.2	24.6	19.7	17.2
127	20.6	25.1	20.1	17.6
128	21.0	25.7	20.6	18.0
129	21.4	26.2	21.0	18.3
130	21.8	26.8	21.4	18.8
131	22.3	27.4	21.9	19.2
132	22.7	28.0	22.4	19.6
133	23.1	28.7	23.0	20.1
134	23.6	29.4	23.5	20.6
135	24.0	30.1	24.1	21.1

Source: FAO, 1990c.

TABLE A15

Weight for height, boys, height 75 to 135 cm

Height (cm)	Weight (kg)			
	-2 SD	Median	80% of median	70% of median
75	7.9	9.9	7.9	6.9
76	8.1	10.1	8.1	7.1
77	8.3	10.4	8.3	7.3
78	8.5	10.6	8.5	7.4
79	8.7	10.8	8.6	7.6
80	8.9	11.0	8.8	7.7
81	9.1	11.2	9.0	7.8
82	9.3	11.5	9.2	8.1
83	9.5	11.7	9.4	8.2
84	9.7	11.9	9.5	8.3
85	9.9	12.1	9.7	8.5
86	10.1	12.3	9.8	8.6
87	10.3	12.6	10.1	8.8
88	10.5	12.8	10.2	9.0
89	10.7	13.0	10.4	9.1
90	10.9	13.3	10.6	9.3
91	11.1	13.5	10.8	9.5
92	11.3	13.7	11.0	9.6
93	11.5	14.0	11.2	9.8
94	11.7	14.2	11.4	9.9
95	11.9	14.5	11.6	10.2
96	12.1	14.7	11.8	10.3
97	12.4	15.0	12.0	10.5
98	12.6	15.2	12.2	10.6
99	12.8	15.5	12.4	10.9
100	13.0	15.7	12.6	11.0
101	13.2	16.0	12.8	11.2
102	13.4	16.3	13.0	11.4
103	13.7	16.6	13.3	11.6
104	13.9	16.9	13.5	11.8
105	14.2	17.1	13.7	12.0
106	14.4	17.4	13.9	12.2
107	14.7	17.7	14.2	12.4
108	14.9	18.0	14.4	12.8
109	15.2	18.3	14.6	12.8
110	15.4	18.7	15.0	13.1
111	15.7	19.0	15.2	13.3
112	16.0	19.3	15.4	13.5
113	16.3	19.6	15.7	13.7
114	16.6	20.0	16.0	14.0
115	16.9	20.3	16.6	14.2
116	17.2	20.7	16.6	14.5
117	17.5	21.1	16.9	14.8
118	17.9	21.4	17.1	15.0
119	18.2	21.8	17.4	15.3
120	18.5	22.2	17.8	15.5
121	18.9	22.6	18.1	15.6
122	19.2	23.0	18.4	16.1
123	19.6	23.4	18.7	16.4
124	20.0	23.9	19.1	16.7

TABLE A15 *(continued)*

Height (cm)	Weight (kg)			
	-2 SD	Median	80% of median	70% of median
125	20.4	24.3	19.4	17.0
126	20.7	24.8	19.8	17.4
127	21.1	25.2	20.2	17.6
128	21.5	25.7	20.8	18.0
129	21.9	26.2	21.0	18.3
130	22.3	26.8	21.4	18.8
131	22.7	27.3	21.8	19.1
132	21.1	27.8	22.2	19.5
133	23.6	28.4	22.7	19.9
134	24.0	29.0	23.2	20.3
135	24.4	29.6	23.7	20.7

Source: FAO, 1990c.

TABLE A16
Standard triceps skinfold, birth to 96 months, by sex (mm)

Age (months)	Male	Female
0	6.0	6.5
6	10.0	10.0
12	10.3	10.2
18	10.3	10.2
24	10.0	10.1
36	9.3	9.7
48	9.3	10.2
60	9.1	9.4
72	8.2	9.6
84	7.9	9.4
96	7.6	10.1

Source: WHO, 1966.

TABLE A17
Percentiles of triceps skinfold thickness, male adolescents, 9 to 18 years (mm)

Age (years)	Percentile						
	5th	10th	25th	50th	75th	90th	95th
9.0	4.8	5.5	6.7	8.4	11.1	14.6	17.8
9.5	4.8	5.5	6.7	8.6	11.5	15.5	18.7
10.0	4.9	5.6	6.8	8.8	11.9	16.4	19.8
10.5	4.9	5.6	6.9	9.0	12.4	17.4	20.8
11.0	4.9	5.6	7.0	9.3	12.8	18.3	21.8
11.5	5.0	5.7	7.0	9.4	13.2	19.1	22.7
12.0	4.9	5.7	7.1	9.6	13.4	19.8	23.4
12.5	4.9	5.6	7.1	9.6	13.6	20.2	23.9
13.0	4.8	5.6	7.0	9.6	13.5	20.3	24.1
13.5	4.6	5.4	6.8	9.4	13.3	20.1	24.0
14.0	4.5	5.3	6.6	9.1	13.0	19.6	23.7
14.5	4.3	5.1	6.4	8.7	12.5	19.0	23.2
15.0	4.1	4.9	6.2	8.4	12.0	18.2	22.7
15.5	3.9	4.7	5.9	8.0	11.5	17.4	22.1
16.0	3.8	4.6	5.8	7.7	11.2	16.8	21.6
16.5	3.8	4.5	5.6	7.4	10.9	16.2	21.3
17.0	3.8	4.5	5.6	7.3	10.9	16.0	21.3
17.5	3.9	4.5	5.7	7.3	11.1	16.1	21.6
18.0	4.2	4.6	5.9	7.5	11.7	16.6	22.3

Source: WHO, 1995. Reference data are based on the Health Examination Survey and the first National Health and Nutrition Examination Survey (NHANES) in the United States.

TABLE A18
Percentiles of triceps skinfold thickness, female adolescents, 9 to 18 years (mm)

Age (years)	Percentile						
	5th	10th	25th	50th	75th	90th	95th
9.0	6.0	6.8	8.4	11.0	14.1	18.5	21.2
9.5	6.0	6.8	8.5	11.2	14.5	19.1	22.0
10.0	6.1	6.9	8.6	11.4	15.0	19.8	22.8
10.5	6.2	7.0	8.8	11.6	15.4	20.4	23.5
11.0	6.3	7.2	9.0	11.9	15.9	21.1	24.2
11.5	6.4	7.3	9.2	12.2	16.4	21.6	24.9
12.0	6.6	7.6	9.5	12.6	16.9	22.2	25.6
12.5	·6.7	7.8	9.8	12.9	17.5	22.8	26.2
13.0	6.9	8.0	10.1	13.3	18.0	23.3	26.8
13.5	7.1	8.3	10.4	13.7	18.5	23.8	27.4
14.0	7.3	8.5	10.7	14.1	19.0	24.2	28.0
14.5	7.5	8.8	11.1	14.5	19.5	24.7	28.5
15.0	7.7	9.1	11.4	14.8	20.0	25.1	29.0
15.5	7.9	9.3	11.8	15.2	20.5	25.5	29.4
16.0	8.0	9.6	12.2	15.6	20.9	25.9	29.8
16.5	8.2	9.8	12.5	16.0	21.3	26.3	30.1
17.0	8.4	10.0	12.8	16.3	21.7	26.7	30.4
17.5	8.5	10.2	13.2	16.6	22.0	27.0	30.7
18.0	8.6	10.4	13.5	17.0	22.2	27.3	30.9

Source: WHO, 1995. Reference data are based on the Health Examination Survey and the first National Health and Nutrition Examination Survey (NHANES) in the United States.

TABLE A19
Triceps skinfold and arm circumference, adults, by sex

Percentage of standard	Triceps skinfold (mm)		Arm circumference (cm)	
	Male	Female	Male	Female
100	12.5	16.5	29.3	28.5
90	11.3	14.9	26.3	25.7
80	10.0	13.2	23.4	22.8
70	8.8	11.6	20.5	20.0
60	7.5	9.9	17.6	17.1

Source: WHO, 1966.

TABLE A20

Mid-upper-arm circumference, boys, 6 to 60 months, median and standard deviations (cm)

Age (months)	-3 SD	-2 SD	-1 SD	Median	+1 SD	+2 SD	+3 SD
6	11.5	12.6	13.8	14.9	16.1	17.3	18.4
7	11.6	12.7	13.9	15.1	16.3	17.5	18.6
8	11.7	12.8	14.0	15.2	16.4	17.6	18.8
9	11.7	12.9	14.2	15.4	16.6	17.8	19.0
10	11.8	13.0	14.2	15.5	16.7	17.9	19.1
11	11.9	13.1	14.3	15.6	16.8	18.0	19.3
12	11.9	13.2	14.4	15.7	16.9	18.1	19.4
13	12.0	12.2	14.5	15.7	17.0	18.2	19.5
14	12.0	13.3	14.5	15.8	17.1	18.3	19.6
15	12.1	13.3	14.6	15.9	17.1	18.4	19.7
16	12.1	13.4	14.6	15.9	17.2	18.5	19.8
17	12.1	13.4	14.7	16.0	17.3	18.6	19.8
18	12.1	13.4	14.7	16.0	17.3	18.6	19.9
19	12.2	13.5	14.8	16.1	17.4	18.7	20.0
20	12.2	13.5	14.8	16.1	17.4	18.7	20.0
21	12.2	13.5	14.8	16.1	17.5	18.8	20.1
22	12.2	13.5	14.9	16.2	17.5	18.8	20.1
23	12.2	13.5	14.9	16.2	17.5	18.9	20.2
24	12.2	13.6	14.9	16.2	17.6	18.9	20.2
25	12.2	13.6	14.9	16.3	17.6	18.9	20.3
26	12.3	13.6	14.9	16.3	17.6	19.0	20.3
27	12.3	13.6	15.0	16.3	17.7	19.0	20.4
28	12.3	13.6	15.0	16.3	17.7	19.1	20.4
29	12.3	13.7	15.0	16.4	17.7	19.1	20.4
30	12.3	13.7	15.0	16.4	17.8	19.1	20.5
31	12.3	13.7	15.1	16.4	17.8	19.2	20.5
32	12.3	13.7	15.1	16.5	17.8	19.2	20.6
33	12.4	13.7	15.1	16.5	17.9	19.2	20.6
34	12.4	13.8	15.1	16.5	17.9	19.3	20.6
35	12.4	13.8	15.2	16.5	17.9	19.3	20.7
36	12.4	13.8	15.2	16.6	18.0	19.3	20.7
37	12.4	13.8	15.2	16.6	18.0	–	–
38	12.4	13.8	15.2	16.6	18.0	–	–
39	12.5	13.9	15.3	16.7	18.1	–	–
40	12.5	13.9	15.3	16.7	18.1	–	–
41	12.5	13.9	15.3	16.7	18.1	–	–
42	12.5	13.9	15.4	16.8	18.2	–	–
43	12.5	14.0	15.4	16.8	18.2	–	–
44	12.5	14.0	15.4	16.8	18.3	–	–
45	12.6	14.0	15.4	16.9	18.3	–	–
46	12.6	14.0	15.5	16.9	18.4	–	–
47	12.6	14.0	15.5	17.0	18.4	–	–
48	12.6	14.1	15.5	17.0	18.4	–	–
49	12.6	14.1	15.6	17.0	18.5	–	–
50	12.6	14.1	15.6	17.1	18.5	–	–
51	12.6	14.1	15.6	17.1	18.6	–	–
52	12.6	14.1	15.6	17.1	18.6	–	–
53	12.6	14.1	15.7	17.2	18.7	–	–
54	12.6	14.2	15.7	17.2	18.7	–	–
55	12.6	14.2	15.7	17.2	18.8	–	–
56	12.6	14.2	15.7	17.3	18.8	–	–
57	12.6	14.2	15.8	17.3	18.9	–	–
58	12.6	14.2	15.8	17.3	18.9	–	–
59	12.6	14.2	15.8	17.4	19.0	–	–
60	12.6	14.2	15.8	17.4	19.0	–	–

Source: WHO, 1995. Reference data are based on the first and second National Health and Nutrition Examination Surveys (NHANES I and II) in the United States.

TABLE A21

Mid-upper-arm circumference, girls, 6 to 60 months, median and standard deviations (cm)

Age (months)	-3 SD	-2 SD	-1 SD	Median	+1 SD	+2 SD	+3 SD
6	10.4	11.5	12.7	13.9	15.0	16.2	17.4
7	10.6	11.8	13.0	14.1	15.3	16.5	17.7
8	10.8	12.0	13.2	14.4	15.6	16.8	18.0
9	11.0	12.2	13.4	14.6	15.8	17.0	18.2
10	11.1	12.3	13.6	14.8	16.0	17.2	18.4
11	11.3	12.5	13.7	15.0	16.2	17.4	18.6
12	11.4	12.6	13.9	15.1	16.4	17.6	18.8
13	11.5	12.7	14.0	15.2	16.5	17.7	19.0
14	11.6	12.8	14.1	15.4	16.6	17.9	19.2
15	11.7	12.9	14.2	15.5	16.7	18.0	19.3
16	11.7	13.0	14.3	15.6	16.8	18.1	19.4
17	11.8	13.1	14.4	15.7	16.9	18.2	19.5
18	11.8	13.1	14.4	15.7	17.0	18.3	19.6
19	11.9	13.2	14.5	15.8	17.1	18.4	19.7
20	11.9	13.2	14.5	15.8	17.2	18.5	19.8
21	11.9	13.3	14.6	15.9	17.2	18.5	19.8
22	12.0	13.3	14.6	15.9	17.3	18.6	19.9
23	12.0	13.3	14.7	16.0	17.3	18.6	20.0
24	12.0	13.4	14.7	16.0	17.4	18.7	20.0
25	12.0	13.4	14.7	16.1	17.4	18.7	20.1
26	12.1	13.4	14.7	16.1	17.4	18.8	20.1
27	12.1	13.4	14.8	16.1	17.5	18.8	20.2
28	12.1	13.4	14.8	16.1	17.5	18.9	20.2
29	12.1	13.5	14.8	16.2	17.5	18.9	20.3
30	12.1	13.5	14.8	16.2	17.6	18.9	20.3
31	12.1	13.5	14.9	16.2	17.6	19.0	20.3
32	12.1	13.5	14.9	16.3	17.6	19.0	20.4
33	12.2	13.5	14.9	16.3	17.7	19.0	20.4
34	12.2	13.6	14.9	16.3	17.7	19.1	20.5
35	12.2	13.6	15.0	16.3	17.7	19.1	20.5
36	12.2	13.6	15.0	16.4	17.8	19.2	20.5
37	12.2	13.6	15.0	16.4	17.8	19.2	–
38	12.2	13.6	15.0	16.4	17.8	19.2	–
39	12.3	13.7	15.1	16.5	17.9	19.3	–
40	12.3	13.7	15.1	16.5	17.9	19.3	–
41	12.3	13.7	15.1	16.6	18.0	19.4	–
42	12.3	13.8	15.2	16.6	18.0	19.4	–
43	12.4	13.8	15.2	16.6	18.1	19.5	–
44	12.4	13.8	15.2	16.7	18.1	19.5	–
45	12.4	13.8	15.3	16.7	18.1	19.6	–
46	12.4	13.9	15.3	16.7	18.2	19.6	–
47	12.4	13.9	15.3	16.8	18.2	19.7	–
48	12.4	13.9	15.4	16.8	18.3	19.8	–
49	12.5	13.9	15.4	16.9	18.3	19.8	–
50	12.5	14.0	15.4	16.9	18.4	19.9	–
51	12.5	14.0	15.5	17.0	18.4	19.9	–
52	12.5	14.0	15.5	17.0	18.5	20.0	–
53	12.5	14.0	15.5	17.0	18.6	20.1	–
54	12.5	14.0	15.6	17.1	18.6	20.1	–
55	12.5	14.1	15.6	17.1	18.7	20.2	–
56	12.5	14.1	15.6	17.2	18.7	20.3	–
57	12.5	14.1	15.7	17.2	18.8	20.3	–
58	12.5	14.1	15.7	17.3	18.8	20.4	–
59	12.5	14.1	15.7	17.3	18.9	20.5	–
60	12.5	14.1	15.7	17.3	18.9	20.5	–

Source: WHO, 1995. Reference data are based on the first and second National Health and Nutrition Examination Surveys (NHANES I and II) in the United States.

<table>
<tr><td colspan="2" align="center">TABLE A22
Average age of dentition, first teeth</td></tr>
</table>

Teeth	Age (months)
Central incisors, lower	7-8
Central incisors, upper	8-9
Lateral incisors, upper	9-11
Lateral incisors, lower	10-12
First molars	12-18
Canines	18-24
Second molars	24-36

<table>
<tr><td colspan="2" align="center">TABLE A23
Average age of dentition, permanent teeth</td></tr>
</table>

Teeth	Age (years)
First molars	6
Central incisors	6-7
Lateral incisors	8
Lower canines	10
First premolars	10
Upper canines	11
Second premolars	11
Second molars	12-14

Annex 3
Nutrient content of selected foods

This annex provides data on the content of energy and of ten important nutrients in some selected foods. The data are based on determinations done by many different scientists in several countries and have been published previously in *Food and nutrition in the management of group feeding programmes* (FAO, 1993b).

The nutrient content is given per 100 g of edible portion of the food listed. It is stressed that foods vary in their nutrient content depending on the particular variety of the food and the conditions under which it is produced, processed, marketed, stored and cooked. For example, one figure is given for the vitamin A content of "tomato, ripe" in these tables, but there are many varieties of tomatoes; some are picked very ripe and others when green; and some are eaten uncooked while others are eaten boiled, fried or cooked in other ways. All of these factors may influence the content of carotene, the precursor of vitamin A. The figure of 113 µg vitamin A per 100 g of tomato consumed has been obtained from many different analyses of different tomato varieties treated under different conditions; it has been judged to be a usual amount of vitamin A of average tomatoes. Although some tomatoes under some conditions may provide only 80 µg per 100 g and others 140 µg, the table shows nevertheless that tomatoes always contain less vitamin A than carrots (listed as 2 813 µg vitamin A per 100 g) and more than bananas (listed as 20 µg per 100 g). Thus the table, used judiciously, is helpful in forming dietary advice and for many other useful purposes.

Readers who need data not included here should consult the source publications.

TABLE A24
Nutrients in 100 g edible portion of food

Food (waste %)[a]	Energy (kcal)	Protein (g)	Fat (g)	Calcium (mg)	Iron (mg)	Vitamin A (µg)	Thiamine (mg)	Riboflavin (mg)	Niacin (mg)	Folate (µg)	Vitamin C (mg)
Cereals											
Barley	350	8.2	1.0	16	2.0	0	0.12	0.05	3.1	20	0
Maize flour, whole	353	9.3	3.8	10	2.5	0	0.30	0.10	1.8	U	0
Maize flour, refined	368	9.4	1.0	3	1.3	50[b]	0.26	0.08	1.0	U	0
Millet, bulrush	341	10.4	4.0	22	3.0	0	0.30	0.22	1.7	U	0
Rice, polished	361	6.5	1.0	4	0.5	0	0.08	0.02	1.5	10	0
Rice, parboiled	364	6.7	1.0	7	1.2	0	0.20	0.08	2.6	11	0
Sorghum	345	10.7	3.2	26	4.5	0	0.34	0.15	3.3	U	0
Wheat, whole	323	12.6	1.8	36	4.0	0	0.30	0.07	5	51	0
Wheat flour, white	341	9.4	1.3	15	1.5	0	0.10	0.03	0.7	22	0
Bread, white	261	7.7	2.0	37	1.7	0	0.16	0.06	1.0	17	0
Pasta	342	12.0	1.8	25	2.1	0	0.22	0.03	3.1	34	0
Cereal products (food aid items)											
Bulgur wheat	354	11.2	1.5	23	7.8	0	0.30	0.1	5.5	38	0
Soy-fortified bulgur wheat	350	17.3	2.0	54	4.7	0	0.25	0.13	4.2	74	0
Maize meal, yellow, degermed	364	7.9	1.2	25	1.1	132	0.14	0.05	1.0	U	0
Soy-fortified maize meal	392	13.0	1.5	178	4.8	228	0.70	0.30	3.1	U	0
Rolled oats	363	13.0	7.0	70	4.0	0	0.60	0.20	1.3	24	0
Soy-fortified sorghum grits	360	16.0	1.0	40	2.0	†	0.20	0.10	1.7	50	0
Soy-fortified rolled oats	380	20.0	6.0	81	5.3	0	0.74	0.14	4.0	U	0
Wheat flour (medium extraction)	350	11.5	1.5	29	3.7	0	0.28	0.14	4.5	U	0
Soy-fortified wheat flour, 6% soy	355	14.0	1.2	0	U	0	U	U	U	U	0
Soy-fortified wheat flour, 11–12% soy	355	16.5	1.4	211	4.8	265	0.65	0.36	4.6	U	0
Blended food and biscuits											
Maize soy milk + wheat soy milk	380	20.0	6.0	1 000	18.0	510	0.80	0.80	8.0	200	40
Instant maize soy milk	380	20.0	6.0	1 000	18.0	510	0.80	0.80	8.0	200	40
Maize soy blend	380	18.0	6.0	513	18.5	500	0.65	0.50	6.8	U	40
Wheat soy blend	360	20.0	6.0	750	20.8	496	1.50	0.60	9.1	U	40
Australian high-protein biscuits	450	20.0	20.0	1 125	25.0	0	2.75	4.08	27.5	U	63
Danish high-protein biscuits	480	20.0	19.0	179	7.2	0	0.25	U	1.0	U	1
Starchy roots and fruits											
Cassava, fresh (26)	149	1.2	0.2	68	1.9	15	0.04	0.05	0.60	24	31
Cassava flour	344	1.6	0.5	66	3.6	0	0.06	0.05	0.90	U	0
Plantain (34)	135	1.2	0.3	8	1.3	390	0.08	0.04	0.60	16	20
Potato, Irish (20)	79	2.1	0.1	7	0.8	0	0.09	0.04	1.50	13	20
Sweet potato (yellow) (19)	105	1.7	0.3	22	0.6	(2 000)[c]	0.07	0.04	0.70	52	23
Yam, fresh (16)	118	1.5	0.2	17	0.5	0	0.11	0.03	0.80	23	17

Table A24 (continued)

Food (waste %)[a]	Energy (kcal)	Protein (g)	Fat (g)	Calcium (mg)	Iron (mg)	Vitamin A (µg)	Thiamine (mg)	Riboflavin (mg)	Niacin (mg)	Folate (µg)	Vitamin C (mg)
Pulses											
Kidney beans, dry	333	23.6	0.8	143	8.2	0	0.5	0.22	2.1	180	5
Mung beans, dry	347	23.9	1.1	132	6.7	11	0.6	0.23	2.3	120	5
Lentils, dry	338	28.1	1.0	51	9.0	4	0.5	0.25	2.6	U	6
Pigeon peas, dry	343	21.7	1.5	130	5.2	3	0.6	0.19	3.0	100	0
Groundnuts, dry	567	25.8	49.2	92	4.6	0	0.6	0.14	12.1	110	0
Soybeans, dry	416	36.5	20.0	277	15.7	2	0.9	0.25	1.6	210	0
Sunflower seeds	605	22.5	49.0	98	6.3	0	1.9	0.14	4.1	U	0
Coconut flesh (27)	376	3.9	36.5	20	2.3	0	0.6	0.80	0.4	U	0
Vegetables											
Carrot (19)	43	1.0	0.2	27	0.5	2813	0.10	0.06	0.9	14	9
Eggplant (17)	26	1.1	0.1	36	0.6	7	0.09	0.02	0.6	18	2
Dark green leaves (spinach) (15)	22	2.9	0.4	99	2.7	672	0.08	0.19	0.7	194	28
Medium-green leaves (Chinese cabbage) (15)	16	1.2	0.2	77	0.3	120	0.04	0.05	0.4	79	27
Light-green leaves (lettuce) (32)	13	1.0	0.2	19	0.5	33	0.05	0.03	0.2	56	4
Onion (8)	34	1.2	0.3	25	0.4	0	0.06	0.10	0.1	20	8
Green pepper (23)	25	0.9	0.5	6	1.3	53	0.09	0.05	0.6	17	128
Red pepper	25	0.9	0.5	6	1.3	530	0.09	0.05	0.6	17	128
Pumpkin (30)	26	1.0	0.1	21	0.8	160	0.05	0.11	0.6	8	9
Tomato, ripe	19	0.9	0.2	7	0.5	113	0.06	0.05	0.6	9	18
Sweet potato leaves	35	4.0	0.3	37	1.0	130	0.16	0.35	1.1	U	11
Amaranth	26	2.5	0.3	215	2.3	292	0.03	0.16	0.7	85	43
Beans, fresh	36	2.5	0.2	43	1.4	375	0.08	0.12	0.5	U	27
Maize, fresh	165	5.0	2.1	2	0.5	28	0.20	0.06	1.7	46	7
Fruits											
Avocado (50)	161	2.0	15.3	11	1.02	61	0.11	0.12	1.9	22	8
Banana (33)	92	1.0	0.5	6	0.30	20	0.05	0.10	0.5	19	9
Orange (28)	47	0.9	0.1	40	0.10	120	0.09	0.04	0.3	30	53
Lime (36)	30	0.7	0.2	33	0.60	1	0.03	0.02	0.2	8	23
Lemon (36)	29	0.6	0.3	26	0.60	3	0.04	0.02	0.1	11	53
Guava (11)	51	0.8	0.6	20	0.30	79	0.05	0.05	1.2	7	184
Mango (31)	65	0.5	0.3	10	0.10	389	0.06	0.06	0.6	7	28
Papaw (28)	39	0.6	0.1	24	0.10	201	0.03	0.03	0.3	1	62
Pineapple (46)	49	0.4	0.4	7	0.40	2	0.09	0.04	0.4	11	15
Watermelon (56)	32	0.6	0.4	8	0.20	37	0.08	0.02	0.2	2	10
Baobab (72)	290	2.2	0.8	284	7.40	70	0.37	0.06	2.1	U	270

TABLE A24 (continued)

Food (waste %)[a]	Energy (kcal)	Protein (g)	Fat (g)	Calcium (mg)	Iron (mg)	Vitamin A (µg)	Thiamine (mg)	Riboflavin (mg)	Niacin (mg)	Folate (µg)	Vitamin C (mg)
Fruits and sugar											
Dried apricots	238	3.7	0.5	45	4.7	724	0.01	0.15	3.0	10	2
Raisins	300	3.2	0.5	49	2.1	1	0.16	0.09	0.8	3	3
Dates, dry (10)	275	2.0	0.5	32	1.2	5	0.09	0.10	2.2	13	0
Marmalade	243	0.4	0	32	2.0	t	t	t	t	t	4
Jam	234	0.4	0	10	2.0	t	0.10	0.10	0.3	t	9
Sugar	400	0	0	0	0	0	0	0	0	0	0
Meat											
Mutton flesh	122	20.4	3.40	12	1.8	U	0.18	0.25	5.8	3	0
Beef flesh	115	22.0	1.90	4	1.9	20	0.23	0.26	7.5	15	0
Beef fat	900	1.5	94.00	0	0	0	0	0	0	0	0
Beef blood	80	17.8	0.13	6	44	21	0.90	0.30	1.0	0	0
Beef liver	123	19.7	3.10	7	7.1	1 500	0.30	2.88	14.7	22	30
Pork flesh	114	22.0	1.90	3	1.0	6	0.90	0.23	5.0	6	2
Goat meat (with fat)	161	19.5	7.90	10	2.0	36	0.15	0.28	4.9	U	0
Corned beef	225	25.3	12.00	14	4.1	0	0.20	0.23	3.2	2	0
Canned pork	536	11.0	51.30	U	U	0	0.60	0.16	2.5	U	0
Poultry (33)	139	19.0	7.00	15	1.5	0	0.10	0.15	9.0	U	0
Fish											
Cod (25)	82	17.7	0.4	24	0.4	10	0.6	0.46	2.3	12	2
Perch (60)	89	18.4	0.8	20	1.0	7	0.8	0.12	1.7	U	0
Fish, dried, salted	225	47.0	7.5	343	2.8	0	0.07	0.11	8.6	U	0
Stock fish (Norway), unsalted (36)	330	79.0	1.4	60	4.3	U	0.9	0.10	3.5	U	0
Sardines (canned in oil)	238	24.1	13.9	330	2.7	58	0.4	0.30	6.5	16	0
Fish protein concentrate, Norse type B	390	73.0	10.0	1 800	26.9	500 IU	0.3	0.73	12.6	U	0
Fish protein concentrate, Astra type A	330	80.0	0.1	300	U	U	U	U	U	U	U
Dairy products and eggs											
Breast milk	70	1.0	4.4	32	0.05	64	0.01	0.04	0.18	5	5
Cows' milk, whole	61	3.3	3.3	119	0.05	31	0.04	0.16	0.10	5	1
Dried whole milk	496	26.3	26.7	912	0.50	280	0.28	1.21	0.60	37	9
Dried skimmed milk	362	36.2	0.8	1 257	1.0	1 500[d]	0.42	1.55	1.00	50	7
Condensed milk, sweetened	321	7.9	8.7	284	0.20	81	0.09	0.42	0.21	11	3
Evaporated milk	134	6.8	7.6	261	0.20	54	0.05	0.32	0.20	8	2
Canned milk	355	22.5	28	630	0.20	120	0.03	0.45	0.20	U	0
Canned cheese (average)	275	19.0	21.0	480	0.60	1 000	0.02	0.14	4.40	38	0
Danish new cheese	475	23.5	23.0	U	U	U	U	U	U	U	U
Milk bars	540	27.0	27.0	U	U	U	U	U	U	U	U
Milk tablets	U	U	U	U	U	U	U	U	U	U	U
Eggs, fresh	158	12.1	11.2	56	2.1	156	0.09	0.30	0.3	65	U
Eggs, dried	594	45.8	41.8	212	7.9	588	0.31	1.17	6.40	184	0

TABLE A24 (continued)

Food (waste %)[a]	Energy (kcal)	Protein (g)	Fat (g)	Calcium (mg)	Iron (mg)	Vitamin A (µg)	Thiamine (mg)	Riboflavin (mg)	Niacin (mg)	Folate (µg)	Vitamin C (mg)
Fats and oils											
Animal fat (lard)	900	0	100.0	0	0	0	0	0	0	0	0
Butter	717	0.9	81.0	24	0.2	754	t	0.04	t	3	0
Ghee	876	0.3	99.5	0	0	925	0	0	0	0	0
Margarine	719	0.9	80.5	30	0	993[d]	0.01	0.04	t	1	0
Palm oil	884	0	100.0	0	0	5 000[e]	0	0	0	0	0
Vegetable oil (maize)	884	0	100.0	0	0	0	0	0	0	0	0
Cooked food											
Rice, polished, boiled	123	2.2	0.3	U	0.2	0	0.01	0.01	0.3	3	0
Kidney beans, boiled	127	8.7	0.5	U	2.9	0	U	U	0.6	129	1
Lentils, boiled	116	9.0	0.4	U	3.3	1	U	U	1.1	180	2
Groundnuts, boiled	318	13.5	22.0	U	1.0	0	U	U	5.3	75	0
Groundnuts, dry roasted	585	23.7	49.7	U	2.3	0	U	U	13.5	45	0
Potatoes, boiled, no skin	86	1.7	0.1	U	0.3	0	0.10	U	1.3	9	7
Spinach, boiled, drained	23	3.0	0.3	U	3.4	819	U	U	0.5	145	10

Sources: USDA, 1976-88; Holland, Unwin and Buss, 1988; Souci, Fachmann and Kraut, 1989; FAO/USDA, 1968, 1972; FAO, 1982; West, Pepping and Temaliwa, 1988.

Notes: All values are for raw food, except in the final section. U = no value could be found for the nutrient; t = a trace of the nutrient is present.

[a] Values for percentage waste are from Souci, Fachmann and Kraut, 1989. Where there is no figure, the food contains no waste.
[b] Yellow maize (FAO, 1982).
[c] Deep-yellow varieties only.
[d] If fortified.
[e] Fresh, unbleached oil.

Annex 4
Reference nutrient densities relevant for developing and evaluating food-based dietary guidelines

The traditional approach to providing dietary guidance and evaluating the nutritional adequacy of diets, which focused on recommended dietary allowances (RDAs) for specific nutrients, has proved inadequate for developing effective nutrition education programmes. The 1995 FAO/WHO Consultation on Preparation and Use of Food-Based Dietary Guidelines used the concept of nutrient density applied to total diet as an alternative to RDA to address better the issues of optimal nutrient intakes.

The concept of nutrient density was originally developed to compare the amount of essential micronutrients provided by a food or diet to the energy provided by that food or diet. Thus, those foods that have a high nutrient density are good sources of micronutrients or protein and are more important as sources of these essential nutrients than as sources of energy.

For use in food-based dietary guidelines (FBDGs), the original nutrient density approach has been modified to include: required nutrient intake (RDA, for example, for protein), desirable nutrient intake (a range from RDA to a higher level that may be protective; for example, a higher level of vitamin C to promote iron absorption or of folic acid to lower the risk of neural tube defects) and population goals (a range of desirable average intakes within the population that may lower the risk of non-communicable diseases, for example, for fat and salt). Because of this comprehensive approach, the concept could be most appropriately used by health professionals or policy-makers in developing dietary goals or targets or for devising FBDGs in relation to the total diet consumed as opposed to individual foods or meals.

In the table, the nutrient density is expressed in relation to 1 000 kcal. This association should not be interpreted as a physiological relationship between the specific nutrients and energy requirements, but as a way of defining the adequacy of a given diet to meet the needs of specific nutrients if sufficient energy is consumed.

TABLE A25
Reference nutrient densities for selected nutrients

Nutrient	Nutrient density (amount of nutrient per 1 000 kcal)	Comments
Energy	See age-, sex- and activity-specific recommendations in Annex 1	For 2-5 years of age: 0.6-0.8 kcal/ml liquid foods; 2 kcal/g solid foods
Protein	20-25 g 25-30 g	8-10% of total energy if protein quality is high 10-12% of total energy if animal protein intake is low
Fats	16-39 g (max)	15-35% of energy; cholesterol <300 mg/day
Saturated fats	<11 g	Up to 10% of total energy intake
Carbohydrates	140-190 g	55-75% of energy
Fibre	8-20 g	Total dietary fibre must be accounted, not only crude fibre
Vitamin A (retinol)	350-500 µg RE	1 retinol equivalent (RE) = 1 µg retinol or 6 µg beta-carotene as provitamin A
Beta-carotene	–	Functions as antioxidant; no RDA for beta-carotene
Vitamin D	2.5-5 µg	Promotes bone health
Vitamin E	3.5-5 mg α-TE	1 mg α-TE = 1 mg α-d-tocopherol; inhibits lipoprotein oxidation
Vitamin K	20-40 µg	
Vitamin C (ascorbic acid)	25-30 mg	Functions as an antioxidant; enhances iron absorption
Thiamine	0.5-0.8 mg	
Riboflavin	0.6-0.9 mg	
Niacin (or equivalent)	6-10 mg	60 mg tryptophan equivalent to 1 mg niacin
Vitamin B_6	0.6-1 mg	
Vitamin B_{12}	0.5-1 µg	Reduces homocysteinaemia
Folate	150-200 µg	Intakes of 400 µg/day associated with reduced risk of neural tube birth defects; reduces hyperhomocysteinaemia
Iron	3.5, 5.5, 11 or 20 mg	For high, intermediate, low and very low bioavailability diets
Zinc	6 or 10 mg	For high and low bioavailability diets
Calcium	250-400 mg	Calcium-rich foods especially for adolescents and lactating pregnant women
Iodine	75 µg	100-200 µg/day in regions free of goitre; salt fortification usually required
Fluoride	0.5-1 mg (max)	If water has ≥1 ppm requirement is met
Sodium as NaCl	<2.5 g	Total sodium as NaCl <6 g/day (population mean)

Source: WHO, 1996.
Note: These nutrient densities refer to total diet; if intake is sufficient to meet energy needs, the diet will also meet the needs of all except possibly infants under two years of age and pregnant and lactating women. Infants up to four to six months of age should be fed exclusively human milk; after this period breastmilk should be complemented with appropriate foods to provide additional energy, protein and specific nutrients.

Annex 5
Conversions

This annex provides approximate values of measurements in the metric and non-metric systems to allow conversion from one to the other. Approximate values are given for easy calculation.

The United States, Canada and the United Kingdom for many years did not use the metric system, whereas most continental European countries did. In the non-industrialized countries the system used up until about 1965 often depended on the main large power that had colonized or influenced that country. Thus in Africa Zaire and Senegal, for example, used the metric system, whereas Nigeria and Zimbabwe did not. Now the United States, Canada and the United Kingdom are increasingly moving to use the metric system, and many countries have followed suit. Nutrition journals largely use the metric system except in some areas. Thus in some countries distances are given in the metric system, but heights of individuals are given in inches rather than centimetres and kilocalories are used rather than joules to express quantities of energy.

Length

1 centimetre (cm) = 0.4 inches (in)
1 metre (m) = 100 cm = 39 in (approximately 3 feet)
1 in = 2.5 cm
1 foot (ft) = 30.5 cm

Weight

100 milligrams (mg) = 1.5 grains (gn)
1 grain = 65 mg
100 grams (g) = 3.6 ounces (oz)
1 ounce = 28.3 g
1 kilogram (kg) = 2.2 pounds (lb)

Fluid measures

1 millilitre (ml) = 17 minims (min)
1 fluid ounce (fl oz) = 30 ml
1 litre = 1.8 pints (pt) = 35.2 fl oz
1 pint = 570 ml
1 teaspoon = 4 ml = 1/8 fl oz
1 tablespoon = 15 ml = 1/2 fl oz

Temperature

Temperature in °C = (Temperature in °F - 32) × 5/9
Temperature in °F = Temperature in °C × 9/5 + 32
Freezing point = 0°C = 32°F
Boiling point = 100°C = 212°F

Energy

1 kilocalorie (kcal) = 1 Calorie = 1 000 calories (cal) = 4 200 joules (J) = 4.2 kilojoules (kJ)
1 kilojoule = 1 000 J = 240 cal = 0.24 kcal = 0.24 Calories

Bibliography

Alleyne, G.A.O., Hay, R.W., Picou, D.I., Stanfield, J.P. & Whitehead, R.G. 1977. *Protein-energy malnutrition*. London, UK, Arnold.

Benenson, A.S. 1990. *Control of communicable diseases in man*. Washington, DC, USA, American Public Health Association Publications.

Berg, A. 1987. *Malnutrition. What can be done? Lessons from the World Bank experience*. Baltimore, Maryland, USA, Johns Hopkins University Press.

Brown, M.L. 1990. *Present knowledge in nutrition*. Washington, DC, USA, International Life Sciences Institute, Nutrition Foundation. 6th ed.

Brun, T.A. & Latham, M.C. 1990. *Maldevelopment and malnutrition*. World Food Issues, Vol. 2. Ithaca, New York, USA, Cornell University, Program in International Agriculture.

Cameron, M. & Hofvander, Y. 1983. *Manual on feeding infants and young children*. Oxford, UK, Oxford University Press. 3rd ed.

Cannon, G.C. 1992. *Food and health: the experts agree. An analysis of one hundred authoritative scientific reports on food, nutrition and public health published throughout the world in thirty years, between 1961 and 1991*. London, UK, Consumers' Association.

Dawson, R.J. & Canet, C. 1991. International activities in street foods. *Food Control*, 2(3): 135-139.

Drummond, T. 1975. *Using the method of Paulo Freire in nutrition education: an experimental plan for community action in Northeast Brazil*. Cornell International Nutrition Monograph Series No. 3. Ithaca, New York, USA, Cornell University.

Dunn, J.T. & van der Haar, F. 1990. *A practical guide to the correction of iodine deficiency*. Technical Manual No. 3. Wageningen, the Netherlands, International Council for Control of Iodine Deficiency Disorders (ICCIDD)/United Nations Children's Fund (UNICEF)/World Health Organization (WHO). 62 pp.

Economic Commission for Africa (ECA)/ FAO. 1978. *Manual on child development, family life and nutrition*, by J.A.S. Ritchie. Addis Ababa, Ethiopia.

Engle, P. 1992. *Care and child nutrition*. Paper for the International Conference on Nutrition. New York, USA, United Nations Children's Fund (UNICEF).

FAO. 1976. *The feeding of workers in developing countries*. FAO Food and Nutrition Paper No. 6. Rome.

FAO. 1977a. *Food and nutrition strategies in national development*. 9th Report of the Joint FAO/WHO Expert Committee on Nutrition, Rome, 1974. FAO Food and Nutrition Series No. 5. Rome.

FAO. 1977b. *Planning and evaluation of applied nutrition programmes*, by M.C. Latham. FAO Food and Nutrition Series No. 16. Rome.

FAO. 1979. *Human nutrition in tropical Africa*, by M.C. Latham. Rome.

FAO. 1981. *Traditional and non-traditional foods*. FAO Food and Nutrition Series No. 2. Rome.

FAO. 1982. *Management of group feeding programmes*. FAO Food and Nutrition Paper No. 23. Rome.

FAO. 1984. *Integrating nutrition into agricultural and rural development projects. A manual*. Rome.

FAO. 1988. *Requirements of vitamin A, iron, folate and vitamin B_{12}*. Report of a joint FAO/WHO expert consultation. Rome.

FAO. 1990a. *Street foods.* Report of an FAO Expert Consultation, Jogyakarta, Indonesia, 5-9 December 1988. FAO Food and Nutrition Paper No. 46. Rome.

FAO. 1990b. *Human energy requirements: a manual for planners and nutritionists.* Oxford, UK, Oxford University Press for FAO.

FAO. 1990c. *Conducting small-scale nutrition surveys: a field manual.* Nutrition in Agriculture No. 5. Rome.

FAO. 1990d. *Bibliography of food consumption surveys.* Rev. 3. Rome.

FAO. 1990e. *Roots, tubers, plantains and bananas.* FAO Food and Nutrition Series No. 24. Rome.

FAO. 1990f. *Women in agricultural development. FAO's Plan of Action.* Rome.

FAO. 1990g. *Women in agricultural development. Gender issues in rural food security in developing countries.* Rome.

FAO. 1992a. *Integrating diet quality and food safety into food security programmes,* by M.F. Zeitlin & L.V. Brown. Nutrition Consultants' Reports Series No. 91. Rome.

FAO. 1992b. *Maize in human nutrition.* Food and Nutrition Series No. 25. Rome.

FAO. 1992c. *Meat and meat products in human nutrition in developing countries.* FAO Food and Nutrition Paper No. 53. Rome.

FAO. 1992d. *The State of Food and Agriculture 1992.* Rome.

FAO. 1993a. *Developing national plans of action for nutrition. Guidelines.* Rome.

FAO. 1993b. *Food and nutrition in the management of group feeding programmes.* Food and Nutrition Paper No. 23, Rev. 1. Rome.

FAO. 1993c. *Integration of consumer interests in food control.* Report of an expert consultation. Rome.

FAO. 1993d. *Rice in human nutrition,* prepared in collaboration with FAO by B.O. Juliano. FAO Food and Nutrition Series No. 26. Rome.

FAO. 1993e. *Guidelines for participatory nutrition projects.* Rome.

FAO. 1994a. *Body mass index. A measure of chronic energy deficiency in adults,* ed. P.S. Shetty & W.P.T. James. FAO Food and Nutrition Paper No. 56. Rome.

FAO. 1994b. *Social communication in nutrition: a methodology for intervention.* Rome.

FAO/United States Department of Agriculture (USDA). 1968. *Food composition tables for use in Africa.* Rome.

FAO/USDA. 1972. *Food composition tables for use in East Asia.* Rome.

FAO/World Health Organization (WHO). 1973. *Energy and protein requirements.* Report of a Joint FAO/WHO Ad Hoc Expert Committee. FAO Food and Nutrition Series No. 7/FAO Nutrition Meetings Report Series No. 52/WHO Technical Report Series No. 522. Rome, FAO/Geneva, Switzerland, WHO.

FAO/WHO. 1985. *FAO/WHO food additives system.* Evaluations by the joint FAO/WHO expert committee on food additives, 1956-1984. Rome.

FAO/WHO. 1992a. *International Conference on Nutrition. Final report of the conference.* Rome.

FAO/WHO. 1992b. *International Conference on Nutrition. Nutrition and development – a global assessment.* Rome.

FAO/WHO. 1994. *Fats and oils in human nutrition.* FAO Food and Nutrition Paper No. 57. Rome.

FAO/WHO/United Nations Environment Programme (UNEP). 1990. *Manuals of food quality control. Food inspection.* Rome.

Gibson, R.S. 1990. *Principles of nutritional assessment.* Oxford, UK, Oxford University Press.

Gopalan, C. & Kaur, H. 1993. *Towards better nutrition – problems and policies.* Special Publication Series No. 9. New Delhi, India, Nutrition Foundation of India.

Gopalan, C., Rao, B.S.N. & Seshadri, S. 1992. *Combating vitamin A deficiency through dietary improvement.* Special Publication Series No. 6. New Delhi, India, Nutrition Foundation of India.

Hetzel, B.S. 1989. *The story of iodine deficiency: an international challenge in nutrition.* New York, USA and Oxford, UK, Oxford University Press.

Holland, B., Unwin, I.D. & Buss, D.H. 1988. *Cereals and cereal products. Third supplement to McCance & Widdowson's The composition of foods.* Nottingham, UK, Royal Society of Chemistry.

International Nutritional Anemia Consultative Group. 1977. *Guidelines for the eradication of iron deficiency anemia.* New York, USA, Nutrition Foundation. 40 pp.

James, W.P.T. & Schofield, E.C. 1990. *Human energy requirements: a manual for planners and nutritionists.* Oxford, UK, Oxford University Press/FAO.

Jelliffe, D.B. & Jelliffe, E.F.P. 1978. *Human milk in the modern world.* Oxford, UK, Oxford Medical Publications, Oxford University Press.

Jelliffe, D.B. & Jelliffe, E.F.P. 1989. *Community nutritional assessment with special reference to less technically developed countries.* Oxford, UK, Oxford Medical Publications, Oxford University Press.

King, F.S. 1992. *Helping mothers to breastfeed.* Nairobi, Kenya, African Medical and Research Foundation. Rev. ed.

King, F.S. & Burgess, A. 1993. *Nutrition for developing countries.* Oxford, UK, Oxford University Press. 2nd ed.

King, M., King, F. & Martodipoero, S. 1979. *Primary child care.* Oxford, UK, Oxford University Press.

Koniz-Booher, P. 1993. *Communication strategies to support infant and young child nutrition.* Proceedings of an international conference. Cornell International Nutrition Monograph Series Nos. 24 and 25. Ithaca, New York, USA, Cornell University.

Lappé, F.A. & Collins, J. 1982. *Food first. Beyond the myth of scarcity.* San Francisco, California, USA, Institute for Food and Development Policy/New York, USA, Ballantine Books.

Latham, M.C., Bondestam, L. & Jonsson, U. 1988. *Hunger and society,* Vols. 1-3. Cornell International Nutrition Monograph Series Nos. 17-19. Ithaca, New York, USA, Cornell University.

Latham, M.C., McGandy, R.B., McCann, M.B. & Stare, F.J. 1980. *Scope manual on nutrition.* Kalamazoo, Michigan, USA, Upjohn Company.

Latham, M.C. & Van Esterik, P. 1982. *The decline of the breast: an examination of its impact on fertility and health, and its relation to socioeconomic status.* Cornell International Nutrition Monograph Series No. 10. Ithaca, New York, USA, Cornell University.

Latham, M.C. & van Veen, M. 1989. *Dietary guidelines.* Proceedings of an international conference, Toronto, Canada, 1988. Cornell International Nutrition Monograph Series No. 21. Ithaca, New York, USA, Cornell University.

Latham, M.C. & Westley, S.B. 1977. *Nutrition planning and policy for African countries.* Summary report of a seminar, Nairobi, Kenya, 2-19 June 1976. Cornell International Nutrition Monograph Series No. 5. Ithaca, New York, USA, Cornell University.

Lawrence, R.A. 1994. *Breastfeeding. A guide for the medical profession.* St Louis, Missouri, USA, Mosby-Yearbook. 4th ed.

Layrisse, M. & Roche, M. 1966. The nature and causes of "hookworm anemia". *Am. J. Trop. Med. Hyg.,* 15: 1031.

Linusson, E., Beaudry, M. & Latham, M. 1994. *The right to food and good nutrition.* Cornell International Nutrition Monograph Series No. 26. Ithaca, New York, USA, Cornell University, Program in International Nutrition.

Maxwell, S. & Frankenberger, T.R. 1992. *Household food security: concepts, indicators, measurements. A technical review.* New

York, USA, United Nations Children's Fund (UNICEF)/International Fund for Agricultural Development (IFAD).

McLaren, D.S. 1983. *Nutrition in the community.* New York, USA, John Wiley and Sons. 2nd ed.

McLaren, D.S., Burmad, D., Belton, N.R. & Williams, N.F. 1991. *Textbook of paediatric nutrition.* Edinburgh, Scotland, UK, Churchill Livingstone. 3rd ed.

Pariser, E.R. 1978. *Postharvest food losses in developing countries.* BOSTID Reports No. 29. Washington, DC, USA, National Academy of Sciences, National Research Council, Board on Science and Technology for International Development, United States Agency for International Development (USAID).

Passmore, R. & Eastwood, M.A. 1986. *Davidson and Passmore human nutrition and dietetics.* Edinburgh, Scotland, UK, Churchill Livingstone. 8th ed.

Pollitt, E., Gorman, K.S., Engle, P.S., Martorell, R. & Rivera, J. 1993. *Early supplementary feeding and cognition.* Monographs of the Society for Research in Child Development, Serial No. 235, Vol. 58, No. 7. Chicago, Illinois, USA, Society for Research in Child Development.

Population Reference Bureau. 1994. *World population: toward the next century.* Washington, DC, USA. 4th ed.

Sanjur, D. 1982. *Social and cultural perspectives in nutrition.* Englewood Cliffs, New Jersey, USA, Prentice-Hall.

Schürch, B. & Scrimshaw, N.S., eds. 1987. *Chronic energy deficiency: consequences and related issues.* Background papers and Working Group reports presented at an IDECG meeting, Guatemala City, Guatemala, 3-7 August 1987. Lausanne, Switzerland, International Dietary Energy Consultative Group (IDECG).

Schürch, B. & Scrimshaw, N.S., eds. 1989. *Activity, energy expenditure and energy requirements of infants and children.* Proceedings of an IDECG workshop, Cambridge, Massachusetts, USA, 14-17 November 1989. Lausanne, Switzerland, International Dietary Energy Consultative Group (IDECG).

Scrimshaw, N.S. & Gleason, G.R., eds. 1992. *RAP – rapid assessment procedures. Qualitative methodologies for planning and evaluation of health related programmes.* Boston, Massachusetts, USA, International Nutrition Foundation for Developing Countries.

Shils, M.E., Olson, J.A. & Shike, M. 1994. *Modern nutrition in health and disease.* Philadelphia, Pennsylvania, USA, Lea and Febiger. 8th ed.

Simmonds, S., Vaughan, P. & Gunn, S.W. 1983. *Refugee community health care.* Oxford, UK, Oxford Medical Publications, Oxford University Press.

Sommer, A. 1982. *Nutritional blindness – xerophthalmia and keratomalacia.* Oxford, UK, Oxford University Press.

Souci, S.W., Fachmann, W. & Kraut, H. 1989. *Food composition and nutrition tables 1989/90.* Stuttgart, Germany, Wissenschaftliche, Verlagsgesellschaft.

Stephenson, L.S. 1987. *Impact of helminth infections on human nutrition.* London, UK, Taylor & Francis.

Stephenson, L.S., Latham, M.C. & Jansen, A. 1983. *A comparison of growth standards: similarities between NCHS, Harvard, Denver and privileged African children and differences with Kenyan rural children.* Cornell International Nutrition Monograph Series No. 12. Ithaca, New York, USA, Cornell University.

United Nations (UN) Administrative Committee on Coordination, Subcommittee on Nutrition (ACC/SCN). 1987. *First report on the world nutrition situation.* Geneva, Switzerland.

UN ACC/SCN. 1989. *Malnutrition and infection. A review,* by A. Tomkin & F. Watson. Geneva, Switzerland.

UN ACC/SCN. 1990a. *Appropriate uses of*

anthropometric indices in children, by G. Beaton, A. Kelly, J. Kevany, R. Martorell & J. Mason. Nutrition Policy Discussion Paper No. 7. Geneva, Switzerland.

UN ACC/SCN. 1990b. *Women and nutrition.* Nutrition Policy Discussion Paper No. 6. Geneva, Switzerland.

UN ACC/SCN. 1991a. *Controlling iron deficiency.* Nutrition Policy Discussion Paper No. 9. Geneva, Switzerland.

UN ACC/SCN. 1991b. *Managing successful nutrition programmes.* Nutrition Policy Discussion Paper No. 8. Geneva, Switzerland.

UN ACC/SCN. 1992a. *Second report on the world nutrition situation*, Vol. 1, *Global and regional results.* Geneva, Switzerland.

UN ACC/SCN. 1992b. *Nutrition and population links. Breastfeeding, family planning and child health.* ACC/SCN symposium report. Nutrition Policy Discussion Paper No. 11. Geneva, Switzerland.

UN ACC/SCN. 1994. *Controlling vitamin A deficiency.* Nutrition Policy Discussion Paper No. 14. Geneva, Switzerland.

United Nations Children's Fund (UNICEF). 1990. *Strategy for improved nutrition of children and women in developing countries. A UNICEF policy review.* New York, USA.

UNICEF. 1991. *Guide for monitoring and evaluation.* New York, USA.

UNICEF. 1994. *The state of the world's children 1994.* Oxford, UK, Oxford University Press.

UNICEF. 1995. *The state of the world's children 1995.* Oxford, UK, Oxford University Press.

United Nations Educational, Scientific and Cultural Organization (UNESCO). 1990. *Malnutrition and infection in the classroom*, by E. Pollit. Paris, France.

United States Agency for International Development (USAID). 1989. *Crucial elements of successful community nutrition programs.* Report of the Fifth International Conference of the International Nutrition Planners Forum, Seoul, Republic of Korea, 15-19 August 1989. Washington, DC, USA, USAID Bureau for Science and Technology, Office of Nutrition.

United States Department of Agriculture (USDA). 1976-88. *Composition of foods.* Agriculture Handbooks Nos. 1, 4, 9, 11, 16. Washington, DC, USA.

United States National Academy of Sciences, Food and Nutrition Board. 1989. *Recommended dietary allowances.* Washington, DC, USA.

Van Esterik, P. 1992. *Women, work and breastfeeding.* Cornell International Nutrition Monograph Series No. 23. Ithaca, New York, USA, Cornell University.

Waterlow, J.C. 1992. *Protein energy malnutrition.* London, UK, Edward Arnold.

Werner, D. 1979. *Where there is no doctor.* Palo Alto, California, USA, Hesperian Foundation.

Werner, D. & Bower, B. 1982. *Helping health workers learn.* Palo Alto, California, USA, Hesperian Foundation.

West, C.E., Pepping, F. & Temaliwa, C.R. 1988. *Composition of foods commonly eaten in East Africa.* Wageningen, the Netherlands, Wageningen Agricultural University.

World Bank. 1993. *World development report. Investing in health.* Oxford, UK, Oxford University Press.

World Bank. 1994. *A new agenda for women's health and nutrition.* Washington, DC, USA.

World Bank. 1994. *Enriching lives. Overcoming vitamin and mineral malnutrition in developing countries.* Washington, DC, USA.

World Food Programme (WFP). 1991. *Food aid in emergencies. Book A: Policies and principles.* Rome.

World Health Organization (WHO). 1966. *The assessment of the nutritional status of the community*, by D.B. Jelliffe. WHO Monograph Series No. 53. Geneva, Switzerland.

WHO. 1975a. *Nutritional anaemias.* WHO

Technical Report Series No. 503. Geneva, Switzerland.

WHO. 1975b. *Health by the people.* Geneva, Switzerland.

WHO. 1976. *Methodology of nutritional surveillance.* Report of a Joint FAO/UNICEF/WHO Expert Committee. WHO Technical Report Series No. 593. Geneva, Switzerland.

WHO. 1982. *Control of vitamin A deficiency and xerophthalmia.* WHO Technical Report Series No. 672. Geneva, Switzerland.

WHO. 1983. *Mass catering,* by R.H.G. Charles. WHO Regional Publications, European Series No. 15. Geneva, Switzerland.

WHO. 1985. *Energy and protein requirements.* Report of a Joint FAO/WHO/UNU Expert Consultation, Rome, 5 October 1981. WHO Technical Report Series No. 724. Geneva, Switzerland.

WHO. 1986a. *Guidelines for training community health workers in nutrition.* WHO Offset Publication No. 59. Geneva, Switzerland.

WHO. 1986b. *The growth chart. A tool for use in infant and child health care.* Geneva, Switzerland.

WHO. 1988a. *Vitamin A supplements. A guide to their use in the treatment and prevention of vitamin A deficiency and xerophthalmia.* Geneva, Switzerland.

WHO. 1988b. *Weaning – from breast milk to family food. A guide for health and community workers.* Geneva, Switzerland.

WHO. 1989. *Dietary management of young children with acute diarrhoea. A practical manual for district programme managers,* by D.B. Jelliffe & E.F.P. Jelliffe. Geneva, Switzerland.

WHO. 1990. *Food for thought: nutrition and school performance.* ACC/SCN News No. 5. Geneva, Switzerland.

WHO. 1993a. *The management and prevention of acute malnutrition. Practical guidelines.* Geneva, Switzerland. 3rd ed.

WHO. 1993b. *Breast-feeding. The technical basis and recommendations for action.* Geneva, Switzerland.

WHO. 1993c. *Educational handbook for nutrition trainers,* by A. Oshaug, D. Benbouzid & J.-J. Guilbert. Geneva, Switzerland.

WHO. 1993d. *Implementation of the global strategy for health for all by the year 2000: second evaluation.* Eighth report on the world health situation. Geneva, Switzerland.

WHO. 1994. *Indicators for assessing iodine deficiency disorders and their control through salt iodization.* Report of a joint WHO, UNICEF, ICCIDD workshop. WHO/NUT/94.6. Geneva, Switzerland.

WHO. 1995. *Physical status: the use and interpretation of anthropometry.* WHO Technical Report Series No. 854. Geneva, Switzerland.

WHO. 1996. *Preparation and use of food-based dietary guidelines.* Report of a joint FAO/WHO Expert Consultation, Nicosia, Cyprus. WHO/NUT/96.6. Geneva, Switzerland.

WHO/United Nations Children's Fund (UNICEF). 1989. *Protecting, promoting and supporting breast-feeding: the special role of maternity services.* A joint WHO/UNICEF statement. Geneva, Switzerland, WHO.

WHO/UNICEF. 1992. *Consensus statement from the WHO/UNICEF Consultation on HIV Transmission and Breastfeeding.* Geneva, 30 April - 1 May 1992. Geneva, Switzerland, WHO.

WHO/UNICEF/International Council for Control of Iodine Deficiency Disorders (ICCIDD). 1993. *Global prevalence of iodine deficiency disorders.* MDIS (Micronutrient Deficiency Information System) Working Paper No. 1. Geneva, Switzerland.

Young, V.R. & Pellett, P.L. 1994. Plant proteins in relation to human protein and amino acid nutrition. *Am. J. Clin. Nutr.,* 59(Suppl.): 1203S-1212S.

Index

Index

A

Acquired immunodeficiency syndrome (AIDS), 11, 28, 71, 72, 142, 207, 217, 230, 342, 359, 380, 382, 387, 413, 433

Acrodermatitis enteropathica, 108, 197, 317

Aflatoxin, 129, 130, 222, 273, 297, 308, 334

Albendazole, 26, 139, 377, 379, 414

Alcoholism, 108, 115, 180, 205, 213, 220, 221, 223, 294

Amino acids, 6, 25, 94-97, 101, 116, 118, 129, 137, 258, 259, 271, 283, 284, 300, 303, 420

Anaemia, 4, 5, 7, 11, 25, 26, 41, 45, 48, 55, 56, 64, 106, 109, 117, 118, 121, 122, 130, 133-136, 139, 142, 147-155, 207, 210, 230, 232, 233, 240, 242, 243, 262, 277, 285, 313, 316, 317, 321, 334, 365, 368, 377, 379, 403, 413-417, 431, 443, 454

Angular stomatitis, 24, 116, 206, 209-211, 309, 310, 316

Anorexia, 25, 28, 129, 136, 142, 197, 230, 316, 355, 379

Anorexia nervosa, 142, 230

Appetite, 25, 26, 52, 53, 56, 83, 84, 108, 121, 128, 133-136, 138, 139, 141, 197, 210, 230, 231, 294, 322, 341, 355, 366, 377, 378, 382, 407, 414, 420

Applied nutrition programmes (ANPs), 6, 7

Ariboflavinosis, 116, 206, 210, 233, 314, 316

Arm circumference, 130, 209, 210, 236, 310, 312

Arteriosclerosis, 56, 92, 93, 122, 213-215, 217, 219, 221, 222, 224, 338, 386, 446

Ascaris lumbricoides – see Roundworm

Ascorbic acid – see Vitamin C

B

Baby Friendly Hospital Initiative (BFHI), 75

Basal metabolic rate (BMR), 47, 86-90, 160, 162, 163

BCG vaccine, 244, 367, 374, 375

Beriberi, 35, 50, 84, 114-116, 177-180, 183, 205, 240, 243, 257, 285, 316

Beta-carotene, 112, 113, 169, 170, 215, 222, 264, 303

Beverages, 33, 105, 181, 261, 274, 293, 294, 298, 331, 422, 423, 425, 426, 432, 435, 436

Bilharzia – see Schistosomiasis

Biotin, 111, 121, 252

Birth control (see also Family planning), 38, 207

Birth weight, 39, 40, 47, 48, 68, 129, 371, 416

Bitot's spots, 171, 172, 176, 209, 210, 310, 316, 402

Body mass index (BMI), 87, 217, 218, 230, 312, 346, 347

Bottle-feeding, 16, 33, 35, 36, 41, 61-63, 71-73, 75, 129, 237, 353, 386, 393, 454

Breastfeeding, 9, 16, 21, 27, 28, 35, 36, 38-42, 49-53, 61-79, 90, 105, 128, 129, 135, 137, 143, 149, 236, 237, 243, 244, 285, 321, 322, 338, 351-356, 359, 367-369, 371, 372, 376, 379, 386, 393, 394, 401, 406, 407, 414, 416, 423, 425, 452, 454

Breastmilk, 36, 39, 41, 49-52, 61-77, 83, 84, 102, 105, 119, 129, 135, 141, 149, 169, 178, 237, 285, 286, 291, 338, 372, 379, 389, 405, 406, 414, 425, 430, 454

Breastmilk substitutes (see also Infant formula), 36, 39, 62-67, 70-75, 237, 286, 338, 389

Burning feet syndrome, 111, 121, 205, 231

WHERE TO PURCHASE FAO PUBLICATIONS LOCALLY
POINTS DE VENTE DES PUBLICATIONS DE LA FAO
PUNTOS DE VENTA DE PUBLICACIONES DE LA FAO

ANGOLA
Empresa Nacional do Disco e de
Publicações, ENDIPU-U.E.E.
Rua Cirilo da Conceição Silva, Nº 7
C.P. Nº 1314-C
Luanda

ARGENTINA
Librería Agropecuaria
Pasteur 743
1028 Buenos Aires
Oficina del Libro Internacional
Av. Córdoba 1877
1120 Buenos Aires

AUSTRALIA
Hunter Publications
P.O. Box 404
Abbotsford, Vic. 3067

AUSTRIA
Gerold Buch & Co.
Weihburggasse 26
1010 Vienna

• **BANGLADESH**
Association of Development
Agencies in Bangladesh
House No. 1/3, Block F,
Lalmatia
Dhaka 1207

• **BELGIQUE**
M.J. De Lannoy
202, avenue du Roi
1060 Bruxelles
CCP 000-0808993-13
E-mail: jean.de.lannoy@infoboard.be

• **BOLIVIA**
Los Amigos del Libro
Av. Heroínas 311, Casilla 450
Cochabamba;
Mercado 1315
La Paz

• **BOTSWANA**
Botsalo Books (Pty) Ltd
P.O. Box 1532
Gaborone

• **BRAZIL**
Book Master Livraria
Rua do Catete 311 lj. 118/119
22220-001 Catete
Rio de Janeiro
Editora da Universidade Federal
do Rio Grande do Sul
Av. João Pessoa 415
Bairro Cidade Baixa 90
040-000 Porto Alegre/RS
Fundação Getúlio Vargas
Praia do Botafogo 190, C.P. 9052
Rio de Janeiro
E-mail: valeria@sede.fgvrj.br
Núcleo Editora da Universidade
Federal Fluminense
Rua Miguel de Frias 9
Icaraí-Niterói 24
220-000 Rio de Janeiro
Fundação da Universidade
Federal do Paraná - FUNPAR
Rua Alfredo Bufrem 140, 30º andar
80020-240 Curitiba

• **CANADA**
BERNAN Associates (ex UNIPUB)
4611/F Assembly Drive
Lanham, MD 20706-4391
Toll-free 800 274-4888
Fax 301-459-0056
Website: www.bernan.com
E-mail: info@bernan.com
Guérin - Editeur
4501, rue Drolet
Montréal, Québec H2T 2G2
Tel. (514) 842-3481
Fax (514) 842-4923

Renouf Publishing
5369 chemin Canotek Road, Unit 1
Ottawa, Ontario K1J 9J3
Tel. (613) 745-2665
Fax (613) 745 7660
Website: www.renoufbooks.com
E-mail: renouf@fox.nstn.ca

• **CHILE**
Librería - Oficina Regional FAO
Calle Bandera 150, 8º Piso
Casilla 10095, Santiago-Centro
Tel. 699 1005
Fax 696 1121/696 1124
E-mail: german.rojas@field.fao.org
Universitaria Textolibros Ltda.
Avda. L. Bernardo O'Higgins 1050
Santiago

• **CHINA**
China National Publications
Import & Export Corporation
16 Gongti East Road
Beijing 100020
Tel. 6506 30 70
Fax 6506 3101
E-mail: cnpiec@public.3.bta.net.cn

• **COLOMBIA**
Banco Ganadero
Vicepresidencia de Fomento
Carrera 9ª Nº 72-21, Piso 5
Bogotá D.E.
Tel. 217 0100

• **CONGO**
Office national des librairies
populaires
B.P. 577
Brazzaville

• **COSTA RICA**
Librería Lehmann S.A.
Av. Central, Apartado 10011
1000 San José

• **CÔTE D'IVOIRE**
CEDA
04 B.P. 541
Abidjan 04

• **CUBA**
Ediciones Cubanas
Empresa de Comercio Exterior
de Publicaciones
Obispo 461, Apartado 605
La Habana

• **CZECH REPUBLIC**
Artia Pegas Press Ltd
Import of Periodicals
Palác Metro, P.O. Box 825
Národní 25
111 21 Praha 1

• **DENMARK**
Munksgaard, Book and
Subscription Service
P.O. Box 2148
DK 1016 Copenhagen K.
Tel. 4533128570
Fax 4533129387
Website: www.munksgaard.dk; E-mail:
subscription.service@mail.munksgaard.dk

• **DOMINICAN REPUBLIC**
CUESTA - Centro del libro
Av. 27 de Febrero, esq. A. Lincoln
Centro Comercial Nacional
Apartado 1241
Santo Domingo

• **ECUADOR**
Libri Mundi, Librería Internacional
Juan León Mera 851
Apartado Postal 3029
Quito
E-mail: librimul@librimundi.com.ec

Universidad agraria del Ecuador
Centro de Información Agraria
Av. 23 de Julio, Apdo 09-01-1248
Guayaquil
Librería Española
Murgeón 364 y Ulloa
Quito

• **EGYPT**
The Middle East Observer
41 Sherif Street, Cairo
E-mail: fouda@soficom.com.eg

• **ESPAÑA**
Librería Agrícola
Fernando VI 2
28004 Madrid
Librería de la Generalitat de
Catalunya
Rambla dels Estudis 118 (Palau Moja)
08002 Barcelona
Tel. (93) 302 6462
Fax (93) 302 1299
Mundi Prensa Libros S.A.
Castelló 37
28001 Madrid
Tel. 431 3399
Fax 575 3998
Website: www.tsai.es/MPRENSA
E-mail: mundiprensa@tsai.es
Mundi Prensa - Barcelona
Consejo de Ciento 391
08009 Barcelona
Tel. 301 8615
Fax 317 0141

• **FINLAND**
Akateeminen Kirjakauppa
Subscription Services
P.O. Box 23
FIN-00371 Helsinki

• **FRANCE**
Editions A. Pedone
13, rue Soufflot
75005 Paris
Lavoisier Tec & Doc
14, rue de Provigny
94236 Cachan Cedex
Website: www.lavoisier.fr
E-mail: livres@lavoisier.fr
Librairie du Commerce
International
10, avenue d'Iéna
75783 Paris Cedex 16
E-mail: pl@net-export.fr
Website: www.cfce.fr

• **GERMANY**
Alexander Horn Internationale
Buchhandlung
Friedrichstrasse 34
D-65185 Wiesbaden
S. Toeche-Mittler GmbH
Versandbuchhandlung
Hindenburgstrasse 33
D-64295 Darmstadt
Uno Verlag
Poppelsdorfer Allee 55
D-53115 Bonn 1

• **GHANA**
SEDCO Publishing Ltd
Sedco House, Tabon Street
Off Ring Road Central, North Ridge
P.O. Box 2051, Accra

• **GREECE**
Papasotiriou S.A.
35 Stournara Str., 10682 Athens
Tel. +301 3302 980
Fax +301 3648254

• **GUYANA**
Guyana National Trading
Corporation Ltd
45-47 Water Street, P.O. Box 308
Georgetown

• **HAÏTI**
Librairie «A la Caravelle»
26, rue Bonne Foi
B.P. 111
Port-au-Prince

• **HONDURAS**
Escuela Agrícola Panamericana
Librería RTAC
El Zamorano, Apartado 93
Tegucigalpa
Oficina de la Escuela Agrícola
Panamericana en Tegucigalpa
Blvd. Morazán, Apts. Glapson
Apartado 93
Tegucigalpa

• **HUNGARY**
Librotrade Kft.
P.O. Box 126
H-1656 Budapest

• **INDIA**
EWP Affiliated East-West
Press PVT, Ltd
G-I/16, Ansari Road, Darya Ganj
New Delhi 110 002
Oxford Book and Stationery Co.
Scindia House
New Delhi 110 001;
17 Park Street
Calcutta 700 016
Oxford Subscription Agency
Institute for Development Education
1 Anasuya Ave, Kilpauk
Madras 600 010
Periodical Expert Book Agency
G-56, 2nd Floor, Laxmi Nagar
Vikas Marg, Delhi 110092

• **IRAN**
The FAO Bureau, International
and Regional Specialized
Organizations Affairs
Ministry of Agriculture of the Islamic
Republic of Iran
Keshavarz Bld, M.O.A., 17th floor
Teheran

• **IRELAND**
Publications Section
Government Stationery Office
4-5 Harcourt Road
Dublin 2

• **ISRAEL**
R.O.Y. International
P.O. Box 13056
Tel Aviv 61130
E-mail: royil@netvision.net.il

• **ITALY**
FAO Bookshop
Viale delle Terme di Caracalla
00100 Roma
Tel. 5225 5688
Fax 5225 5155
E-mail: publications-sales@fao.org
Libreria Commissionaria Sansoni
S.p.A. - Licosa
Via Duca di Calabria 1/1
50125 Firenze
E-mail: licosa@ftbcc.it
Libreria Scientifica Dott. Lucio de
Biasio "Aeiou"
Via Coronelli 6
20146 Milano

• **JAPAN**
Far Eastern Booksellers
(Kyokuto Shoten Ltd)
12 Kanda-Jimbocho 2 chome
Chiyoda-ku - P.O. Box 72
Tokyo 101-91
Maruzen Company Ltd
P.O. Box 5050
Tokyo International 100-31
E-mail: h_sugiyama@maruzen.co.jp

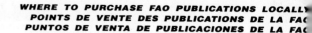

• **KENYA**
Text Book Centre Ltd
Kijabe Street
P.O. Box 47540
Nairobi

• **LUXEMBOURG**
M.J. De Lannoy
202, avenue du Roi
1060 Bruxelles (Belgique)
E-mail: jean.de.lannoy@infoboard.be

• **MADAGASCAR**
Centre d'Information et de
Documentation Scientifique et
Technique
Ministère de la recherche appliquée
au développement
B.P 6224 Tsimbazaza
Antanarivo

• **MALAYSIA**
Electronic products only:
Southbound
Sendirian Berhad Publishers
9 College Square
01250 Penang

• **MALI**
Librairie Traore
Rue Soundiata Keita X 115
B.P. 3243
Bamako

• **MAROC**
La Librairie Internationale
70 Rue T'ssoule
P.O. Box 302 (RP)
Rabat
Tel. (07) 75-86-61

• **MEXICO**
Librería, Universidad Autónoma de
Chapingo
56230 Chapingo
Libros y Editoriales S.A.
Av. Progreso Nº 202-1º Piso A
Apdo. Postal 18922
Col. Escandón
11800 México D.F.

• **NETHERLANDS**
Roodveldt Import b.v.
Brouwersgracht 288
1013 HG Amsterdam
E-mail: roodboek@euronet.nl
Swets & Zeitlinger b.v.
P.O. Box 830, 2160 Lisse
Heereweg 347 B, 2161 CA Lisse

• **NEW ZEALAND**
Legislation Services
P.O. Box 12418
Thorndon, Wellington
E-mail: gppmjxf@gp.co.nz

• **NICARAGUA**
Librería HISPAMER
Costado Este Univ. Centroamericana
Apdo. Postal A-221
Managua
Universidad centroamericana
Apartado 69
Managua

• **NIGERIA**
University Bookshop (Nigeria) Ltd
University of Ibadan
Ibadan

• **NORWAY**
NIC Info A/S
Bertrand Narvesens vei 2
P.O. Box 6512, Etterstad
0606 Oslo 6
Tel. (+47) 22-57-33-00
Fax (+47) 22-68-19-01

• **PAKISTAN**
Mirza Book Agency
65 Shahrah-e-Quaid-e-Azam
P.O. Box 729, Lahore 3

• **PARAGUAY**
Librería Intercontinental
Editora e Impresora S.R.L.
Caballero 270 c/Mcal Estigarribia
Asunción

• **PERU**
INDEAR
Jirón Apurimac 375, Casilla 4937
Lima 1
Peruvian Book Central S.r.l.
Jr. Los Lirios 520 - A.P. 733
Lima
Universidad Nacional "Pedro Ruiz
Gallo"
Facultad de Agronomía, A.P. 795
Lambayeque (Chiclayo)

• **PHILIPPINES**
International Booksource Center,
Inc.
Room 720, Cityland 10 Tower 2
H.V. de la Costa, Cor. Valero St
Makati, Metro Manila

• **POLAND**
Ars Polona
Krakowskie Przedmiescie 7
00-950 Warsaw

• **PORTUGAL**
Livraria Portugal, Dias e Andrade
Ltda.
Rua do Carmo 70-74
Apartado 2681
1200 Lisboa Codex

• **SINGAPORE**
Select Books Pte Ltd
03-15 Tanglin Shopping Centre
19 Tanglin Road
Singapore 1024

• **SLOVAK REPUBLIC**
Institute of Scientific and
Technical
Information for Agriculture
Samova 9
950 10 Nitra
Tel. +42 87 522 185
Fax +42 87 525 275
E-mail: uvtip@nr.sanet.sk

• **SOMALIA**
Samater
P.O. Box 936, Mogadishu

• **SOUTH AFRICA**
David Philip Publishers (Pty) Ltd
P.O. Box 23408
Claremont 7735
Tel. Cape Town (021) 64-4136
Fax Cape Town (021) 64-3358

• **SRI LANKA**
M.D. Gunasena & Co. Ltd
217 Olcott Mawatha, P.O. Box 246
Colombo 11

• **SUISSE**
Buchhandlung und Antiquariat
Heinimann & Co.
Kirchgasse 17
8001 Zurich
UN Bookshop
Palais des Nations
CH-1211 Genève 1
Website: www.un.org
Van Diermen Editions Techniques
ADECO
41 Lacuez
CH-1807 Blonzy

• **SURINAME**
Vaco n.v. in Suriname
Domineestraat 26, P.O. Box 1841
Paramaribo

• **SWEDEN**
Books and documents:
C.E. Fritzes
P.O. Box 16356
103 27 Stockholm
Subscriptions:
Information Services AB
P.O. Box 1305
171 25 Solna

• **THAILAND**
Suksapan Panit
Mansion 9, Rajdamnern Avenue
Bangkok

• **TOGO**
Librairie du Bon Pasteur
B.P. 1164, Lomé

• **TUNISIE**
Société tunisienne de diffusion
5, avenue de Carthage
Tunis

• **TURKEY**
Kultur Yayiniari is - Turk Ltd Sti.
Ataturk Bulvari Nº 191, Kat. 21
Ankara
Bookshops in Istanbul and Izmir
DUNYA INFOTEL
Basin Yayin Haberlesme
Istikal Cad. Nº 649
80050 Tunel, Istanbul
Tel. 0212 251 9196
Fax 0212 251 9197

• **UNITED KINGDOM**
The Stationery Office
51 Nine Elms Lane
London SW8 5DR
Tel. (0171) 873 9090 (orders)
(0171) 873 0011 (inquiries)
Fax (0171) 873 8463
and through The Stationery Office
Bookshops
Website: www.the-stationery-office.co.uk
Electronic products only:
Microinfo Ltd
P.O. Box 3, Omega Road
Alton, Hampshire GU34 2PG
Tel. (01420) 86848
Fax (01420) 89889
Website: www.microinfo.co.uk
E-mail: emedia@microinfo.co.uk

• **URUGUAY**
Librería Agropecuaria S.R.L.
Buenos Aires 335, Casilla 1755
Montevideo C.P. 11000

• **UNITED STATES**
Publications:
BERNAN Associates (ex UNIPUB)
4611/F Assembly Drive
Lanham, MD 20706-4391
Toll-free 1-800-274-4447
Fax 301-459-0056
Website: www.bernan.com
E-mail: info@bernan.com
Periodicals:
Ebsco Subscription Services
P.O. Box 1943
Birmingham, AL 35201-1943
Tel. (205) 991-6600
Telex 78-2661
Fax (205) 991-1449
The Faxon Company Inc.
15 Southwest Park
Westwood, MA 02090
Tel. 6117-329-3350
Telex 95-1980
Cable FW Faxon Wood

• **VENEZUELA**
Fundación La Era Agrícola
Calle 31 Junín Qta Coromoto 5-49
Apartado 456
Mérida
Fundación para la Investigación
Agrícola
San Javier
Estado Yaracuy
Apartado Postal 182
San Felipe
Fax 054 44210
E-mail: damac@diero.conicit.ve
Fudeco, Librería
Avenida Libertador-Este
Ed. Fudeco, Apartado 254
Barquisimeto C.P. 3002, Ed. Lara
Tel. (051) 538 022
Fax (051) 544 394
Telex (051) 513 14 FUDEC VC
Librería FAGRO
Universidad Central de Venezuela
(UCV)
Maracay
Librería Universitaria, C.A.
Av. 3, entre 29 y 30 Nº 29-25
Edif. EVA
Mérida
Fax 074 52 09 56
Tamanaco Libros Técnicos S.R.L.
Centro Comercial Ciudad Tamanaco
Nivel C-2
Caracas
Tel. 261 3344/261 3335/959 0016
Tecni-Ciencia Libros S.A.
Torre Phelps-Mezzanina
Plaza Venezuela
Apartado Postal 20.315
1020 Caracas
Tel. 782 8697/781 9945/781 9954
E-mail: tchlibros@ibm.net
Tecni-Ciencia Libros, S.A.
Centro Comercial
Av. Andrés Eloy, Urb. El Prebo
Valencia, Ed. Carabobo
Tel. 222 724

• **ZIMBABWE**
Grassroots Books
100 Jason Moyo Avenue
P.O. Box A 267, Avondale
Harare;
61a Fort Street
Bulawayo

• **Other countries/Autres pays/
Otros países**
Sales and Marketing Group
Information Division, FAO
Viale delle Terme di Caracalla
00100 Rome, Italy
Tel. (39-6) 52251
Fax (39-6) 5225 3360
Telex 625852/625853/610181 FAO I
E-mail: publications-sales@fao.org